T0292637

Respiratory Medicine

Series editor

Sharon I.S. Rounds, Providence, RI, USA

More information about this series at http://www.springer.com/series/7665

Atul C. Mehta · Prasoon Jain
Thomas R. Gildea
Editors

Diseases of the Central Airways

A Clinical Guide

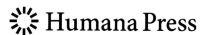 Humana Press

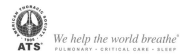

Editors
Atul C. Mehta, MD, FACP, FCCP
Professor of Medicine
Lerner College of Medicine
Buoncore Family Endowed Chair
  in Lung Transplantation
Respiratory Institute, Cleveland Clinic
Cleveland, OH
USA

Thomas R. Gildea, MD, MS, FCCP, FACP
Pulmonary, Allergy, Critical Care Medicine
  and Transplant Center
Respiratory Institute, Cleveland Clinic
Cleveland, OH
USA

Prasoon Jain, MBBS, MD, FCCP
Pulmonary and Critical Care
Louis A Johnson VA Medical Center
Clarksburg, WV
USA

ISSN 2197-7372   ISSN 2197-7380 (electronic)
Respiratory Medicine
ISBN 978-3-319-29828-3   ISBN 978-3-319-29830-6 (eBook)
DOI 10.1007/978-3-319-29830-6

Library of Congress Control Number: 2016931430

Printed on acid-free paper

This Humana Press imprint is published by SpringerNature
The registered company is Springer International Publishing AG Switzerland

To my teachers who taught me how to hold the bronchoscope

—Atul C. Mehta

To my mother and father

—Prasoon Jain

To my patients

—Thomas R. Gildea

Foreword

Open up one of the major textbooks of pulmonary medicine, and it readily becomes apparent that the central airways of the lung garner little attention beyond an obligatory chapter. Comprised of the trachea and proximal bronchi, the central airways are viewed largely as a conduit for airflow. As such, they tend to become clinically relevant when there is critical narrowing, as occurs in the setting of neoplastic disease or iatrogenic strictures from prior endotracheal or tracheostomy tubes. Those most familiar with the central airways are members of the burgeoning field of interventional pulmonology, who on a daily basis venture into the central airways to biopsy, dilate, laser, stent, and ultrasound, place valves and coils, and apply thermal energy. It is these practitioners who have called attention to the many and varied disorders that can affect the central airways, beyond the tumors and strictures that have conventionally populated the textbook chapters.

This scholarly monograph highlights the full spectrum of inflammatory, autoimmune, infectious, neoplastic, and idiopathic disorders that affect the central airways. The editors of this monograph, all practitioners of interventional pulmonology, are to be commended for focusing on the cognitive rather than the technical aspects of their field. Their message is clear: Those who hold a bronchoscope must be diagnosticians first and technicians second. Importantly, this monograph is relevant not only to those who practice interventional pulmonology but for all clinicians who want to learn from the insights that this field has provided into the diversity of disorders that affect the central airways.

Robert M. Kotloff
Department of Pulmonary Medicine
Respiratory Institute, Cleveland Clinic
Cleveland
OH, USA

Herbert W. Wiedemann
Respiratory Institute, Cleveland Clinic
Cleveland
OH, USA

Preface

As 2016 dawns, Interventional Pulmonology has become an essential component of pulmonary medicine, as vital and as widely accepted as Interventional Cardiology. This subspecialty is extremely attractive to most pulmonologists, and the establishment of national and international organizations, myriad scholarly contributions to the literature, and well-attended scientific seminars provide definitive evidence of its worldwide favor. One possible reason for this widespread interest is that endobronchial procedures often yield important results and positively impact patients' well-being. For example, a successful lung transplantation cannot be achieved without the contributions of a bronchoscopist. Similarly, there is no doubt about the contributions bronchoscope has made in the diagnosis and staging of lung cancer. In fact, there are only a handful of pulmonary ailments that a bronchoscope cannot diagnose, palliate, or cure.

Interventional pulmonary medicine thrives within the penumbra of multiple specialties: Bronchoscopists provide the transitional step from the unknown to the known, from lesion to cancer, from wheezes to granulomatosis with polyangiitis, and from treatment to palliation. Interventional pulmonologists are uniquely positioned to improve many fields because bronchoscopy offers the best access to lung tissue.

The modern day interventional pulmonologist has a dual commitment: to be a competent endoscopist and to demonstrate a thorough knowledge of diseases involving the central airways, as well as other systemic diseases that can affect the central airways. This body of knowledge must also include the understanding of symptoms that are not associated with airways disease.

The objective of this monograph is to illuminate the fact that Interventional Pulmonology offers more than mere interventions. The bronchoscopist should be able to recognize aspiration in the absence of a foreign body and perhaps diagnose inflammatory bowel disease before it involves the gastrointestinal tract. The interventional pulmonologist should be able to differentiate when a cardiac or pulmonary embolism evaluation should be considered, rather than a bronchoscopy. One must consider the patient as an individual, not an endobronchial tree. With appropriate training, anyone can perform a procedure, but the editors strongly believe that "a good bronchoscopist is the one who knows when not to perform the procedure."

The optimal application of bronchoscopy arises from the coalescence of medical science and prudence, and the editors vehemently assert that reducing the cost of health care is a civic responsibility. However, the current directives of Interventional Pulmonology, to a significant degree, are based upon expert opinion, not evidence. In addition, the cost-effectiveness of new elective bronchoscopy procedures has not been well documented. Therefore, the interventionalist must rise above his or her technical abilities and consider noninvasive therapeutic options, then perform an unnecessary procedure. The bronchoscopist should be a technology savant, not a technology servant.

We, the editors, have made a sincere effort to focus only on the conditions that require limited or no technical interventions within the purview of Interventional Pulmonology. Although we do not claim this book encompasses the subject in its entirety, we offer our attempt to illuminate the noninterventional aspects of our subspecialty. We applaud all the authors for their support and timely contributions to this project; the credit is theirs to claim. Our ultimate objective is the well-being of patients suffering with central airways diseases, through the safe and cost-effective practice of Interventional Pulmonology.

Atul C. Mehta
Prasoon Jain
Thomas R. Gildea

Contents

Contributors

Francisco Aécio Almeida, MD, MS Pulmonary Medicine, Respiratory Institute, Cleveland Clinic, Cleveland, OH, USA

Andrea Valeria Arrossi, MD Anatomic Pathology, Cleveland Clinic, Cleveland, OH, USA

Debabrata Bandyopadhyay Department of Thoracic Medicine, Geisinger Medical Center, Danville, PA, USA

Joseph Cicenia Pulmonary Medicine, Respiratory Institute, Cleveland Clinic, Cleveland, OH, USA

Daniel A. Culver Department of Pulmonary Medicine, Respiratory Institute, Cleveland Clinic, Cleveland, OH, USA; Department of Pathobiology, Lerner Research Institute, Cleveland Clinic, Cleveland, OH, USA

Gustavo Cumbo-Nacheli Pulmonary and Critical Care Division, Spectrum Health Medical Group, Grand Rapids, MI, USA

Abigail D. Doyle Department of Internal Medicine, Metro Health Hospital, Wyoming, MI, USA

Yaser Abu El-Sameed Respiratory Institute, Cleveland Clinic Abu Dhabi, Abu Dhabi, United Arab Emirates

Carol Farver Department of Pathology, Cleveland Clinic, Cleveland, OH, USA

Erik Folch Division of Thoracic Surgery and Interventional Pulmonology, Beth Israel Deaconess Medical Center, Harvard Medical School, Boston, MA, USA

Shekhar Ghamande Department of Medicine/Division of Pulmonary and Critical Care, Baylor Scott and White Healthcare, Temple, TX, USA; Texas A&M University, College Station, TX, USA

Thomas R. Gildea Respiratory Institute, Cleveland Clinic, Cleveland, OH, USA

Umur Hatipoğlu Respiratory Institute, Cleveland Clinic, Cleveland, OH, USA

Kristin B. Highland Respiratory Institute, Cleveland Clinic, Cleveland, OH, USA

Prasoon Jain Pulmonary and Critical Care, Louis A Johnson VA Medical Center, Clarksburg, WV, USA

Satish Kalanjeri Section of Pulmonary, Critical Care and Sleep Medicine, Louisiana State University Health Sciences Center, Shreveport, LA, USA

Demet Karnak Department of Chest Disease, Ankara University School of Medicine, Ankara, Turkey

Danai Khemasuwan Interventional Pulmonary and Critical Care Medicine, Intermountain Medical Center, Murray, UT, USA

Pyng Lee Division of Respiratory and Critical Care Medicine, National University Hospital, National University of Singapore, Singapore, Singapore

Michael S. Machuzak Respiratory Institute, Cleveland Clinic, Cleveland, OH, USA

Atul C. Mehta, MD, FACP, FCCP Professor of Medicine, Lerner College of Medicine, Buoncore Family Endowed Chair in Lung Transplantation, Respiratory Institute, Cleveland Clinic, Cleveland, OH, USA

Claudio F. Milstein Head and Neck Institute, Cleveland Clinic, Cleveland, OH, USA

Tathagat Narula Respiratory Critical Care and Sleep Medicine Associates, Baptist South, Baptist Medical Center, Jacksonville, FL, USA

Tanmay S. Panchabhai, MD, FACP, FCCP Advanced Lung Disease and Lung Transplant Programs, Norton Thoracic Institute, St. Joseph's Hospital and Medical Center, Phoenix, AZ, USA

Hardeep S. Rai Respiratory Institute, Cleveland Clinic, Cleveland, OH, USA

Jose F. Santacruz Bronchoscopy and Interventional Pulmonology, Houston Methodist Lung Center, Houston, TX, USA

Sonali Sethi Respiratory Institute, Cleveland Clinic, Cleveland, OH, USA

Nirosshan Thiruchelvam, MD Hospitalist, Department of Pulmonary Medicine, Respiratory Institute, Cleveland Clinic Foundation, Cleveland, OH, USA

Pichapong Tunsupon Division of Pulmonary, Critical Care, and Sleep Medicine, Department of Internal Medicine, University of Buffalo, Buffalo, NY, USA; Amherst, NY, USA

Chapter 1
Diseases of Central Airways: An Overview

Prasoon Jain and Atul C. Mehta

Introduction

Central airways are involved in a variety of neoplastic and non-neoplastic disorders causing non-specific symptoms such as chronic cough, dyspnea, wheezing, and hemoptysis [1–4]. Establishing early diagnosis of less common diseases poses a unique challenge because in many instances the clinical presentation closely simulates the more common disorders such as asthma and COPD. Because these disorders have received less-than-adequate attention in the medical literature, the practicing physicians are less aware of these entities than more common diseases of the central airways. Due to the delay in establishing the diagnosis for extended periods, it is not unusual for the correct pathology to be identified in advanced stages of the disease. For an individual patient, it prevents timely institution of appropriate treatment placing them at high risk of adverse clinical outcome. In many instances, such delay in diagnosis may lead to cartilage damage may lead to cartilage damage, advanced fibrotic strictures that not only cause considerable morbidity but also defy optimal outcome even with appropriate medical interventions. With a mistaken diagnosis of treatment-resistant asthma, many patients have inappropriately received oral corticosteroids for a prolonged period of time, exposing them to the well-known risks associated with such treatment. Sometimes,

P. Jain (✉)
Pulmonary and Critical Care, Louis A Johnson VA Medical Center,
Clarksburg, WV, USA
e-mail: prasoonjain.md@gmail.com

A.C. Mehta
Lerner College of Medicine, Buoncore Family Endowed Chair in Lung Transplantation,
Respiratory Institute, Cleveland Clinic, Cleveland, OH, USA
e-mail: Mehtaa1@ccf.org

A.C. Mehta
Pulmonary Medicine, Respiratory Institute, Cleveland Clinic, Cleveland, OH, USA

© Springer International Publishing Switzerland 2016
A.C. Mehta et al. (eds.), *Diseases of the Central Airways*,
Respiratory Medicine, DOI 10.1007/978-3-319-29830-6_1

failure to identify the underlying process leads to advanced central airway obstruction and it is not unusual for a patient to present for the first time with acute respiratory distress, imminent suffocation, and devastating clinical outcome.

In this chapter, we provide an overview of the clinical presentation and diagnostic approach to the diseases of central airways. We discuss the role of pulmonary function tests, airway imaging, and bronchoscopy in diagnosis of these disorders. We also discuss the basic principles that govern the therapeutic approach in patients with diseases of central airways. A detailed discussion on individual disease processes is left to the individual chapters.

Etiology

Central airways are a target for a wide variety of disease processes. There is no uniformly accepted classification, but it is useful to divide these disorders according to underlying etiology. Broadly, the diseases of central airways are classified as neoplastic and non-neoplastic disorders (Table 1.1). Neoplastic disorders of central airways are further divided into malignant tumors, which include primary tracheal tumors, direct extension of tumors into the airways, metastatic cancers, central airway lymphoproliferative diseases, and benign tumors. The etiology of non-neoplastic disorders of central airways includes congenital disorders, infections, iatrogenic injuries, systemic inflammatory diseases, and a wide range of miscellaneous causes. In the following section, we highlight a few important points pertaining to the etiology of central airway diseases. Details are covered in individual chapters.

Primary tumors of trachea and central bronchi are uncommon, accounting for 1–2 % of all respiratory tract malignancies [5]. Malignant tumors are more common in adults and arise from airway epithelium or salivary glands in the airways. In contrast, the benign central airway tumors are more common in pediatric age-group and arise from the tissues of mesenchymal origin [6]. A delay in diagnosis by as much as 2–4 years is common in both adults and pediatric patients, and symptoms are most often attributed to bronchial asthma before the correct diagnosis is identified [7, 8]. Tracheal tumors must be considered in any patient who is newly diagnosed with adult-onset asthma, or has unexplained hemoptysis, wheezing, dyspnea, and hoarseness in the presence of a normal chest radiograph. Further testing with MDCT and bronchoscopy must be pursued in order to identify the correct diagnosis at an early stage in such patients [4] (Fig. 1.1).

Papillomas are the most common benign tumors. Multiple squamous cell papillomas of the tracheobronchial tree or juvenile laryngotracheal papillomatosis is most often diagnosed in pediatric age-group, but there are increasing reports of this disorder among adults [9]. The disease is caused by infection with human papilloma viruses (HPV) 6 and 11 and is acquired either at birth or by sexual transmission [10]. Larynx is the most common location of papillomas [11] (Fig. 1.2). Failure of early diagnosis and treatment leads to involvement of distal airways and lung parenchyma where the lesions manifest as multiple lung nodules with central

Table 1.1 Diseases of central airways

1. **Non-neoplastic diseases**	g. *Miscellaneous*
a. *Infections*	• Tracheobronchopathia osteochondroplastica
• Bacterial, including actinomycosis, rhinoscleroma	• Mounier–Kuhn syndrome
• Mycobacterial	• Brancholiths
• Viral	• Anthracofibrosis
• Fungal	• Foreign body
• Parasitic	• Airway trauma
	• Tracheal polyps
b. *Systemic disorders*	• Inflammatory pseudotumor
• Granulomatosis with polyangiitis	• Blood clot
• Relapsing polychondritis	• Mucus plug
• Inflammatory bowel disease	• Hypertrophied bronchial arteries
• Amyloidosis	**2. Neoplastic diseases**
• Sarcoidosis	**Malignant tumors**
c. *Extrinsic compression*	a. *Tracheal tumors*
• Goiter	• Squamous cell cancer
• Lymphoma	• Adenoid cystic cancer
• Mediastinal masses and tumors	• Carcinoid tumors
• Aberrant blood vessel	• Mucoepidermoid tumors
• Cervical osteophytes	• Chondrosarcoma
• Mediastinal hematoma	b. *Bronchogenic carcinoma*
d. *Airway stenosis*	c. *Metastatic cancers*
• Post-intubation	• Colon
• Post-tracheostomy	• Renal
• Post-transplant	• Thyroid
• Post-radiation	• Melanoma
• Postoperative	• Breast
• Post-traumatic	• Ovarian
• Post-infectious	d. *Local infiltration*
• Idiopathic subglottic stenosis	• Esophageal cancer
e. *Tracheobronchomalacia*	• Thyroid cancer
• Genetic	• Lung cancer
• Mounier–Kuhn syndrome	• Laryngeal cancers
• Chronic obstructive pulmonary disease	e. *Miscellaneous*
• Relapsing polychondritis	• Lymphoma
• Post-intubation	• Kaposi sarcoma
• Post-tracheostomy	**Benign tumors**
• Post-lung transplant	• Hamartoma
• Extrinsic tracheal compression	• Lipoma
• Vascular rings	• Schwannoma
f. *Congenital disorders*	• Papillomatosis
• Tracheal bronchus	• Hemangioma
• Accessory cardiac bronchus	

cavitation [12, 13] (Fig. 1.3). Close surveillance with CT and bronchoscopy is indicated because there is risk of malignant transformation of these lesions, especially when associated with HPV-11 infection [14, 15].

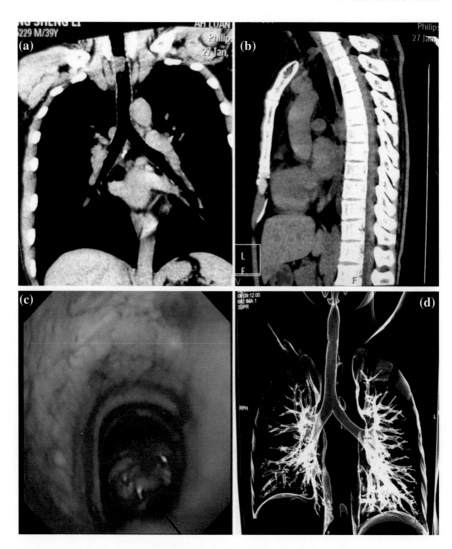

Fig. 1.1 Multiplanar computed tomography (*CT*) and bronchoscopic images from a patient with tracheal adenoid cystic carcinoma. Coronal (**a**) and sagittal (**b**) reconstructed CT images reveal irregular tumor within tracheal lumen (*red arrow*). There is no increase in the thickness of tracheal wall. Bronchoscopic image (**c**) shows tracheal tumor causing near-total obstruction of trachea (*black arrow*). 3D reconstruction image (**d**) after tracheal resection and end-to-end anastomosis shows that wound is healed and there is no residual tumor. Reprinted from Li [273]. With the permission from Springer Science+Business Media

Congenital disorders of tracheobronchial tree are uncommon in adult patients. The most common abnormalities are tracheal bronchus and accessory cardiac bronchus [16]. Tracheal bronchus is a displaced bronchus that most commonly arises from the right lateral wall of trachea within 2 cm of carina and supplies the right

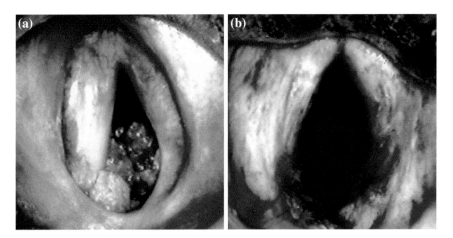

Fig. 1.2 Glottic and subglottic cauliflower-like tumors due to recurrent papillomatosis (**a**). A marked improvement is noted after laser treatment (**b**). Reprinted from Bugalho [274]. With the permission from Springer Science

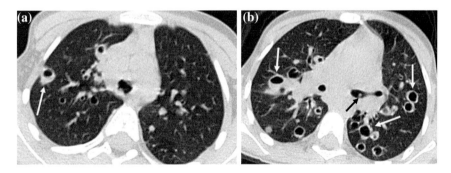

Fig. 1.3 Computed tomography images showing the presence of multiple cavitary lesions (*white arrows*) in a patient with juvenile recurrent papillomatosis. Note the presence of intraluminal tumors in trachea (**a**) and left-main bronchus (black arrow) (**b**). Reprinted from Acar et al. [275]. With the permission from Springer Science

upper lobe apical segment (Figs. 1.4 and 1.5). In a study of 9781 MDCT examination, tracheal bronchus was discovered in 30 patients for an incidence of 0.31 % [17]. Sometimes, the entire right upper lobe bronchus arises from the lateral wall of trachea, when it is called a "pig bronchus" [18]. Tracheal bronchus may be associated with other congenital anomalies. For example, in one study, the incidence of tracheal bronchus was 3.74 % with and 0.29 % without underlying congenital heart disease [19]. Accessory cardiac bronchus is a supranumerary bronchus that arises from the inner wall of right main bronchus or bronchus intermedius and advances toward pericardium [20] (Figs. 1.6 and 1.7). Its lumen is usually filled with debris, ending either into a soft tissue mass or ventilated lung parenchyma. In a study of 11159 CT examinations, accessory cardiac bronchus was detected in 9 patients for

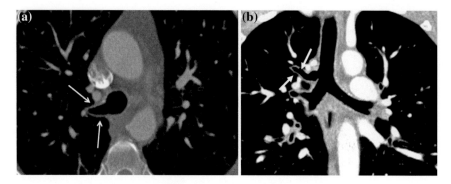

Fig. 1.4 Tracheal bronchus: Axial (**a**) and coronal (**b**) CT images of a patient with tracheal bronchus. Reprinted from Acar et al. [275]. With the permission from Springer Science

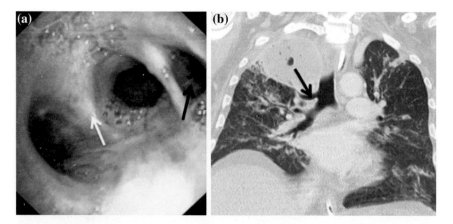

Fig. 1.5 Bronchoscopic image (**a**) and corresponding CT image (**b**) of tracheal bronchus (*black arrow*). *White arrow* indicates primary carina. Reprinted from Holland [276]. With the permission from Springer Science+Business Media

an incidence of 0.08 % [21]. Both tracheal bronchus and accessory cardiac bronchus are usually discovered as asymptomatic radiological or bronchoscopic findings, but recurrent infections and hemoptysis may develop in some patients [22].

Endobronchial tuberculosis is the most important infectious disease of central airways [23]. Involvement of central airways is reported in 10–40 % of patients with pulmonary tuberculosis. Most common anatomic sites of involvement are trachea and proximal bronchi. Submucosal granuloma, hyperplastic changes, ulceration, and necrosis of mucosal wall are hallmark of active disease [24]. Healing occurs with concentric scarring that leads to residual stenosis, atelectasis, and recurrent pneumonia [25]. A normal chest radiograph does not exclude the diagnosis. In fact, 10 % of patients had no chest radiographic findings to suggest pulmonary tuberculosis in one series of 121 patients with endobronchial

Fig. 1.6 Axial (**a**) and coronal (**b**) CT images of a patient with accessory cardiac bronchus (*black arrow*). Reprinted from Sirajuddin [277]. With the permission from Springer Science

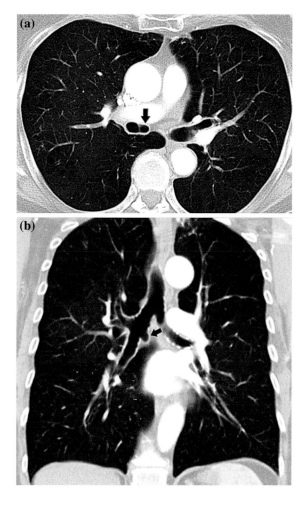

tuberculosis [26]. Bronchoscopy is indicated in sputum-negative patients suspected to have endobronchial tuberculosis.

Endobronchial fungal infections are less common but are increasingly recognized in recent times with the increasing use of bronchoscopy for the evaluation of patients with underlying immunosuppression and stem cell or solid organ transplantation (Fig. 1.8). In an extensive review of the literature, Karnak and associates provide a detailed account of 228 cases of endobronchial fungal infections [27]. The causative organisms were Aspergillus species ($n = 121$), Coccidioides immitis ($n = 38$), Zygomycetes ($n = 31$), Candida species ($n = 14$), Cryptococcus neoformans ($n = 13$), Histoplasma capsulatum ($n = 11$), and Pseudallescheria boydii ($n = 1$). Bronchial washings, brushing, bronchoalveolar lavage, and endobronchial biopsies provided diagnosis in majority of patients. Unfortunately, complete cure was achieved in only 38 % of reported cases. Early diagnosis and institution of appropriate antifungal agents are essential for optimal outcome.

Fig. 1.7 Accessory cardiac
bronchus (*ACB*). RLL denotes
right lower lobe bronchus.
Reprinted from Barreiro
[278]. With the permission
from Springer Science
+Business Media

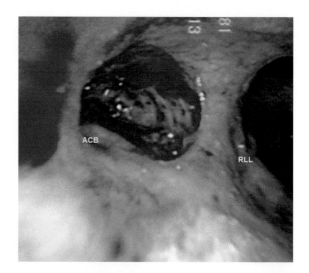

Fig. 1.8 Bronchoscopic
findings of a patient with
Aspergillus
tracheaobronchitis. Notice the
presence of severe
inflammation and thick
mucus. All abnormalities
resolved after 3 months of
treatment with itraconazole

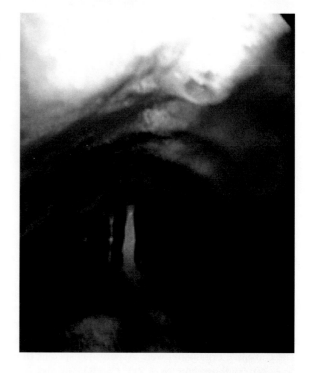

Rhinoscleroma is a progressive granulomatous disease caused by Klebsiella
rhinoscleromatis [28]. The disease is endemic in tropical and subtropical climates
and mainly involves nasal mucosa, but trachea and bronchi can also be involved in
some cases. Untreated, the disease progresses slowly with periods of remissions and
relapses. Four overlapping stages of the disease are (1) catarrhal stage, associated

with prominent symptom of purulent nasal discharge, (2) atrophic stage, associated with mucosal atrophy and crusting, (3) granulomatous phase, associated with nodular changes in nose and other parts of respiratory tract, and (4) sclerotic stage, associated with the formation of dense fibrosis of the involved tissues [29]. Bronchoscopy is helpful in diagnosis [30]. Antimicrobial therapy with tetracyclines or fluoroquinolone agents is recommended for a period of 6 months.

Endobronchial involvement in actinomycosis is uncommon but is occasionally reported [31–33]. Bronchoscopy may show irregular granular thickening and partial occlusion of bronchi or exophytic mass with purulent material raising concern for endobronchial tumor. Characteristic histology with sulfur granules clinches the diagnosis [34]. The majority of cases of endobronchial actinomycosis have been reported in association with airway foreign bodies [35], broncholiths [36], or airway stents [37].

Central airways are also involved with a wide variety of systemic inflammatory disorders. Central airway disease contributes significantly to morbidity and mortality in these diseases. The central airways are involved in 20–50 % of patients with relapsing polychondritis (RP) [38–40]. Initial symptoms in 50 % of RP patients are due to the tracheobronchial involvement. Presenting symptoms include dyspnea, wheezing, stridor, hoarseness, and laryngeal or tracheal tenderness [39]. Airway inflammation and progressive cartilage destruction in initial stages are associated with dynamic airway collapse. These are followed by fibrotic changes that cause subglottic and tracheobronchial stenosis [41]. There are no specific serum markers for the diagnosis. Bronchoscopy reveals airway inflammation, tracheobronchomalacia (TBM), and focal airway stenosis, but biopsies do not disclose any distinctive findings (Fig. 1.9).

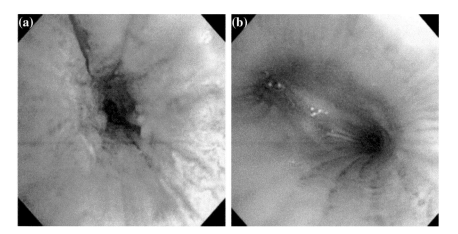

Fig. 1.9 Bronchoscopic findings of relapsing polychondritis. The tracheal lumen is markedly narrowed due to the destruction of cartilage and mucosal edema (**a**). Severe narrowing of both main-stem bronchi is readily appreciated with near-total collapse of left-main bronchus (**b**). Reprinted from Hong [236]. With the permission from Springer Science+Business Media

Fig. 1.10 Subglottic stenosis in granulomatosis with polyangiitis. Notice the inflammatory tissue circumferentially narrowing the subglottis. Reprinted from Bugalho [274]. With the permission from Springer Science

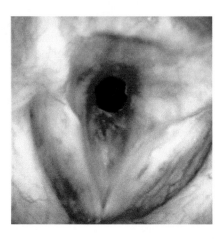

Central airway involvement in granulomatosis with polyangiitis (GPA) typically occurs in conjunction with involvement of other organs, but in some instances, it is the sole presenting feature of the disease [42]. Overall, airway involvement occurs in 15–55 % of patients with GPA [43]. Typical airway involvement includes mucosal inflammation, ulceration, hemorrhage, subglottic stenosis (Fig. 1.10), localized or complex tracheobronchial stenosis, inflammatory pseudotumors, and TBM [42]. The tracheobronchial manifestation may develop in patients who seem to have achieved complete remission of other systemic symptoms with appropriate immunosuppressive therapy, sometimes progressing to advanced airway scarring and stenosis [44]. Cough, dyspnea, wheezing, hoarseness, hemoptysis, and epistaxis are the usual symptoms. Delay in diagnosis is a common problem [45]. A positive antineutrophil cytoplasm antibody (ANCA) test supports the diagnosis, but ANCA levels are undetectable in 25 % of patients with GPA limited to the respiratory tract [46].

Isolated involvement of central airways with amyloidosis is uncommon [47]. Submucosal amyloid deposits cause focal or diffuse plaques and narrowing of airway lumen (Fig. 1.11). Posterior tracheal membrane is not spared, which differentiates it from tracheobronchopathia osteochondroplastica (TO) (Fig. 1.12). In rare instances, a masslike lesion (called amyloidoma) is encountered raising concern for airway malignancy [48]. Simultaneous involvement of pulmonary parenchyma and tracheobronchial tree is uncommon [49]. Clinical presentation is non-specific, and as with other disorders of central airways, patients are treated with a mistaken diagnosis of asthma and COPD for prolonged periods before correct diagnosis is established [50]. Diagnosis requires bronchoscopy with endobronchial biopsies. Congo-red stain of endobronchial biopsies reveals apple green birefringence under polarized light.

Involvement of central airways is reported in up to two-thirds of patients with sarcoidosis [51]. The anatomic abnormalities in the airways may include mucosal airway edema, mucosal granularity, nodular changes, cobblestone appearance, and friability. Yellowish mucosal plaques and nodules measuring 2–4 mm are the most classical finding in endobronchial sarcoidosis. In later stages, fibrotic scarring leads to luminal narrowing and fixed stenosis, predominantly involving lobar or segmental

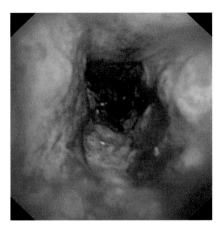

Fig. 1.11 Bronchoscopic appearance of laryngotracheal amyloidosis. Notice extensive involvement of posterior tracheal membrane. Reprinted from Bugalho [274]. With the permission from Springer Science

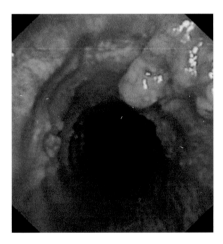

Fig. 1.12 Tracheobronchopathia osteochondroplastica. Notice the nodules projecting from the anterior and lateral walls of trachea with sparing of posterior membranous wall. Reprinted from Holland [276]. With the permission from Springer Science+Business Media

bronchi [52]. Single or multiple segmental or lobar stenoses were observed in 8 % of patients in a study of 99 patients with sarcoidosis [53]. Involvement of trachea and main-stem bronchi is reported but is less common than involvement of more distal airways [54, 55]. Larynx and supraglottic airways are involved in up to 6 % of patients [56]. Definitive diagnosis of endobronchial involvement is established by the demonstration of non-caseating granuloma on endobronchial biopsies.

Central airway is the most common site of respiratory involvement in inflammatory bowel disease (IBD) [57, 58]. In a review of 155 patients from 55 case series, large airway disease accounted for 39 % of respiratory involvement in IBD [59]. The anatomic site of involvement includes the vocal cords, subglottic region, and tracheobronchial tree. Isolated involvement of larynx is uncommon [60–62]. Acute respiratory failure requiring immediate intubation and mechanical ventilation due to severe tracheobronchitis has been reported in a few case reports [63, 64]. Stenosis of large airways has also been reported. Bronchoscopy is helpful in establishing diagnosis, but there are no distinctive pathological changes on endo-bronchial biopsies.

TO is an uncommon disorder characterized by the development of multiple cartilaginous and bony nodules in the submucosal layer of central airways [65, 66]. The clinical presentation is non-specific with chronic cough, sputum production, intermittent hemoptysis, and breathlessness. In many instances, the diagnosis is discovered as an incidental finding on CT or bronchoscopy performed for unrelated indications. The most characteristic finding is the presence of multiple bony or cartilaginous nodules arising from the anterior and lateral walls of the airways, usually sparing the posterior tracheal membrane [67, 68] (Fig. 1.12).

Tracheobronchomegaly or Mounier–Kuhn syndrome is characterized by thinning of the muscularis mucosa due to atrophy of elastic fibers and longitudinal muscles of airways [69]. Both cartilaginous and membranous portions of trachea and bronchi are involved. In many cases, tracheal or bronchial diverticula are formed due to the protrusion of redundant tissue between the cartilaginous rings. On bronchoscopy, there is increase in tracheal diameter with prominent finding of TBM [70]. Typically, patients present after 3rd or 4th decade of life with a striking male predominance. Symptoms are non-specific and are mainly related to recurrent bronchopulmonary suppuration, dyspnea, and, occasionally, hemoptysis. In one series of 10 patients, the diagnosis was discovered in 7 patients as an incidental finding on radiological studies [71].

Broncholithiasis is characterized by the presence of calcified material within the lumen of the bronchi, most commonly originating from the adjacent calcified lymph nodes [72]. Aspiration of bone tissue, calcification of aspirated foreign body, and extrusion of ossified bronchial cartilage may also cause broncholithiasis. Cough and hemoptysis are the most common presenting symptoms [73]. Dyspnea, lithoptysis, and wheezing are also reported. Histoplasmosis and tuberculosis are the leading causes of broncholithiasis. Actinomycosis and silicosis have also been associated with broncholithiasis in isolated reports. Diagnosis is established with chest CT and bronchoscopy (Fig. 1.13).

Bronchial anthracofibrosis is an uncommon entity associated with inflammatory bronchial stenosis with the deposition of anthracotic pigment visible on broncho-scopic examination, without a significant history of smoking or coal worker's pneumoconiosis [74] (Fig. 1.14a). The black pigment in the bronchial wall is derived from carbon particles in the adjacent lymph nodes (Fig. 1.14 b). The majority of the patients are elderly women presenting with cough, sputum, and dyspnea, and the right middle lobe is the most common site of involvement. An association with tuberculosis was suggested in one report, but the exact etiology remains unknown [75]. CT reveals bronchial narrowing with peribronchial soft

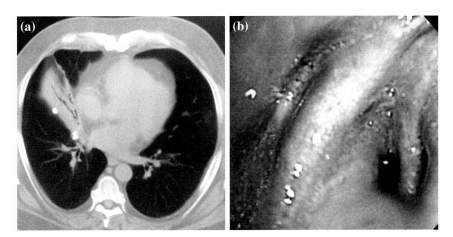

Fig. 1.13 CT and bronchoscopic images from a patient with right middle lobe syndrome presenting with recurrent pneumonia and hemoptysis. CT image (**a**) shows right middle lobe atelectasis due to broncholithiasis. Bronchoscopy (**b**) showed near-total obstruction of right middle lobe bronchus with purulent secretions and inflammatory swelling. Bronchoscopic biopsies showed non-specific chronic inflammatory changes. Patient underwent right middle lobectomy with complete resolution of symptoms

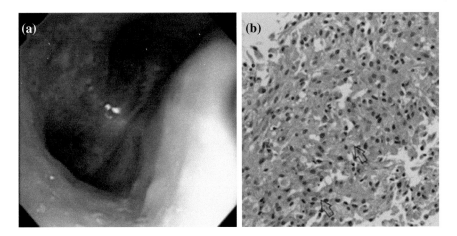

Fig. 1.14 **a** Bronchoscopic image showing anthracotic pigmentation in the right upper bronchus and bronchus intermedius with stricture. **b** Microscopic examination of subcarinal lymph node showing chronic granulomatous inflammation with black pigmentation (*arrow*). Reprinted from Choi et al. [279]. With the permission from Springer Science)

tissue thickening and surrounding calcified or non-calcified lymph nodes [76] (Fig. 1.15). Bronchoscopy is required to differentiate anthracofibrosis from tuberculosis and malignancy.

Airway complications are encountered in 10–15 % of lung transplant recipients and are associated with morbidity and mortality rates of 2–3 % [77]. Important

Fig. 1.15 Axial (**a**) and coronal (**b**) CT images in a patient with anthracofibrosis showing narrowing of right upper lobe bronchus and enlarged subcarinal and hilar lymph nodes. Reprinted from Choi et al. [279]. With the permission from Springer Science

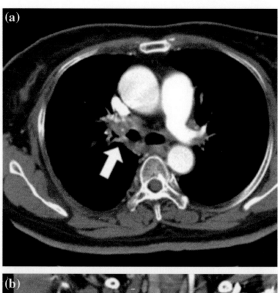

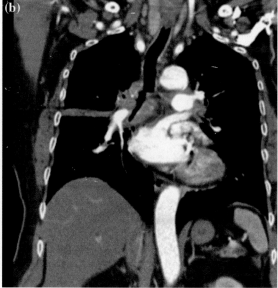

airway complications are anastomotic and non-anastomotic bronchial stenosis, necrosis and dehiscence, exophytic granulation tissue, diffuse tracheobronchial and focal bronchial malacia at anastomotic site, fistula, and anastomotic infections [78]. Common presenting symptoms of airway complications are increasing dyspnea, cough, sputum, and declining spirometry parameters. Rapid development of bacteremia, systemic sepsis, bronchopleural fistula, and mediastinal abscess are ominous findings suggestive of anastomotic dehiscence or development of fistula.

Fig. 1.16 Subglottis stenosis as a cicatricial sequela of endotracheal intubation. Reprinted from Monnier [280]. With the permission from Springer Verlag

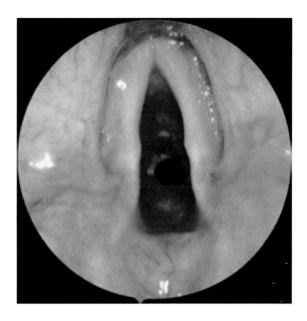

Bronchoscopy and multidetector CT are most helpful in the initial evaluation and treatment planning.

Iatrogenic airway stenosis is most often due to the prior endotracheal intubation or tracheostomy [79] (Fig. 1.16). Post-intubation stenosis most often occurs in subglottic area where endotracheal tube cuff makes contact with the inner tracheal wall. Mucosal ischemia due to the high pressure of endotracheal balloon is the initiating event for the development of post-intubation stenosis. Later, there is softening and fragmentation of tracheal cartilage which causes localized tracheo-malacia. This phase is followed by the development of granulation tissue, and eccentric or concentric thickening of the tracheal wall. The incidence of post-intubation stricture has decreased to 1 % since the introduction of low-pressure cuffs and with routine monitoring of cuff pressures [80]. Post-tracheostomy stenosis occurs most often at the level of stoma and less commonly at the site where the tip of tracheostomy tube makes contact with the tracheal wall. Tracheal stenosis has been reported in 30 % of patients with long-standing tracheostomy [81]. The symptoms of tracheal obstruction can occur immediately after extubation, but it is more usual for patients to present with dyspnea, wheezing, hoarseness, and cough, months to years after the initial insult.

TBM refers to the excessive collapsibility of trachea and bronchi due to the structural damage and weakness of the airway cartilage (Fig. 1.17). A related condition is excessive dynamic airway collapse (EDAC) in which there is excessive bulging of posterior membranous wall into the airway lumen. Both TBM and EDAC produce symptoms due to the expiratory flow limitation [82]. Important causes of TBM are listed in Table 1.1 [83, 84]. TBM and EDAC are reported to occur in 12 % of patients with respiratory diseases [85]. Many patients are

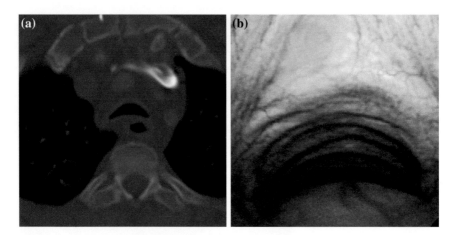

Fig. 1.17 CT and bronchoscopic findings in tracheobronchomalacia. **a** CT shows significant narrowing of trachea with bulging of posterior tracheal membrane. **b** Bronchoscopy shows near opposition of anterior and posterior walls of trachea during normal expiration. A complete tracheal obstruction was seen during coughing

asymptomatic, and some studies have shown a poor correlation between the tracheal collapsibility and expiratory flow limitation [86]. The symptoms of TBM include "barking" type of cough, dyspnea, wheezing, stridor, recurrent chest infections, and respiratory failure [87].

Thus, central airways are involved in a wide range of disease processes. A thorough clinical evaluation is a good starting point to identify the underlying disease at an early stage. Important aspects of history and physical examination are discussed in the following section.

Clinical Assessment

The clinical presentation depends on the cause and severity of central airway disease. Many patients have no symptoms in the early stages of disease. In other cases, the presentation is non-specific and provides no strong persuasion to consider central airway disease as a diagnostic possibility. As a consequence, and not unexpectedly, the diagnosis is often delayed. In majority of instances, the patient receives treatment for bronchial asthma or COPD for several months to years before the correct underlying pathology is identified. Atypical clinical features, lack of clinical response to asthma therapies, and appearance of extrapulmonary symptoms suggest a rapid and rigorous need to consider disorders of central airways in differential diagnosis. In the following section, we discuss the general symptoms of diseases of central airways. Details of individual disease process are covered in the subsequent chapters.

Signs and symptoms of central airway disorders are summarized in Table 1.2. Cough and dyspnea are the most common presenting symptoms. Depending on the underlying cause, cough can be dry or productive. It is not unusually for patients with central airway diseases to develop superimposed bacterial infection due to the airway obstruction, abnormal ciliary function, and underlying bronchiectasis. Many such patients require frequent courses of antibiotics for repeated bouts of respiratory infections. It is a sound practice to suspect the presence of a structural disorder of central airways in such patients. Chronic sputum production must also raise suspicion for infectious diseases such as tuberculosis or fungal infections in appropriate clinical settings. History of lithoptysis or expectoration of stones is rarely volunteered by the patients with broncholithiasis without being asked by the physicians [88].

Table 1.2 Common symptoms and physical findings in central airway diseases

Symptoms
• Cough
• Sputum production
• Dyspnea
• Wheezing
• Hemoptysis
• Lithoptysis
• Fever
• Weight loss
Physical examination
(a) *Common findings*
• Tachypnea
• Tachycardia
• Use of accessory muscles of respiration
• Cyanosis
• Clubbing
• Distended neck veins
• Deviation of trachea
• Generalized or localized wheezing
• Stridor
• Crackles
• Findings of atelectasis or pneumonia
(b) *Findings in specific diseases*
• Papules, nodules, lupus pernio: sarcoidosis
• Palpable purpura: GPA
• Erythema nodosum: sarcoidosis
• Pyoderma gangrenosa: IBD
• Arthritis: sarcoidosis, IBD, GPA, RP

(continued)

Table 1.2 (continued)

• Lymphadenopathy: sarcoidosis, TB, fungal infections, lymphoma
• Uveitis: sarcoidosis, IBD
• Proptosis: GPA
• Chondritis (ear, laryngotracheal, nose, costal cartilage): RP
• Saddle nose deformity: GPA, RP
• Ozanae: TO, rhinoscleroma
• Icterus: sarcoidosis, IBD
• Myopathy: sarcoidosis, prolonged steroid use
• Neuropathy: sarcoidosis, amyloidosis
• Mononeuritis multiplex: GPA
• Restrictive cardiomyopathy: amyloidosis, sarcoidosis

Abbreviations: *IBD* Inflammatory bowel disease, *RP* Relapsing polychondritis, *GPA* Granulomatosis with polyangiitis, *TO* Tracheobronchopathia osteochondroplastica

Dyspnea on exertion usually does not develop until the trachea is narrowed to about 8 mm or 50 % of diameter. Dyspnea at rest can be expected when the lumen is narrowed to about 5 mm or 25 % of diameter. Accordingly, the majority of patients who experience dyspnea already have an advanced airway disease at the time of presentation. Airway narrowing of this magnitude further increases their susceptibility to develop complete airway obstruction from mucus plugging, blood clots, or airway inflammation. Hence, it is not surprising that acute respiratory distress is the presenting symptom in many patients with diseases of central airway.

Hemoptysis is an important symptom of diseases of central airways. Hemoptysis can be a presenting symptom in both neoplastic and non-neoplastic disorders of central airways. The majority of central airway diseases tend to cause chronic, intermittent, and mild hemoptysis. Massive hemoptysis is unusual but can be encountered in patients with underlying bronchiectasis, tuberculosis, fungal infections, GPA, and broncholiths.

Other symptoms of central airway obstruction are hoarseness, wheezing, and stridor. Chronic hoarseness must immediately raise suspicion for laryngeal pathology which can coexist with nearly every disorder of central airways. "All that wheezes is not asthma" is a clinical dictum that has withstood the test of time. Associated upper airway symptoms such as nasal discharge, sore throat, and epistaxis may be observed in many central airway diseases such as GPA, sarcoidosis, and rhinoscleroma.

Because many central airway diseases are a part of a systemic disorder, the presence of extrapulmonary symptoms should immediately alert clinicians to look for correct underlying disease. Extrapulmonary symptoms such as fever, anorexia, weight loss, joint pain, and ocular disease provide valuable clues to the presence of underlying systemic disease. Unfortunately, due to their non-specific nature, these symptoms play a limited role in differentiating one airway disorder from the other.

Distinctive clinical features of diseases such as IBD (chronic bloody diarrhea), RP (auricular, nasal, and laryngotracheal chondritis), and GPA (epistaxis, hematuria, glomerulonephritis) are more helpful in this regard. History of travel to areas endemic for tuberculosis, fungal infections, and parasitic diseases must be sought in appropriate clinical setting.

A thorough clinical evaluation for comorbid conditions such as immunocompromised state, prior chemotherapy or radiation therapy, organ transplantation, heart disease, coagulopathy, renal failure, obstructive sleep apnea, and cervical arthritis is essential in every patient suspected to have disorder of central airways. It is also important to seek any prior history of problems during intubation or attempted bronchoscopy as it will alert the treating team to maintain a heightened state of readiness to deal with difficult airways during the interventional procedures.

Physical examination may provide many valuable clues (Table 1.2), but it may be underwhelming in the early stages of central airway disorders. Chest examination may reveal evidence of tracheal deviation, stridor, localized or diffuse wheezing, coarse crackles, decreased breath sounds, and signs of pneumonia. Localized wheezing is an important clinical sign of focal large airway narrowing at the level of main-stem or lobar bronchus. Tumors and foreign bodies are the most common causes of localized wheezing, although it can be found in any disease process associated with localized bronchostenosis.

Stridor is a high-pitched musical sound that is most prominent during inspiration and is best heard over the neck [89]. It must be differentiated from wheezing, which is best heard over the chest during both inspiration and expiration. Often, the sound is readily audible from a distance without the aid of a stethoscope. The sound is produced by turbulent airflow through narrowed central airways. Prominent stridor during inspiratory phase indicates obstruction at the level of larynx or extrathoracic part of the trachea. Common causes include vocal cord dysfunction, laryngeal tumors, inhaled foreign body, anaphylaxis, epiglottitis, airway edema, thyroiditis, subglottic stenosis, and tracheal tumors. Variable obstruction of the intrathoracic trachea can cause expiratory stridor and fixed central airway obstruction can cause both inspiration and expiration stridor. The common causes include mediastinal or tracheal tumors, lymphoma, and large retrosternal goiter.

Certain findings on physical examination also provide valuable clues toward underlying etiology of central airway diseases (Table 1.2). In rare instances, patients present with subcutaneous emphysema or superior vena cava syndrome with facial and upper extremity edema and dilated superficial veins over the chest wall. Active use of accessory muscles of respiration, tachycardia, tachypnea, pulsus paradoxus, diaphoresis, and restlessness should raise immediate suspicion of critical airway narrowing. Bradycardia, cyanosis, and obtundation are more ominous and suggest that the airway lumen is severely compromised. Immediate intervention is needed in these patients in order to avoid imminent asphyxia and death.

Pulmonary Function Tests (PFTs)

Pulmonary function tests are routinely performed for the detection of airflow obstruction in diseases of central airways. Unfortunately, standard spirometry parameters such as forced expiratory volume in first second (FEV1) and the ratio of FEV1 to forced vital capacity (FVC) have a low sensitivity for the early detection of central airway obstruction. Miller and Hyatt have shown that FEV1 remains above 90 % of predicted until a 6-mm orifice is introduced into the breathing circuit [90]. The decrease in the diameter of airway lumen reduces maximal flows near-total lung capacity before airflows at lower lung volumes are affected. With decreasing orifice size, a progressive decrease in airflows occurs over an increasing portion of vital capacity, readily appreciated on flow volume loop. It is therefore not surprising that FEV1 and FEV1/FVC often fail to provide an early indication of central airway disease in many patients. In contrast, flow volume loop helps define the location of obstruction at an earlier stage providing invaluable clinical information in many such patients.

The characteristic abnormalities on flow volume loop depend on two major factors [91].

First is the anatomic location of maximal airway narrowing. The obstruction is extrathoracic when it is located above the thoracic inlet and intrathoracic when it is located below this level. What surrounds the affected portion of airway is atmospheric pressure in extrathoracic obstruction and intrapleural pressure in intrathoracic obstruction. The second key factor that determines the abnormality on flow volume loop is the dynamic behavior of airway wall (and therefore overall airway lumen) in response to changes in transmural pressure with maximum inspiration and expiration. In fixed obstruction, there is no change in the cross-sectional area of airways, whereas in variable obstruction, the airway lumen changes in response to changes in transmural pressure differences generated during forced inspiratory and expiratory maneuvers.

In a study of 43 patients, Miller and Hyatt identified 3 patterns of abnormalities on flow volume loop which correlated with the location and the type of central airway obstruction [92]. In patients with variable extrathoracic obstruction, the expiratory curve is normal, but there is a plateau in the inspiratory component of the flow volume loop (Fig. 1.18a). This pattern is most commonly caused by vocal cord paralysis, extrathoracic goiter, and laryngeal tumors. In these cases, the intratracheal pressure becomes significantly lower than the atmospheric pressure during forced inspiration. As a result, the obstruction is increased during inspiration, which causes the flow volume loop to show a plateau during inspiration. With forced expiration, the intratracheal pressure increases relative to atmospheric pressure so that the obstruction to airflow is reduced and the expiratory curve remains relatively unaffected.

In variable intrathoracic obstruction, there is a flattening of the expiratory limb of the loop, but the inspiratory component remains unaffected (Fig. 1.18b). Common causes include tracheobronchomalacia and tracheal tumors. In this situation,

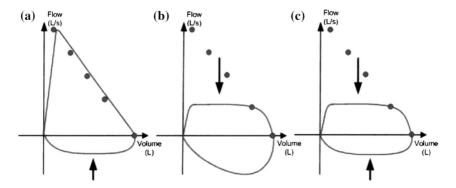

Fig. 1.18 Flow volume loop abnormalities in central airway obstruction. In variable extrathoracic obstruction, there is a plateau in the inspiratory component of the flow volume loop, with normal expiratory loop (**a**). In variable intrathoracic obstruction, there is a flattening of the expiratory limb of the loop, but the inspiratory component remains unaffected (**b**). In fixed large airway obstruction, there is flattening of both the inspiratory and expiratory flow volume loops (**c**). Reprinted from Hadique et al. [281]. With the permission from Springer Science+Business Media

a negative intrapleural pressure during inspiration tends to reduce the degree of obstruction, whereas a positive intrapleural pressure during forced expiration tends to decrease the diameter of the airways, further increasing the degree of obstruction.

Third pattern is seen in fixed large airway obstruction due to tracheal stenosis or to tracheal compression by large tumors that demonstrate flattening of both the inspiratory and expiratory phases of the flow (Fig. 1.18c). Regardless of the location (intra- or extrathoracic), the airway diameter remains unaffected by changes in transmural pressures with forced inspiration or expiration in these cases.

Flow volume loop may suggest the presence of prominent dynamic collapse of airways in some patients with COPD. Usually, the flow volume loop in COPD shows a decrease in expiratory flows over the entire range of vital capacity without showing an initial spike. In some COPD patients, a different pattern is observed in which there is a sharp decrease in expiratory flow rate at high lung volume [93]. This biphasic morphology of expiratory component is reported in up to 20 % of patients with TBM [94]. The inflection point is observed at less than 50 % of peak flow rate, and it occurs within first 25 % of expired vital capacity [95] (Fig. 1.19). The low flow rates persist all the way to residual volume. Inspiratory limb of flow volume loop is normal. This pattern suggests the presence of dynamic airway collapse and loss of elastic recoil in patients with COPD. Interestingly, this pattern of flow volume loop changes to usual curvilinear pattern in some COPD patients after treatment with inhaled bronchodilators.

Unilateral narrowing of the main-stem bronchus is sometimes associated with a biconcave abnormality in flow volume loop (Fig. 1.20). Several authors have reported this finding in association with bronchial stenosis after unilateral lung transplantation [96, 97]. In these instances, normal initial flows during both inspiration and expiration are followed by a plateau giving a unique biconcave

Fig. 1.19 Flow volume loop in severe dynamic airway collapse. Notice a sharp decrease in expiratory curve with inflection point (*arrow*) at less than 50 % of peak flow and less than 25 % of forced vital capacity. *Red curve* represents prebronchodilator, and *blue curve* represents post-bronchodilator maneuver

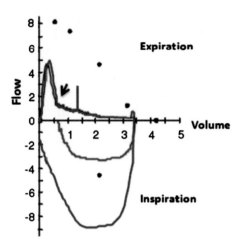

Fig. 1.20 Flow volume loop in unilateral main-stem obstruction sometime shows a biphasic expiratory and inspiratory flow volume loop. Notice a biconcave appearance of both expiratory (*black arrow*) and inspiratory (*green arrow*) curves

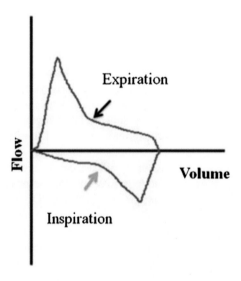

appearance to the flow volume loop. This abnormality most likely reflects inspiration and expiration of two lungs with different respiratory time constants. The initial portion of curve seemingly represents air movement in and out of the normal side, and the flat portion of the curve represents the airflow through the narrowed main-stem bronchus. Resolution of abnormality in flow volume loop has been observed after placement of airway stent for correction of bronchial stenosis.

Flow volume loop sometimes discloses flow oscillations which are reproducible sequence of accelerations alternating with decelerations in airflows giving a sawtooth appearance to the inspiratory and expiratory curves [98] (Fig. 1.21). Sawtooth pattern on flow volume loop suggests the presence of a structural or functional disorder of central and upper airways. This finding was initially described in

Fig. 1.21 Flow volume loop
showing oscillations in
airflows giving a sawtooth
appearance to the expiratory
curve (*black arrow*) in a
patient with
tracheobronchomalacia

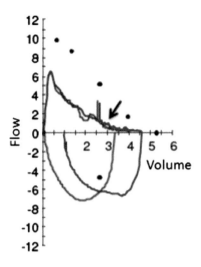

patients with obstructive sleep apnea [99]. Subsequently, it has been reported in upper airway stenosis [100], upper airway burns [101], extrapyramidal disorders such as Parkinson's disease [102], neuromuscular disorders with bulbar involvement [103], TBM [94, 104], and central airway tumors [105, 106].

Flow volume loop must be carefully examined in every patient suspected to have upper airway pathology. Some investigators have also found it to be useful in acute care setting for differentiating central airway disorder from more common disease processes such as asthma exacerbation [107]. Unfortunately, a high-quality flow volume loop is difficult to obtain in a patient with acute respiratory distress. Flow volume loop also provides a convenient noninvasive tool to monitor the course of central airway diseases after therapeutic interventions. Improvement in flow volume loop is readily apparent after therapeutic bronchoscopy in central airway obstruction due to strictures and tumors [108]. In a study of 25 patients with bulky mediastinal Hodgkin's disease, although FEV1 was normal in every patient, flow volume loop was abnormal in 14 (56 %) of patients prior to the therapy. After chemotherapy, the flow volume loop remained abnormal in only 6 (24 %) of patients [109].

Although there can be no doubt that examination of flow volume provides critical information, there is very limited information on sensitivity and specificity of flow volume loops in patient with central airway diseases. In a study of 144 patients with goiter, flow volume loop had a sensitivity of 100 % and a specificity of 78 % in the detection of upper airway obstruction [110]. Two studies have found flow volume loop to have low sensitivity in patients with central airway obstruction. In the first study, the visual inspection of flow volume loop had a sensitivity of 5.5 % and a specificity of 93.8 % in 36 patients with mixed causes of upper airway obstruction [111]. In the second study, flow volume loop had a sensitivity of 30.6 % and a specificity of 93.5 % in patients with confirmed central airway obstruction [112]. Therefore, in patients with suspected central airway disease, it is important

Table 1.3 Quantitative
criteria to detect upper airway
obstruction

• Ratio of FEV_1 to PEF > 10 ml/L/min
• Ratio of FEV_1 to PEF > 8 ml/L/min
• Ratio of $FEF_{50\%}$ to $FIF_{50\%}$ < 0.3 or > 1.0
• $FIF_{50\%}$ < 100 L/min
• Ratio of FEV_1 to $FEV_{0.5}$ > 1.5

Abbreviations: FEV_1 Forced expiratory volume in 1 s, $FEV_{0.5}$ Forced expiratory volume in 0.5 s, *PEF* Peak expiratory flow, $FEF_{50\%}$ Forced expiratory flow at 50 % of vital capacity, $FIF_{50\%}$ Forced inspiratory flow at 50 % of vital capacity

for clinicians to pursue further evaluation with imaging and/or direct bronchoscopic examination even if the flow volume loop is normal.

Quantitative analyses of flow volume loop and spirometry parameters are proposed to be helpful in the detection of central airway obstruction in some patients. The most commonly used quantitative criteria to detect upper airway obstruction are summarized in Table 1.3 [92, 113–115]. Incorporation of quantitative analysis seems to improve the sensitivity in the range of 69–91 % but tends to reduce the specificity to 30–91 % for the detection of upper airway obstruction [92, 113–115]. It is clear that there are many instances in which both qualitative and quantitative parameters fail to detect involvement of central airway with a disease process.

Many other limitations of spirometry and flow volume loop in these patients must be highlighted. The presence of severe airflow obstruction due to a disease process such as COPD or asthma significantly reduces the ability to identify central airway obstruction on flow volume loop [116, 117]. Furthermore, in a recent study, the flow volume loop was only 45 % accurate in differentiating variable from fixed central airway obstruction [118]. In practical terms, adequate pulmonary function tests and flow volume loops cannot be performed in every patient with central airway disease. Many patients are too ill to follow instructions and are unable to make a maximum effort during pulmonary function testing. In some instances, the clinician may choose not to pursue pulmonary function testing since forced expiratory maneuvers have potential to worsen the airflow obstruction in the presence of critical narrowing of large airways.

There is some interest in impulse oscillometry as an alternative to spirometry and flow volume loop in the physiologic assessment of patients with central airway obstruction. In this technique, an oscillating pressure signal of different frequencies is superimposed over the tidal breathing at airway opening using a loudspeaker or a mechanical piston [119, 120]. The resulting change in pressure and flow is analyzed to derive the resistive, elastic, and inertial properties of the respiratory system [121].

Preliminary studies have reported encouraging results with the application of impulse oscillometry in the assessment of patients with central airway diseases. In one report, impulse oscillometry was found to be useful for assessing patency of a tracheal stent in a patient with complicated tracheal strictures [122].

A recent study found impulse oscillometry to be more accurate than spirometry and flow volume loop in differentiating variable from fixed airway obstruction in 20 patients with central airway disorders [118]. Impulse oscillometry was also found useful in the objective assessment of patients after interventional bronchoscopy procedures. Dyspnea scores after therapeutic bronchoscopy correlated with impulse oscillometry parameters but not with spirometry parameters in this study. Encouraging results from this study need independent validation by others interested in this field.

Impulse oscillometry has an intuitive appeal in the assessment of patients with central airway obstruction [123]. Because the test is conducted during tidal breathing, it is easier to perform than the conventional spirometry and the results are not dependent on the patient's effort. The most attractive feature of this technique is its ability to provide a reasonable assessment of airway resistance in patients who are unable to cooperate with or perform conventional spirometry, such as pediatric patients and patients with underlying neurological deficits [124]. Limitations of impulse oscillometry must also be noted. It is difficult to differentiate variable central airway obstruction from severe COPD using this technique [118, 125]. As with other physiological tests, the precise anatomic location of the narrowest segment of airway that defines the choke point for airflow limitation cannot be determined using this technique. Finally, lack of familiarity and non-availability of technology in majority of clinical settings are important practical problems that have prevented more widespread application of impulse oscillometry in these patients. Many of these issues need to be sorted out before this technique can be adopted in routine care of patients with central airway obstruction.

Chest Imaging

Imaging studies play a pivotal role in the diagnosis and the treatment of central airway disorders. Chest radiograph has low sensitivity but a significant narrowing (Fig. 1.22) or an enlargement of the tracheal air column (Fig. 1.23), and tracheal distortion or significant deviation (Fig. 1.24) should raise the suspicion for central airway disease. Indirect signs of airway disease on plain radiographs are unilateral hyperlucency (Fig. 1.25), atelectasis, mediastinal widening, and presence of calcified lymph nodes. Smooth calcification of tracheobronchial cartilage is a common variant on chest radiograph, especially in elderly females (Fig. 1.26). However, pathological calcification of tracheal cartilage seen in conditions such as TO, tracheobronchial amyloidosis, and RP is better shown on CT imaging than on plain chest radiograph. Still, many clues of central airway disease on chest radiographs are missed due to the failure to examine the plain films in sufficient details.

Chest computed tomography (CT) is the mainstay of noninvasive imaging of the central airways. There should be a low threshold to perform CT in any patient suspected to have a central airway disease. Unfortunately, CT imaging may not be

Fig. 1.22 A chest radiograph demonstrating a significant narrowing of tracheal air column (*black arrow*). Reprinted from Hayden [282]. With the permission from Springer Science

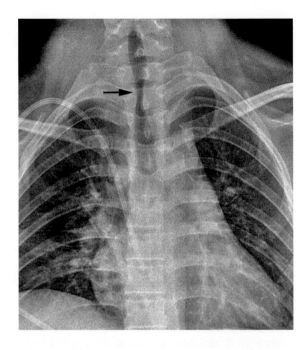

Fig. 1.23 Marked widening of tracheal air column due to the enlargement of trachea in a patient with Mounier–Kuhn syndrome

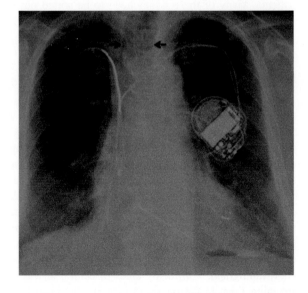

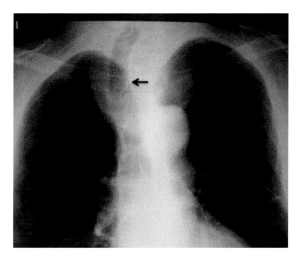

Fig. 1.24 Significant rightward tracheal deviation (*arrow*) due to the extrinsic compression from a large retrosternal goiter

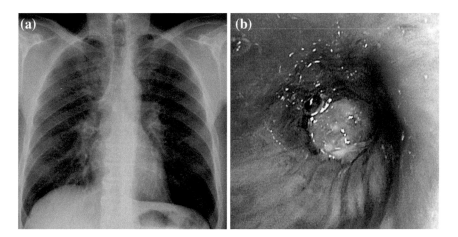

Fig. 1.25 a Hyperlucency of left lung on chest radiograph, most prominent in left lower lobe. **b** Bronchoscopy revealed near-total obstruction of left lower lobe bronchus with a tumor

feasible in acutely ill patients who are unable to hold breath or lay supine for the image acquisition.

The advent of multidetector helical CT scanners has dramatically reduced the scanning time and improved the spatial resolution of CT images. By providing isotropic data set in which the spatial resolution is same in axial, coronal, and sagittal planes and by reducing the motion artifacts, MDCT has allowed two- or three-dimensional reconstruction of high-quality images that provide valuable

Fig. 1.26 Benign
calcification of
tracheobronchial cartilage,
commonly observed in elderly
females. Reprinted from
Sirajuddin [277]. With the
permission from Springer
Science

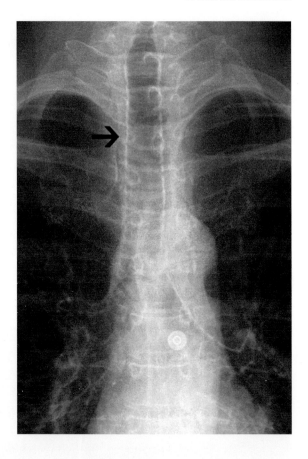

additional information [126] (Fig. 1.27a–f). With the latest CT scanners, thin section images of the central airways can be obtained during a short breath hold. The advances in CT imaging have greatly improved the ability to detect the diseases of central airways at an early stage. An important advantage of CT imaging is its ability to demonstrate the status of airways distal to the stenosis beyond which the bronchoscope cannot be passed. Intravenous contrast is not essential but is recommended for the assessment of the enlarged mediastinal and hilar lymph nodes, tracheal tumors, atelectasis, and vascular malformations. Enhancement of tracheal wall after intravenous administration of iodinated contrast suggests ongoing active infection or inflammation in disorders such as endobronchial tuberculosis, GPA, and RP.

At the outset, it is important to point out the limitations of axial CT in the assessment of the central airway diseases. The most important limitation of axial images is underestimation of the craniocaudal extent of the disease involving the central airways. This is an important limitation because it is a key information that determines the preferred therapeutic approach. Second, axial CT has a limited ability to detect subtle and early airway stenoses. Third, axial imaging is inadequate

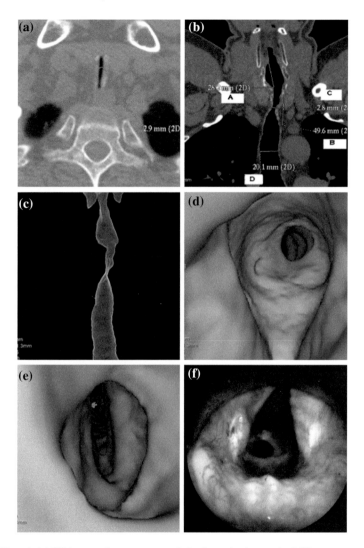

Fig. 1.27 a Axial CT images show a severe subglottic tracheal stenosis. **b** The reconstructed 2D coronal images provide further useful information such as length from vocal cords (*A*), length of planned segmental resection of trachea (*B*), diameter of tracheal stenosis (*C*), and diameter of normal trachea (*D*). **c** 3D shaded surface display shows narrowed tracheal column. Virtual bronchoscopy shows concentric narrowing of the airways from the proximal (**d**) and distal (**e**) sides of stenosis. **f** Direct visual inspection shows high-grade tracheal stenosis, but in such a patient, the length of the narrowed tracheal segment and the status of airways distal to stenosis are difficult to ascertain during bronchoscopy. Complimentary information from multiplanar reconstruction and virtual bronchoscopy is very helpful in the treatment planning of such challenging patients. Reprinted from Morshed et al. [283]. With the permission from Springer Science

for imaging of airways oriented at an oblique angle. Finally, complex three-dimensional relationships between the obstructing lesion and the airway are difficult to assess on axial CT [127].

Multiplanar and 3D reconstruction of CT images provide solution to some of the aforementioned limitations and provide complimentary information in these patients [128, 129] (Fig. 1.27b, c).

Two-dimensional multiplanar images can be displayed in coronal, sagittal, and oblique planes. The length and craniocaudal extent of central airway stenosis is better appreciated with 2D multiplanar images than with axial CT [130]. This information is most helpful in patient with airway stenosis and central airway tumors prior to interventional and surgical therapies [131] (Fig. 1.27b). Reconstructed images are also very helpful in selecting the length and size of airway stents [132]. Several studies have also established the usefulness of MDCT with the reconstruction in the evaluation of stent-related complications [133, 134]. 2D MPR is also useful in the imaging of congenital anomalies such as tracheal or cardiac bronchus.

There are two fundamental types of 3D reconstruction: external rendering and internal rendering. External 3D-rendered images demonstrate the external surface of the airway and its relationship to adjacent structures (Fig. 1.27c). In one study, addition of 3D external rendering to axial imaging provided further information on the shape, length, and degree of airway stenosis in one-third of patients with non-malignant tracheobronchial stenosis and corrected the interpretation of axial CT in 10 % of patients [135].

Internal rendering or virtual bronchoscopy uses the helical CT data to produce images of the internal lumen of the airway as seen during conventional bronchoscopy [136] (Fig. 1.27d, e]). Virtual bronchoscopy allows evaluation of airways beyond the high-grade lesions that are not accessible with standard bronchoscopy [137, 138]. In one study, virtual bronchoscopy images of diagnostic quality could be obtained in 19 of 20 patients with high-grade airway stenosis, but the subtle external compression was underestimated in 25 % of patients [139]. Comparison with conventional bronchoscopy in one study showed virtual bronchoscopy to have a sensitivity of 90–100 % for endoluminal or obstructive lesions, but only 16 % for the detection of mucosal abnormalities [140]. In another study, virtual bronchoscopy was superior to flexible bronchoscopy in evaluating the airways distal to the obstructing lesion but was inferior to flexible bronchoscopy in detecting the early tumor infiltration and subtle mucosal alterations [141]. In recent times, virtual bronchoscopy has also emerged as an important navigational tool to improve the diagnostic yield of bronchoscopy in peripheral lung lesions [142].

The most obvious limitation of virtual bronchoscopy is that it is an imaging tool and conventional bronchoscopy is still needed to obtain the biopsy and culture specimens. The utility of virtual bronchoscopy is also limited by false-positive results because thick secretions or blood clots can be mistaken for endobronchial pathology [143]. Nevertheless, the false-positive result with virtual bronchoscopy is more of a problem for the segmental and smaller bronchi than for the central airways where the majority of interventional procedures are needed [144].

Table 1.4 Dimensions of normal trachea

	Average dimensions (range)
Length (cm)	11.8 (10–13)
Coronal diameter	
Males (cm)	2.3 (1.3–2.5)
Females (cm)	2.0 (1–2.1)
Sagittal diameter	
Males (cm)	1.8 (1.3–2.7)
Females (cm)	1.4 (1–2.3)
Cartilaginous rings	18–24

While reconstruction of CT data is useful in selected clinical situation, most relevant clinical information is obtained from axial CT images in patients with diseases of central airways. Axial CT provides valuable information regarding the size and shape of central airways. Normal trachea has a round, oval, or pear shape during inspiration [145, 146]. Due to the invagination of posterior tracheal membrane into the lumen, trachea assumes horseshoe appearance during expiration. Dynamic CT studies have shown as much as 30 % decrease in the anteroposterior diameter of trachea with expiration [147]. Normal dimensions of trachea are given in Table 1.4 [148].

Several conditions are associated with the abnormal shape and size of tracheobronchial tree. Saber sheath trachea is a common abnormality characterized by a decrease in the coronal and increase in the sagittal diameter of intrathoracic part of trachea (Fig. 1.28). The coronal diameter of saber sheath trachea is two-third or less than sagittal diameter at the same level without any evidence of extrinsic compression [149]. Saber sheath trachea is most commonly seen in COPD patients and is strongly associated with pulmonary hyperinflation [150, 151]. Excessive strain on lateral part of tracheal cartilage is thought to play an important role in the development of saber sheath trachea [152]. Abnormal increase in the size of trachea and main-stem bronchi is most commonly observed in Mounier–Kuhn syndrome (Fig. 1.29). The tracheal diameter measured 2 cm above the aortic arch is more than

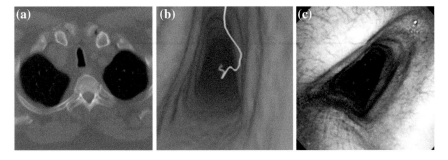

Fig. 1.28 Axial CT image (**a**), virtual bronchoscopy (**b**), and bronchoscopic findings (**c**) in saber sheath trachea

Fig. 1.29 Axial CT image showing marked tracheal enlargement in Mounier–Kuhn syndrome

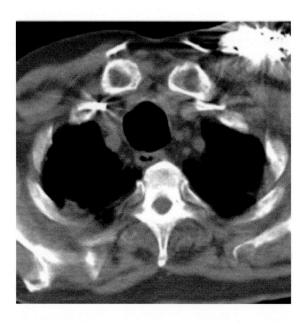

3 cm, and right and left-main bronchi are more than 2.4 and 2.3 cm, respectively, in this disorder [153]. Associated findings include tracheal or bronchial diverticuli, bronchiectasis, and dynamic airway collapse [71]. Abnormal increase in tracheo-bronchial dimensions is also reported in pulmonary fibrosis, cystic fibrosis, ankylosing spondylitis, Marfan syndrome, Ehler–Danlos syndrome, and cutis laxa.

Important CT findings in diseases of central airways are listed in Table 1.5. The most important abnormality to recognize on axial CT is abnormal thickness of tracheal wall. Normally, the anterior and lateral walls of trachea are 1–3 mm thick, delineated by externally by mediastinal fat or lung and internally by tracheal air column. The tracheal wall appears denser than the surrounding soft tissues on CT imaging due to the presence of cartilage. Mucosa and submucosa cannot be delineated from tracheal cartilage with the current CT resolution. The posterior tracheal wall is thinner than the anterior and lateral walls due to the lack of cartilage. Calcification of tracheal cartilage is not unusual in older patients, particularly in women.

Apart from the abnormal thickening of airway wall, central airway diseases are associated with a variable combination of focal or diffuse narrowing of tracheal lumen, calcification, and focal or generalized TBM (Table 1.5). In the following section, we briefly discuss the important CT findings in various disorders of central airways. Details are covered in the subsequent chapters.

CT findings in tuberculosis depend on the clinical stage of the disease process. In active phase of endobronchial tuberculosis, CT shows irregular lumen narrowing with thickened wall, most often involving distal trachea and main-stem bronchi [154, 155] (Fig. 1.30). Contrast enhancement of airway wall and ring enhancement of mediastinal lymph nodes are important clues to the underlying diagnosis. In later

Table 1.5 Chest computed tomography findings in central airway diseases

1. **Direct signs**	g. *Tracheobronchomalacia*
a. *Airway wall thickening*	h. *Tracheal diverticulum*
• Amyloidosis	• Mounier–Kuhn syndrome
• Sarcoidosis	• TB
• RP	• GPA
• TO	i. *Calcification within airway lumen*
• TB	• Broncholiths
• Fungal infections	• Foreign bodies
• GPA	• Calcified tumors, e.g., carcinoid tumor
• IBD	• TO
• Tracheobronchitis	2. **Indirect signs**
• Rhinoscleroma	• Tracheal deviation
b. *Focal mass*	• Atelectasis
• Tracheal tumors	• Post-obstructive pneumonia
• Polyps	• Unilateral hyperlucency
• Papillomatosis	• Air trapping
• GPA	• Mediastinal lymphadenopathy
• Sarcoidosis	• Fibrosing mediastinitis
• Anthracofibrosis	• Focal bronchiectasis
• Broncholiths	• Mucocele
c. *Calcification of tracheal wall*	3. **Associated parenchymal disease**
• TO	• GPA
• RP	• Sarcoidosis
• Amyloidosis	• TB
• TB	• Fungal infections
• GPA	• Amyloidosis
• Advanced age	• Laryngotracheal papillomatosis
• Warfarin therapy	• IBD
d. *Mucosal irregularities or ulcerations*	
• TO	
• TB	
• Fungal infections	
• GPA	
• Amyloidosis	
e. *Airway stenosis*	
• Post-intubation	
• Post-tracheostomy	
• Postoperative	
• Post-transplant	
• Post-radiation	
• Post-traumatic	
• Post-infectious	
• GPA	
• IBD	
• RP	
• Sarcoidosis	
f. *Sparing of posterior membrane*	
• TO	
• RP	

Abbreviations: *GPA* Granulomatosis with polyangiitis, *IBD* Inflammatory bowel disease, *RP* Relapsing polychondritis, *TB* Tuberculosis, *TO* Tracheobronchopathia osteochondroplastica

Fig. 1.30 Axial CT image in endobronchial tuberculosis showing a left hilar soft tissue mass obstructing left-main bronchus (*arrow*). Reprinted from Acar et al. [275]. With the permission from Springer Science

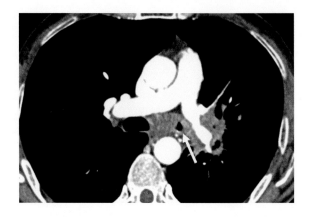

stages, inflammatory changes are replaced by fibrostenosis, which is seen on CT as smooth narrowing of airway lumen with minimal wall thickness. Bronchial stenosis usually involves a long segment (>3 cm) of bronchus, most often affecting the left-main bronchus [156].

Smooth or nodular tracheobronchial wall thickening is observed in fungal tracheobronchitis, but these findings are non-specific and diagnosis requires direct airway examination and isolation of causative agent [157, 158]. Same is true for the rhinoscleroma in which CT can reveal diffuse nodular thickening of airway wall, luminal narrowing, mediastinal lymphadenopathy, and, in late stages, concentric strictures of the trachea and bronchi, similar to those seen in tuberculosis [159]. Because this entity has same geographic distribution as tuberculosis, it is essential to establish diagnosis with appropriate cultures and biopsy.

CT findings in airway disease associated with sarcoidosis mainly involve the main-stem and lobar bronchi, causing distortion, displacement, and bronchial stenosis due to the mural thickening [160, 161]. Trachea is less commonly involved [162]. Confirmation of endobronchial involvement in direct bronchoscopic examination is essential because airway findings on CT can be false positive in some of these patients [163].

In tracheobronchitis associated with IBD, CT findings include irregularity of airway mucosa, concentric thickening of airway wall, narrowing, and large airway stenosis [164–167]. Although non-specific, these findings strongly suggest airway involvement in patients already known to have IBD.

The characteristic CT findings in RP are smooth tracheal or bronchial wall thickening with increased airway wall attenuation [168] (Fig. 1.31). Posterior membrane of trachea is spared. Airway wall calcification is common. Dynamic collapse of airway lumen and air trapping on expiratory CT are additional important findings in RP [169]. In advanced cases, circumferential wall thickening and destruction of airway cartilage lead to fibrotic stenosis.

The most common CT finding in TO is the presence of multiple calcified and non-calcified nodules arising from inner anterolateral wall of trachea and projecting

Fig. 1.31 Imaging in relapsing polychondritis. Axial CT image (**a**) from trachea shows calcification and thickening of tracheal wall (*arrow*) with sparing of posterior tracheal membrane (*arrowhead*). Coronal reformatting image (**b**) in another patient shows diffuse thickening of trachea and bronchi with smooth long-segment luminal narrowing. **a** Reprinted from Acar et al. [275]. With the permission from Springer Science. **b** Reprinted from Hayden [282]. With the permission from Springer Science

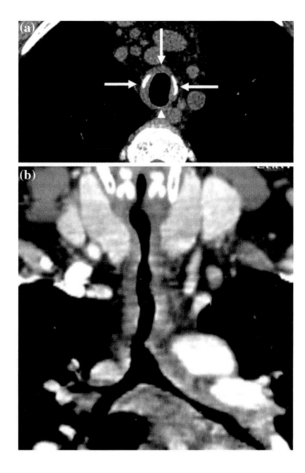

into the lumen without involving the posterior wall [170–173] (Fig. 1.32). Although diffuse or focal narrowing of central airways can occur, TBM is not seen.

TO needs to be differentiated from tracheobronchial amyloidosis in which CT reveals circumferential thickening of tracheobronchial wall due to submucosal nodules and plaques with prominent mural calcification [174, 175]. However, the posterior membrane is not spared in amyloidosis (Fig. 1.33). Associated calcified or non-calcified hilar and mediastinal lymph node enlargement may also be seen [176, 177]. Localized deposition of amyloid material called amyloidoma in the tracheobronchial tree may raise suspicion for neoplasm in some cases.

Involvement of trachea with GPA manifests as 2- to 4-cm-long smooth or irregular circumferential narrowing, swelling of airway wall, and ulceration most frequently involving the subglottic trachea [178, 179] (Fig. 1.34). Tracheal cartilage may be thickened and calcified. Distal involvement of segmental and subsegmental bronchi with inflammation and wall thickening was reported in 73 % of patients in one report [180]. Bronchial stenosis may lead to lobar atelectasis or consolidation.

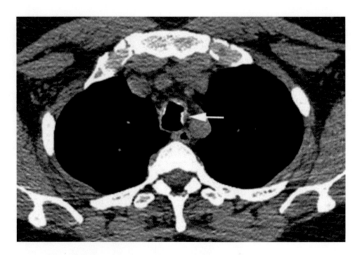

Fig. 1.32 Axial CT imaging in tracheobronchopathia osteochondroplastica showing calcified nodular thickening of tracheal wall, sparing the posterior membrane. Reprinted from Hayden [282]. With the permission from Springer Science

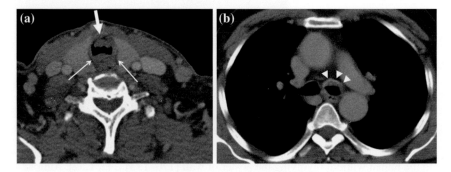

Fig. 1.33 Axial CT images of trachea (**a**) and subcarinal region (**b**) in RP, showing mucosal thickening of trachea (*thick arrow*) and left-main bronchus (*arrowheads*). Note that posterior tracheal membrane is also involved (*thin arrows*). Reprinted from Acar et al. [275]. With the permission from Springer Science

CT also provides useful information of focal diseases involving the central airways. CT findings in primary tracheal tumors depend on underlying histology. In squamous cell cancers, CT may disclose an intraluminal lobulated or polypoid filling defect, a focal sessile lesion, circumferential wall thickening, or eccentric narrowing of the airway lumen [181]. CT in adenoid cystic carcinomas (ACC) reveals a smooth intraluminal mass that seems to infiltrate the airway wall and the surrounding mediastinal fat (Fig. 1.35) [182, 183]. Submucosal extension of tumor tends to cause the circumferential narrowing of tracheobronchial wall. Multiplanar reconstruction is more accurate than axial CT in assessing the longitudinal extent of airway wall involvement in ACC. Mucoepidermoid cancers tend

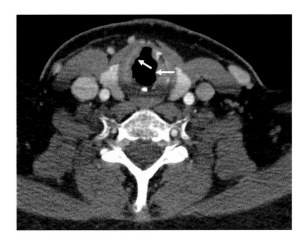

Fig. 1.34 CT imaging in granulomatosis with polyangiitis showing thickening and irregularity at the tracheal mucosal surface (*arrows*). Reprinted from Acar et al. [275]. With the permission from Springer Science

to develop in lobar or segmental bronchi rather than in trachea, manifesting as intraluminal nodule with distal atelectasis or post-obstructive pneumonia [184]. Similar to mucoepidermoid tumors, the most common CT finding in carcinoid tumor is an intraluminal ovoid nodule with lobulated borders causing distal atelectasis [185]. However, a characteristic feature of carcinoid tumors is marked enhancement after administration of intravenous contrast. In some instances, the intraluminal component is much smaller in size as compared to the bulk of the tumor, representing the tip of the iceberg. Calcification is seen in 25 % of carcinoid tumors. Lymph node enlargement may be observed in atypical carcinoid tumors.

Benign tumors of central airways are rare, and CT usually demonstrates a smooth and well-demarcated intraluminal rounded mass less than 2 cm in size [186]. Endobronchial hamartomas are suggested by the presence of fat or popcorn calcification. Detection of fat density is helpful in diagnosing the tracheobronchial lipoma on CT imaging [187].

CT in laryngotracheal papillomatosis shows multiple nodules projecting into airway lumen or nodular thickening of airway wall. Lung parenchyma may reveal multiple thin-walled cavitating lung nodules [188–190] (Fig. 1.3). In primary tracheal lymphoma, CT may reveal solitary mass or polypoid thickening of tracheobronchial wall, but these findings are non-specific [191].

Subglottic region is the principle site of benign strictures of airways due to the endotracheal intubation. Post-tracheostomy strictures occur either at stoma or at the site where the tip of tracheostomy tube impinges against airway wall. Axial CT reveals concentric or eccentric airway wall thickening with luminal narrowing involving 1.5–2.5 cm of tracheal wall in longitudinal direction. Multiplanar reconstruction is more accurate in assessing the craniocaudal extent of benign stenosis and usually shows an hourglass configuration [130] (Fig. 1.27). In some instances, CT shows a weblike stenosis of trachea or bronchi. Axial CT and virtual bronchoscopy can also detect focal narrowing at bronchial anastomotic site in lung transplant recipients [191].

Fig. 1.35 Axial (**a**) and
coronal (**b**) CT images
showing a soft tissue lesion in
the right lateral wall of
trachea (*arrow*), obstructing
the tracheal lumen.
Pathological diagnosis was
adenoid cystic carcinoma.
Reprinted from Acar et al.
[275]. With the permission
from Springer Science

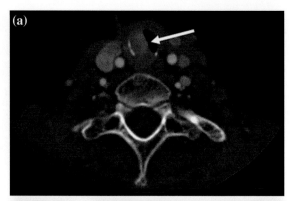

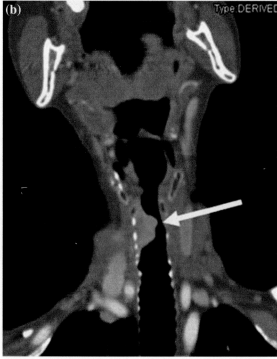

CT images obtained during expiratory phase are routinely used to demonstrate
TBM (Fig. 1.17). Earlier studies used end-inspiratory and end-expiratory CT
images to detect TBM [192]. Several recent studies have shown CT images
obtained during active expiration to be more effective in demonstrating the extent of
airway collapse [193, 194]. In one of these studies, dynamic expiratory CT identified 28 of 29 (97 %) patients who had dynamic airway collapse on bronchoscopic
examination [193].

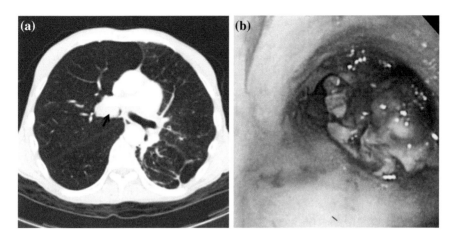

Fig. 1.36 CT (**a**) and bronchoscopic (**b**) images from a patient with near-total occlusion of right main bronchus with squamous cell lung cancer (*arrow*). Right lung is hyperlucent compared to left lung due to the severe right-sided expiratory limitation and air trapping

It is also important to look for indirect signs of central airway diseases on chest CT. The presence of unilateral hyperlucency and expiratory air trapping may be observed in patients with incomplete obstruction of main-stem or lobar bronchi (Fig. 1.36). Similarly, obstructing lesions of bronchi can manifest to atelectasis, recurrent pneumonia, mucoceles, and focal bronchiectasis on chest CT. In some instances, these indirect signs are the only CT manifestations of underlying airway disease. In many diseases such as tuberculosis, sarcoidosis, GPA, IBD, and laryngotracheal papillomatosis, associated CT findings such as localized lung infiltrates, cavitary nodules, bronchiectasis, and mediastinal lymphadenopathy may prompt the clinicians to carefully examine the airways for involvement in the disease process. There must be a low threshold to perform bronchoscopy if any thickening, nodularity, or narrowing of central airways are suspected on CT in these patients.

Apart from providing the diagnostic information, CT is also helpful in assessing the disease progression and effectiveness of therapy in selected cases. Follow-up CT for this purpose is found useful in tuberculosis [155], GPA [180], RP [195], and TBM after surgical treatment [196]. Although a routine radiologic follow-up is unnecessary, CT examination is also found useful in the detection of stent-related complications [133, 197]. In one study, MDCT was performed to evaluate stent-related complications in 21 patients with metallic ($n = 11$) and silicone ($n = 10$) stents [134]. MDCT detected 29 of 30 (97 %) of complications diagnosed with direct bronchoscopic examination. There were no false-positive stent-related complications on MDCT.

Magnetic Resonance Imaging

Magnetic resonance imaging (MRI) is mainly used in the assessment of central airways in pediatric patient population [198]. The use of MRI minimizes the exposure to ionizing radiation in these patients. MRI is most suitable for the study of aberrant vascular anatomy, which is a common cause of airway compression in pediatric patient [199]. Cine MRI is also useful in the assessment of TBM in children [200].

There is limited information on the usefulness of MRI in the assessment of central airway diseases in adult patients. MRI has an established role in the detection of tracheal invasion by thyroid carcinoma [201]. In isolated reports, airway imaging with MRI has also provided useful information in congenital anomalies of trachea [202], tracheobronchial amyloidosis [203], GPA [204], fibrosing mediastinitis [205], and TO [206], but further work is needed to understand the clinical value of MRI in these conditions.

FDG-PET Scan

Main application of 18 fluorodeoxyglucose positron emission tomography (FDG-PET) in diseases of central airways is in patients with tumors of central airways (Fig. 1.37). At FDG-PET, malignant tumors usually have a high uptake, whereas the benign tumors usually have a little or no uptake [207]. FDG-PET can be false negative in patients with carcinoid tumors [208]. Airway inflammation may be associated with a high FDG-PET activity in many non-malignant disorders of airways. In most situations, it is not helpful, but there is an emerging role of

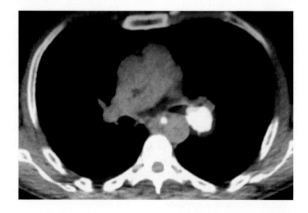

Fig. 1.37 PET-CT image from a patient with a hypermetabolic tumor with a high standardized uptake value (SUV) blocking left lower lobe bronchus

FDG-PET in patients with RP (Fig. 1.38). Preliminary studies suggest that initial FDG-PET is helpful in determining the extent of the disease and follow-up studies are useful in the assessment in response to therapy in these patients [209]. Abnormal FDG-PET activity in RP is observed at several cartilaginous sites including tracheal and bronchial cartilages in untreated patients, which tends to resolve after 3–6 months of systemic corticosteroid therapy [210] (Fig. 1.39).

Bronchoscopy

Bronchoscopy is the key diagnostic test in patients suspected to have diseases of central airways. There should be a low threshold to perform bronchoscopy in these patients. As a general rule, chronic cough resistant to usual initial measures, unexplained dyspnea, wheezing, and hemoptysis should prompt clinicians to suspect diseases of central airway and perform airway examination. Bronchoscopy is also indicated in patients with indirect indicators of central airway pathology such as recurrent pneumonia and unexplained atelectasis on chest radiographs.

Direct visualization not only identifies the lesion but also provides important information regarding the severity and extent of airway involvement. Bronchoscopy allows the operator to assess the extent of mucosal infiltration and detect extrinsic compression of the airways. In addition, it provides valuable specimen for culture and histological examination for tissue diagnosis.

Bronchoscopy provides critical information on location and severity of airway stenosis, which is a common manifestation of several diseases of central airways. Cotton–Myer classification is a commonly used grading system to assess the severity of central airway stenosis [211]. According to this scheme, the airway stenosis is divided into 4 grades: grade I ≤ 50 % obstruction; grade II 51–70 % obstruction; grade III > 70 % obstruction; and grade IV complete obstruction. This description does not provide any information regarding the possible underlying etiology, location, or the length of the lesion. Furthermore, this classification does not apply to lower trachea or bronchi. Freitag and associates have proposed a more comprehensive classification of airway stenosis based on structural changes (Fig. 1.40), variation with respiratory cycle, anatomic location within the tracheobronchial tree, severity of obstruction (Fig. 1.41), and transition between healthy and diseased areas (Table 1.6) [212]. According to this scheme, exophytic, intraluminal, benign, or malignant tumors, or granulation tissue is classified as type I stenosis. Extrinsic compression of airways due to mediastinal tumors, thyroid enlargement, lymph nodes, or aberrant blood vessels is designated as class II stenosis. Distortion, kinking, bending, or buckling of central airways as seen in post-pneumonectomy syndrome, sleeve resection, lung transplant, or massive pleural effusion is classified as type III stenosis. Airway strictures due to the prior intubation, tracheostomy, thermal burns, chemical injury, or surgery, etc., are classified as type IV stenosis. Although no classification can include every possible endoscopic findings encountered with diseases of central airways, it is a helpful

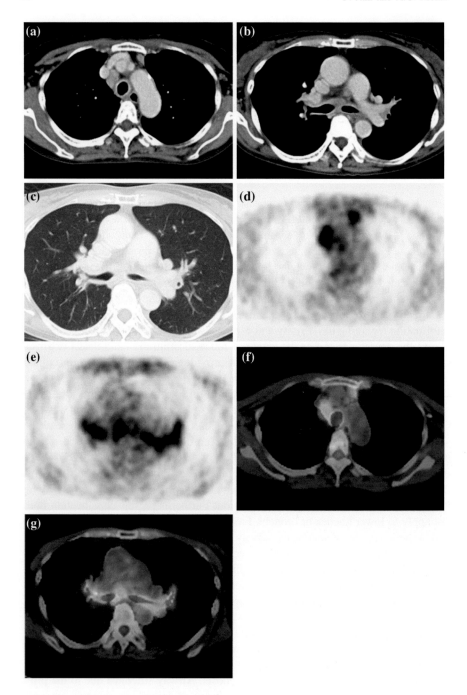

◄ **Fig. 1.38** Contrast-enhanced CT (**a–c**) showing smooth tracheal and bronchial wall thickening with calcification and airway narrowing in a patient with relapsing polychondritis. The airway wall thickening is most predominant in the anterior and lateral walls with sparing of the posterior membranous wall. Axial PET and fusion images showed moderate FDG accumulation in the tracheal and bronchial walls and in several rib cartilages (**d–g**). CT also demonstrated multiple, bilateral, cervical, supraclavicular, and mediastinal lymph node enlargement with homogeneous contrast enhancement (**a**) and moderate FDG accumulation (**d–g**). Reprinted from Sato et al. [284]. With the permission from Springer Science

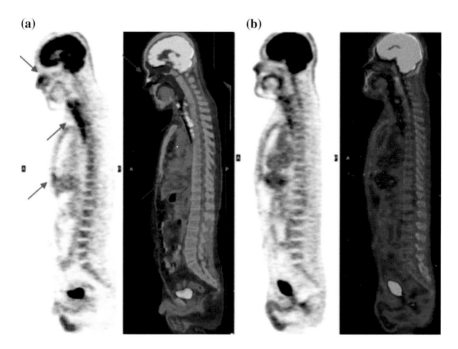

Fig. 1.39 Role of FDG-PET/CT in the assessment of response to therapy in relapsing polychondritis. The initial PET/CT (**a**) showed numerous cartilage foci of pathological tracer uptake including tracheal cartilages, nasal cartilage, costal cartilages, and arytenoid cartilage (*red arrows*). Ten months after the steroid treatment, the 18F-FDG uptake was significantly decreased or disappeared (**b**). Reprinted from Wang et al. [285]. With the permission from Springer Science

starting point when comparing outcome with different therapeutic modalities across the studies.

From therapeutic standpoint, it is most relevant during bronchoscopy to distinguish a weblike stenosis from a long and irregular complex airway stenosis which is typically associated with a significant cartilage involvement and fibrotic reaction. Patients with weblike stenosis have a short (<1 cm) circumferential stenosis and have no evidence of significant cartilage damage, or TBM. Such lesions are better suited for endoscopic therapy and have a better long-term outlook than complicated stenoses with associated cartilage damage and fibrotic reaction [213].

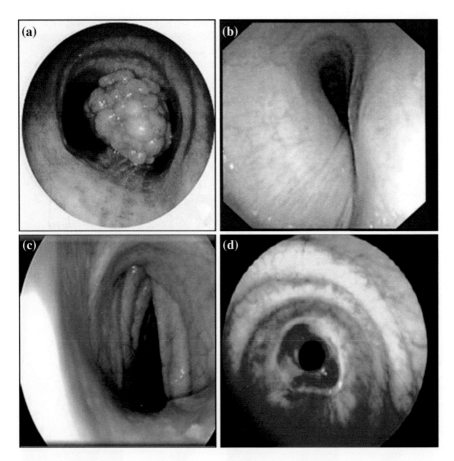

Fig. 1.40 Classification of structural airway stenosis: **a** type I stenosis—from intraluminal papillomatosis, **b** type II stenosis—extrinsic compression from a vascular sling, **c** type III stenosis —distortion in an A-shaped post-tracheostomy stricture, and **d** type IV stenosis—due to the scar from idiopathic tracheal stenosis. Reprinted from Anantham [286]. With the permission from Springer Science

A thorough assessment for the presence of TBM and EDAC is an important aspect of bronchoscopy in diseases of central airways [214] (Fig. 1.17). Bulging of posterior tracheobronchial membrane into the lumen leading to a greater than 50 % decrease in cross-sectional area during expiratory phase of tidal breathing indicates the presence of excessive airway collapse during bronchoscopy. EDAC is most commonly observed in severe COPD and obesity. TBM is due to the weakness or destruction of cartilage of central airways. On bronchoscopy, it may be classified as crescent-type TBM when anterior wall is weakened, saber sheath trachea when lateral walls are collapsing into the lumen or circumferential type when both anterior and lateral walls are collapsing, as seen in RP [214]. Some investigators suggest performing bronchoscopy under noninvasive positive pressure ventilation

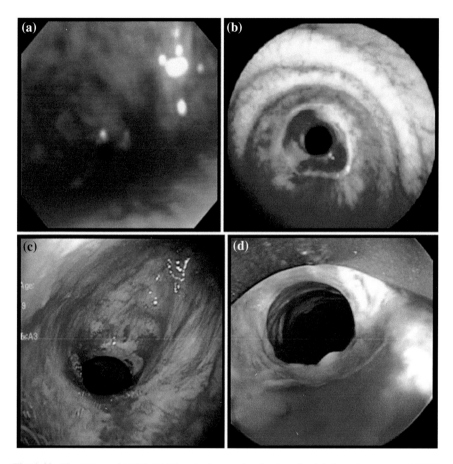

Fig. 1.41 The degree of endoluminal occlusion as visualized on flexible bronchoscopy as **a** 90 %, **b** 75 %, **c** 50 %, and **d** 25 %. Reprinted from Anantham [286]. With the permission from Springer Science

to determine the optimal continuous positive airway pressure (CPAP) or bilevel positive airway pressure (BiPAP) required to maintain airways open during the expiratory phase [215]. The stated goal is to maintain airway lumen during expiration at least 50 % of that during inspiration with positive pressure breathing [216]. Merit of such approach in routine clinical practice needs to be examined in future prospective studies.

In some instances, a localized area of severe TBM secondary to focal destruction of cartilage is observed during airway examination. The causes of focal TBM include infection (e.g., tuberculosis), inflammation (e.g., GPA and RP), radiation (external beam or brachytherapy), stent-related complications, and malignancy. This finding usually indicates advanced airway involvement in the aforementioned

Table 1.6 Proposed classification of central airway stenosis

Structural type of stenosis
1: Exophytic or intraluminal
2: Extrinsic
3: Distortion
4: Scar or stricture

Dynamic behavior with respiration
1: Tracheomalacia—damaged cartilage
2: Floppy posterior tracheal membrane

Degree of stenosis—decrease in cross-sectional area
1: 25 %
2:50 %
3:75 %
4:90 %

Location
I: Upper third of trachea
II: Middle third of trachea
III: Lower third of trachea
IV: Right main bronchus
V: Left-main bronchus

Transition zone
1: Abrupt
2: Gradual

disease processes, needing consideration for airway stent placement or surgical correction.

In certain disorders, diagnosis is evident on direct visual inspection and biopsies are not essential for diagnosis (Table 1.7). Examples of such disease processes include TO, broncholiths, airway foreign body, post-intubation tracheal stenosis, and TBM. In some disorders, bronchoscopic findings are strongly suggestive, but biopsy or culture evidence is needed to confirm the diagnosis. Examples of such disorders include infections such as endobronchial tuberculosis, fungal tracheo-bronchitis, central airway tumors, and systemic disorders such as sarcoidosis and tracheobronchial amyloidosis. In many disorders, neither visual inspection nor the biopsy or cultures establish the diagnosis, but bronchoscopy provides evidence of airway involvement in a disease process already diagnosed on the basis of overall clinical presentation. Some examples of such disorders include airway involvement in GPA, RP, and IBD. In some instances, the presence of active infection may preclude the detection of actual underlying disease. A repeat procedure after treatment with appropriate antibiotics is strongly advised in those cases.

Bronchoscopy is frequently performed to evaluate central airways in patients with tracheal and esophageal cancers. Bronchoscopic findings may lead to a more extensive surgery in some cases and preclude surgery in other cases [217]. Bronchoscopic findings depend on the extent of airway invasion with surrounding mediastinal tumors. In some instances, there is a direct invasion of tumor into the airway lumen, which is readily visible to the bronchoscopist. More commonly, the

Table 1.7 Diagnostic role of bronchoscopy in central airway diseases

1. **Provide diagnosis with airway examination**
• TO
• Stenosis
• TBM
• Foreign body
• Broncholiths
• Congenital diseases, e.g., tracheal bronchus
• Extrinsic compression
2. **Provide diagnosis with airway examination and sampling procedure**
• Amyloidosis
• Sarcoidosis
• TB
• Fungal infections
• Parasitic infections
• Actinomycosis
• Rhinoscleroma
• Anthracofibrosis
• Papillomatosis
• Tumors
3. **Provide supportive evidence**
• WG
• IBD
• RP
• Mounier–Kuhn syndrome

Abbreviations: *IBD* Inflammatory bowel disease, *RP* Relapsing polychondritis, *TB* Tuberculosis, *TO* Tracheobronchopathia osteochondroplastica, *TBM* Tracheobronchomalacia, *WG* Wegener's granulomatosis

evidence of airway wall invasion with surrounding tumors is more subtle, indicated by localized mucosal redness, telangiectasia, mucosal edema, and mucosal erosions [218, 219]. Confirmation with biopsy and brush is essential due to the low positive predictive value of early macroscopic findings in these patients.

Considerable experience is needed to achieve proficiency in identifying a wide variety of abnormalities in diseases of central airways. Bronchoscopy in these patients is not without risks. There is potential for patients to develop complete airway obstruction due to the physical presence of the bronchoscope in the critically narrowed central airways. Local bleeding and mucosal trauma during bronchoscopy may further compromise the airway lumen increasing the risk of sudden development of acute respiratory failure and asphyxiation. Higher-than-average risk of bleeding is reported with bronchoscopic biopsy in patients with carcinoid tumors and endobronchial amyloidosis. Massive bleeding is sometimes encountered after attempted removal of broncholiths during bronchoscopy. Therefore, it is essential that the procedure is performed with utmost care by the most experienced operator with ready access to full resuscitation capabilities.

In some instances, the standard bronchoscope cannot be negotiated through the critically narrowed central airways. As a matter of common sense, no attempts must be made to force the bronchoscope through such lesions. Immediate consultations with interventional pulmonologist, otolaryngologist, and thoracic surgeon must be obtained in these patients. High-quality bronchoscopic images are very helpful in further treatment planning in such patients. In less dire situations, examination of distal airways can be accomplished using ultrathin bronchoscopes, which have a diameter of 2.8–3.5 mm [220]. Successful inspection of distal airway with ultrathin bronchoscopes was possible in more than 80 % of cases in which standard bronchoscope could not be passed beyond the obstructing lesion in one study [221]. Unfortunately, an ultrathin bronchoscope is not available in majority of bronchoscopy facilities.

Radial Probe Endobronchial Ultrasound

Radial probe endobronchial ultrasound (RP-EBUS) has an emerging role in selected patients with diseases of central airways. In this technique, a flexible 20-MHz probe fitted within a balloon is introduced through the working channel of flexible bronchoscope. Endobronchial ultrasound is performed after inflation of balloon with sterile water. The layers of tracheobronchial wall and structures in immediate vicinity can be visualized with this technique. RP-EBUS is highly accurate in estimating the depth of invasion of the tracheobronchial wall in patients with endobronchial tumors [222]. This information is helpful in selecting patients with central airway tumors most suitable for bronchoscopic therapies with curative intent [223].

In one series, EBUS was used for selecting the most appropriate airway location for the placement of airway stents in large airway obstruction due to inoperable cancers [224]. EBUS was also found useful in patients undergoing therapeutic bronchoscopy for advanced central airway obstruction. In a large study, guidance from EBUS influenced the therapeutic approach in 43 % of cases [225]. The most common management changes were adjustment of size of the stent and termination of procedure after finding a large blood vessel in close proximity. In some instances, EBUS findings suggested need for surgical interventions rather than endoscopic therapy.

Endobronchial ultrasound is highly reliable in differentiating airway compression from actual infiltration by the tumors from surrounding organs. In one study, the sensitivity, specificity, and accuracy of 89, 100, and 94 %, respectively, for endobronchial ultrasound were much higher than 75, 28, and 51 % for chest CT for this purpose [226]. Many others have independently validated these results and have shown EBUS to be the most accurate modality in detecting infiltration of airway wall from thyroid and esophageal cancers [227–229]. This information has important implication in preoperative staging and treatment planning of such patients.

Evidence is also emerging for usefulness of endobronchial ultrasound in the assessment of TBM [214]. In EDAC, EBUS is associated with intact tracheal cartilage but reveals thinning of the posterior membrane, presumably due to the loss of elastic fibers. In TBM due to RP, the cartilage appears thick and irregular, while the posterior membrane is spared. In tracheomalacia associated with post-inflammatory strictures, both cartilage and posterior membrane are involved with the disease process [230]. EBUS images have also shown thickening of bronchial wall and destruction of bronchial cartilage in patients with endobronchial tuberculosis. Demonstration of cartilaginous involvement and instability is useful in deciding whether or not to place an airway stent in these patients [231].

There are isolated reports of the application of EBUS in other disorders of central airways. In some reports, EBUS has demonstrated cartilage abnormalities and swelling of airway wall in patients with RP [232]. These abnormalities seem to resolve with corticosteroid therapy [233]. One report also suggests a potential role of EBUS in differentiating graft infection from graft rejection, but independent validation of these data is needed [234].

Overall, EBUS appears to be a promising tool, but more work is also needed to define its role in diagnosis and therapeutic monitoring of disorders of central airway diseases. Non-availability of equipment and lack of training in this area have precluded its more widespread application in these patients.

Diagnosis

Identifying a disease of central airway in a timely fashion is a formidable challenge. A major impediment to early diagnosis is non-specific nature of symptoms. There is no simple test to establish a direct causative link between the symptoms and the underlying disease. High index of clinical suspicion is the key to an early diagnosis. It is not unusual for patients to ignore early symptoms and become increasingly accustomed to dyspnea on exertion by imposing a gradual limitation to their physical activity.

Majority of these patients carry a diagnosis of asthma or COPD with recurrent exacerbation, and many have already experienced important adverse effects from prolonged and frequent use of corticosteroids. Every instance of atypical and medically refractory adult-onset asthma, frequent COPD exacerbation, and chronic unexplained hemoptysis should raise the suspicion of central airway.

A thorough history and a detailed physical examination are essential initial steps. The role of clinician is to identify early clues of central airway diseases and evaluate these patients with pulmonary function tests, MDCT, and bronchoscopy as deemed appropriate. The details of diagnostic findings in individual disorders will be discussed in the subsequent chapters.

Treatment

A wide array of treatments is available for the management of diseases of central airways (Table 1.8). The choice of treatment depends not only on underlying diagnosis but also on the severity of symptoms and airway involvement, disease activity, the presence or absence of fixed airway stenosis and cartilage damage, cardiopulmonary reserve, and patient's preference. The management of individual disorders is covered in the subsequent chapters. Here, we want to highlight ten basic principles that guide the treatment choices and patient management in diseases of central airways.

Table 1.8 Treatment options for central airway diseases

1. **General measures**
• Supplemental oxygen
• Humidification
• Bronchodilators
• Inhaled and systemic corticosteroids
• Heliox
• Mechanical ventilation
2. **Antimicrobial agents (systemic or local)**
• Antibacterial agents: post-obstructive pneumonia, tracheobronchitis, actinomycosis, rhinoscleroma
• Antitubercular agents
• Antifungal agents
• Antiviral agents
• Antiparasitic agents
3. **Corticosteroids and immunosuppressive agents**
• Sarcoidosis
• IBD
• GPA
• RP
4. **Biologic agents**
• GPA
• IBD
• Sarcoidosis
• RP
• Lymphoma
5. **Chemotherapy**
• Lymphoma
• Malignant tumors

(continued)

Table 1.8 (continued)

6. Radiation therapy
• Lymphoma
• Malignant tumors
• Amyloidosis
7. Noninvasive positive pressure ventilation
• TBM
• RP
8. Interventional bronchoscopy procedures
• Foreign body
• Airway stenosis
• TBM
• Airway tumors
• Polyps
• Broncholiths
• Amyloidosis
• Extrinsic compression
• Management of hemoptysis
9. Surgery
• Airway stenosis
• TBM
• Broncholiths
• Airway tumors
• Massive hemoptysis

Abbreviations: *IBD* Inflammatory bowel disease, *RP* Relapsing polychondritis, *TBM* Tracheobronchomalacia, *GPA*, Granulomatosis with polyangiitis

Principles of Therapy in Diseases of Central Airway

1. *Early diagnosis is essential*

   Early identification of diseases of central airways is an essential prerequisite for an optimal patient outcome. In early stages, the disease process may be more amenable to simple therapeutic measures such as antibiotics, steroids, and immunosuppressive medications. Timely institution of medical therapies is clearly associated with better outcome in infectious disorders such as tuberculosis and fungal infections and in airway disease associated with systemic inflammatory disorders such as sarcoidosis, IBD, and RP [235, 236]. Early diagnosis and treatment are clearly useful in GPA, but the airway pathology may continue to progress despite institution of appropriate medical interventions [237, 238]. Valuable opportunity for definitive surgical treatments may be missed if tracheal tumors are not identified in early stages.

   Early diagnosis also provides valuable opportunity to obtain further diagnostic tests, seek specialty consultations, and study natural progression of the disease.

Such thoughtful approach and meticulous planning may not be feasible in patient presenting with acute and life-threatening central airway obstruction.

2. *Early referral and multidisciplinary involvement*
   Managing disorders of central airways is a complicated task at hand. These disorders are uncommon. Most practicing physicians have little or no experience managing these diseases, and with very little evidence-based literature to guide, there is high risk of suboptimal care and adverse patient outcome. For examples, audits have shown inappropriate management in majority of patients with a resectable primary tracheal tumor [239]. There are other reasons to obtain an early consultation from advanced medical centers. The type of equipment and ancillary support required for appropriate care of these patients are not available in majority of community medical centers. Further, expertise required for appropriate management of these disorders crosses the boundaries of many medical and surgical specialties. An optimal care to these patients is a joint effort of pulmonologist, interventional bronchoscopist, otolaryngologist, thoracic surgeon, experienced anesthesiologist, and interventional radiologist from the outset. Such collaboration and experience are only available in a handful of centers of excellence which specialize in disorders of central airways. Many such centers have developed protocols and treatment pathways to provide a standardized care as much as possible. Early referral is clearly essential for optimal outcome in these patients.

3. *Secure the airway*
   Unfortunately, it is not uncommon for patients with central airway diseases to present for the first time with severe respiratory distress and impending asphyxiation [240]. Managing these patients is very challenging. In acute distress, ventilating the patient with a secure airway is the top priority. In the presence of severe airway narrowing, no attempts should be made to force the endotracheal tube past the obstruction as it can further traumatize the airways resulting in airway swelling and bleeding, which can lead to a complete loss of airways. In emergency room setting, the options in these patients are to ventilate with an endotracheal tube placed above the obstruction, to place laryngeal mask airway, or to perform an emergent tracheostomy. Unfortunately, tracheostomy performed in such extreme situations is a difficult proposition and is associated with many delayed complications that may limit the future surgical options in patients with pre-existing high tracheal or subglottic stenosis.
   Rigid bronchoscopy is very helpful in unstable patients with significant airway compromise. Rigid bronchoscopy provides the most reliable airway for ventilation and interventional procedures [241]. As much as possible, otolaryngology and thoracic surgery consultants should be in attendance in the operation room during this time, not only for airway management but also for a rapid assessment of central airway disease in order to establish a definitive therapeutic plan. Unfortunately, expertise in rigid bronchoscopy is not available in many acute care settings.

Common medical measures in these patients include supplemental oxygen, airway humidification, and inhaled bronchodilators. Racemic epinephrine and intravenous corticosteroids are commonly administered, but with exception of croup in children, there is virtually no evidence to support their use in patients with critical airway obstruction from other causes. There are several reports of usefulness of heliox [helium–oxygen mixture] in patients with respiratory distress due to the severe airflow obstruction. Helium has a lower density than nitrogen. Inhalation of a mixture of helium and oxygen reduces the work of breathing by reducing the turbulence and promoting the laminar airflow across the critically narrowed air passages [242]. Temporary relief in symptoms with heliox provides a valuable opportunity to perform a more thorough medical and consultative assessment and allows a better therapeutic planning in these patients [243–245].

4. *Bronchoscopists must be prepared to manage complications*
Natural history of disease is very unpredictable and poorly understood in many disorders of central airways. However, every patient with underlying central airway disease is at high risk of developing respiratory failure with superimposed respiratory infection, airway manipulation, bleeding, mucus plugging, or worsening airway inflammation. Although bronchoscopy has an exception safety record, it is prudent to approach these patients with great caution because serious problems do arise during diagnostic or therapeutic bronchoscopy. The key to a safe procedure is to anticipate the problem and be in a state of readiness to deal with it. Equipment and expertise must be in place to manage serious complications such as hemorrhage or pneumothorax during bronchoscopy. It is helpful to have a clear contingency plan in the event of a major complication. A safe procedure requires a dedicated team of workers with sufficient education, training, and experience to deal with any catastrophic complication. Support from anesthesia, thoracic surgery, and intensive care units should be readily available whenever needed.

5. *Treat the patient and not the image*
Every disease of central airways does not need immediate medical or interventional therapy. Close observation is the most appropriate therapeutic choice in some patients. For example, many asymptomatic patients with TO, broncholiths, Mounier–Kuhn syndrome, amyloidosis, and post-inflammatory stricture do not need any immediate therapy [246–248]. No therapy is needed for asymptomatic patients who found to have TBM on CT performed for unrelated indications. In contrast, early institution of appropriate medical or surgical therapies is always indicated regardless of the symptoms in disorders such as tuberculosis, fungal infections, RP, GPA, and airway tumors.
Thus, the decision to treat must be based on a thorough assessment, natural history of disease, severity of airway involvement, and patient's preference. Every CT or bronchoscopic image that appears abnormal does not automatically become an indication to intervene. In the absence of clear indications, every effort must be made to avoid potentially harmful therapies such as

systemic corticosteroids, repeated courses of antibiotics, and immunosuppressive therapies. Many additional therapies (e.g., biologic agents) that entail high cost to the society may be effective in active disease but provide limited or no benefit in advanced and inactive phase of the disease such as post-inflammatory strictures. Similarly, appropriate patient selection is also critical for favorable results with bronchoscopic interventions and airway surgeries [249].

6. *Medical therapies are highly effective in many disorders of central airways*
Medical therapy is the mainstay of treatment in several disorders of central airways. Highly effective therapies are available for infections such as tuberculosis, fungal infections, actinomycosis, rhinoscleroma, sarcoidosis, IBD-associated airway disease, RP, and GPA. Having technical skills in interventional bronchoscopy procedures is never an appropriate reason to choose bronchoscopic therapies over less invasive and more appropriate medical therapies. For example, in TBM associated with COPD, aggressive medical measures and a trial of positive airway pressure are always advisable before subjecting patients to more invasive therapies such as airway stents or surgery [250].

7. *Intervene only when intervention is essential*
At the outset, it must be understood that the primary role of bronchoscopy is in establishing the diagnosis and not in the treatment of diseases that affect central airways. Still, interventional bronchoscopy is highly effective in certain situations. Important point is to understand the appropriate indication and timing of the interventional bronchoscopic procedure. The main indications for therapeutic bronchoscopy in central airway disease are as follows: (1) immediate restoration of critically narrowed airways, (2) palliative treatment of advanced airway obstruction due to malignant tumors, (3) management of postoperative complications such as granulation tissue and post-lung-transplant anastomotic complications, (4) removal of obstructing foreign bodies, loose broncholiths, tenacious secretions and mucus plugs, and blood clots from airways, and (5) management of airway stenosis when airway surgery either is not indicated or is not feasible due to the extent of disease or medical reasons. A wide range of ablative procedures such as Nd:YAG laser, electrocautery, argon plasma coagulation, cryotherapy, brachytherapy, and balloon dilation have been applied in patients with central airway diseases [231, 251]. Airway stents have been placed for symptomatic relief in patients with extrinsic compression, severe TBM, and airway stenosis [252]. In some instances, immediate relief of obstructive symptoms with the successful application of interventional procedure may pave way to a more definitive therapy or an elective surgery at a later date. Care must be taken to avoid extensive airway manipulations and airway stents in such patients [253].
However, choosing a right interventional procedure for a right indication is not as easy as it seems. A deep understanding of the correct indication, timing, and choice of an interventional procedure is a difficult skill to acquire. Technical aspects are easier to learn with an appropriate training. A decision to perform an

interventional procedure must be based on a thorough assessment and thoughtful planning. Unfortunately, we are aware of many instances in which poor choice of initial bronchoscopic intervention has seriously jeopardized the prospects of a more definitive and potentially curative surgical therapy. In disorders of central airways, the aim of the treatment is to achieve cure, whereas in advanced malignant obstruction, the primary goal of treatment is palliation of symptoms. The majority of interventional bronchoscopy procedures are better suited to provide palliation of symptoms than to provide a permanent cure. It is also important to point out that interventional bronchoscopy for central airway diseases is a high-risk procedure. In a multi-institutional study, therapeutic bronchoscopy was associated with a complication rate of 19.8 % and a 30-day mortality of 7.8 % [254]. Although complication rate with interventional procedure was higher in patients with underlying malignant disease, a significant proportion of patients (15 %) with a benign disorder also experienced procedure-related complication in this study.

8. *Primum non nocere: Do not place metallic stents in non-malignant disorders*
Airway stents have an important palliative role in advanced airway obstruction due to intrathoracic malignancies. Fully covered metallic stents are preferred in these patients due to the relative ease of placement using flexible bronchoscope [255]. Stent placement is also needed in some patients with non-malignant airway obstruction. Generally, stents for non-malignant disorders are placed in one of the two situations: (1) when more definitive therapies such as surgery are not a treatment option and (2) when a stent is placed with an intention to remove it at a later date after it has served its purpose. Examples of latter indication include airway stent placement for post-tuberculosis airway strictures [256] and a stent trial prior to tracheoplasty operation for severe TBM [257]. Airway stents can be associated with many serious complications. Three main complications are stent migration, formation of biofilms causing recurrent respiratory tract infections, and formation of granulation tissue. Migration is more likely with silicone stents than with metallic stents. Granulation tissue is more common with metallic stents. Development of excessive amounts of granulation tissue can cause severe airway narrowing which requires repeated bronchoscopic procedures to restore the airway lumen [258]. Many factors such as direct airway irritation from broken wires, mucosal ischemia, overgrowth of bacteria, and galvanic currents from metallic wires are said to contribute to the development of exuberant granulation tissue [259]. Formation of granulation after placement of self-expanding metallic stent is a common problem in benign airway diseases [260, 261]. Removal of metallic stents may not feasible once the stent is fully embedded in the airway wall and overgrowth of respiratory epithelium has developed [262]. Removal of metallic stents may be associated with significant hemorrhage and requires experience in rigid bronchoscopy [263]. Frequent reports of this complication and difficulties in removal of metallic stents have prompted FDA to issue a specific blackbox warning against placement of metallic stent in non-malignant disorders of airways in 2005.

At present, metallic stents cannot be recommended for non-malignant disorders, with rare exceptions when all other measures to correct the underlying pathology have been tried unsuccessfully, leaving no other viable treatment option [264, 265].

 9. *Surgery is beneficial in selected patients:*
    Surgery is the only chance for cure in patients with primary tracheal tumors [266, 267]. The diagnostic evaluation and appropriate surgical consultation must be expedited in these patients. Surgery is also preferred over interventional therapies in patients with bronchial carcinoids and benign tracheal tumors [268, 269]. Among non-neoplastic disorders, surgery is the treatment of choice in the management of complex post-intubation and post-tracheostomy strictures [270]. Repeated failed attempts of bronchoscopic interventions only serve to delay and complicate the surgical therapy. Tracheoplasty has been performed in selected patients with severe TBM with good results, but its indications and benefits remain poorly defined. Bronchoscopic interventions have a role in some patients with broncholiths [271], but surgical treatment is the standard of care in symptomatic patients with large broncholiths adhered to airway wall [247, 272]. In some patients, surgical intervention is needed for the management of post-inflammatory airway strictures secondary to tuberculosis, fungal infections, sarcoidosis, IBD, and TO. Severe bleeding, repeated lung infections, and atelectasis due to the severe disease of central airways may require lobectomy and pneumonectomy in some cases.

10. *Regular follow-up is essential*
    A long-term follow-up is essential in every patient with disorder of central airways. The main goals are to assess the therapeutic response and to detect the disease progression or relapse at an early stage. Individual clinical scenario should dictate the frequency of follow-up visits. Apart from a thorough clinical assessment, a physiological assessment with PFTs and flow volume loop is an important component of ongoing care. In selected situations, repeat imaging with MDCT provides valuable clinical information. A decision to reexamine the airway with bronchoscopy should be based on underlying diagnosis and clinical symptoms. With few exceptions, there are little data to guide physicians in this regard. A clear action plan must be in place in the event of an emergency.

Conclusion

Central airways are involved in a wide variety of disorders, ranging from infections, to malignancies, systemic inflammatory disorders, and iatrogenic diseases. The correct diagnosis is usually delayed due to the non-specific presentation and low sensitivity of routine pulmonary function tests and chest radiographs. Careful examination of flow volume loops is very helpful, but it appears to have a low sensitivity in the detection of central airway diseases. Patients are often misdiagnosed as having asthma or COPD and are treated inappropriately for a prolonged periods before the actual diagnosis is identified. Valuable opportunity to treat patient with simple medical measures is sometimes lost due to the delay in diagnosis. Early diagnosis requires high index of suspicion and keen awareness of these disease processes. Multidetector chest computed tomography is the most useful radiological investigation in patients suspected to have diseases of central airways. Axial images are most useful, but in selected situation, two- or three-dimensional multiplanar reconstructions provide additional clinical information. Bronchoscopy is the key diagnostic test. Apart from the direct airway examination, biopsy and culture specimens provide pathological and microbiologic confirmation of underlying diagnosis. Bronchoscopy is also essential before selecting patients for intervention and surgical therapies. The treatment of these disorders is complicated and often requires a multidisciplinary approach. Due to the complex nature of the underlying disease, high demand for equipment, expertise, and multispecialty consultations, majority of these patients are best managed in medical centers which specialize in complex airway disorders.

References

1. Grenier PA, Beigel-Aubry C, Brillet P-Y. Non-neoplastic tracheal and bronchial stenosis. Thorac Surg Clin. 2010;20:47–64.
2. Barros CD, Fernandez-Bussy S, Folch E, Flades AJ, Majid A. Non-malignant central airway obstruction. Arch Broncopneomol. 2014;50:345–54.
3. Puchalski J, Musani AI. Tracheobronchial stenosis. Causes and advances in management. Clin Chest Med. 2013;34:557–67.
4. Honing J, Gaissert HA, van der Heijden HFM, Verhagen ADFMT, Kaanders JHAM, Marres HAM. Clinical aspects and treatment of primary tracheal malignancies. Acta Otolaryngol. 2010;130:763–72.
5. Ferretti GR, Bithigoffer C, Righni CA, Arbib F, Lantuejoul S, Jankowski A. Imaging of tumors of the trachea and central bronchi. Thorac Surg Clin. 2010;20:31–45.
6. Macchiarini P. Primary tracheal tumors. Lancet Oncol. 2006;7:83–91.
7. Gaissert HA, Grillo HC, Shadmehr MB, Wright CD, Gokhale M, Wain JC. Long term survival after resection of primary adenoid cystic and squamous cell carcinoma of trachea and carina. Ann Thorac Surg. 2004;78:1889–97.
8. Licth PB, Friis S, Pettersson G. Tracheal cancers in Denmark: a nationwide study. Eur J Cardiovasc Surg. 2001;19:339045.
9. Venkatesan NN, Pine HS, Underbrink MP. Recurrent respiratory papillomatosis. Otolaryngol Clin North Am. 2012;45:671–94.
10. Kashima HK, Mounts P, Shah K. Recurrent respiratory papillomatosis. Obstet Gynecol Clin North Am. 1996;23:699–706.
11. Derkay CS, Waitrak B. Recurrent respiratory papillomatosis: a review. Laryngoscope. 2008;118:1236–47.
12. Blackledge FA, Anand VK. Tracheobronchial extension of recurrent respiratory papillamatosis. Ann Otol Rhinol Laryngol 2000;109:812–8.
13. Soldatski IL, Onufrieva EK, Steklov AM, Schepin NV. Tracheal bronchial and pulmonary papillomatosis in children. Laryngoscope. 2005;115:1848–54.

14. Schraff S, Derkay CS, Burke B, et al. American society of pediatric otolaryngology members' experience with recurrent respiratory papillomatosis and the use of adjuvant therapy. Arch Otolaryngol Head Neck Surg. 2004;130:1039–42.
15. Cook JR, Hill DA, Humphrey PA, Pfeifer JD, El-Mofty SK. Squamous cell carcinoma arising in recurrent respiratory papillomatosis with pulmonary involvement: emerging common patterns of clinical features and human papilloma serotype association. Mod Pathol. 2000;13:914–8.
16. Desir A, Ghaye B. Congenital abnormalities of intrathoracic airways. Radiol Clin North Am. 2009;47:203–25.
17. Suzuki M, Matsui O, Kawashima H, et al. Radioanatomical study of a true tracheal bronchus using multidetector computed tomography. Jpn J Radiol. 2010;28:188–92.
18. Ghaye B, Szapiro D, Fanchamps JM, Dondelinger RE. Congenital bronchial abnormalities revisited. Radiographics. 2001;21:105–19.
19. Ming Z, Lin Z. Evaluation of tracheal bronchus in Chinese children using multidetector CT. Pediatr Radiol. 2007;37:1230–4.
20. Yildiz H, Ugurel S, Soylu K, Tesar M, Somuncu I. Accessory cardiac bronchus and tracheal bronchus anomalies: CT bronchoscopy and CT-bronchography findings. Surg Radiol Anat. 2006;28:646–9.
21. Ghaye B, Kos X, Dondelinger RF. Accessory cardiac bronchus: 3D CT demonstration in 9 cases. Eur Radiol. 1999;9:45–8.
22. McGuinness G, Naidich DP, Garay SM, Davis AL, Boyd AD, Mizrachi HH. Accessory cardiac bronchus: CT features and clinical significance. Radiology. 1993;189:563–6.
23. Shim YS. Endobronchial tuberculosis. Respirology 1996;1:95–106.
24. Lee JH, Chung HS. Bronchoscopic, radiologic and pulmonary function evaluation of endobronchial tuberculosis. Respirology. 2000;5:411–7.
25. Chung HS, Lee JH. Bronchoscopic assessment of the evolution of endobronchial tuberculosis. Chest. 2000;117:385–92.
26. Lee JH, Park SS, Lee DH, Shin DH, Yang SC, Yoo BM. Endobronchial tuberculosis. Clinical and bronchoscopic features in 121 cases. Chest. 1992;102:990–4.
27. Karnak D, Avery RK, Gildea TR, Sahoo D, Mehta AC. Endobronchial fungal disease: an unrecognized entity. Respiration. 2007;74:88–104.
28. Miller RH, Shulman JB, Canlais RF, Ward PH. Klebsiella rhinoscleromatis: a clinical and pathogenic enigma. Otolaryngol Head Neck Surg. 1979;87:212–21.
29. Amolis CP, Shindo ML. Laryngotracheal manifestations of rhinoscleroma. Ann Otol Rhinol Laryngol. 1996;105:336–40.
30. Soni NK. Scleroma of lower respiratory tract: a bronchoscopic study. J Laryngol Otol. 1994;108:484–5.
31. Farrokh D, Rezaitalab F, Bakhshoudeh B. Pulmonary actinomycosis with endobronchial involvement: a case report and literature review. Tanaffos. 2014;13:52–6.
32. Broquetas J, Aran X, Moreno A. Pulmonary actinomycosis with endobronchial involvement. Eur J Clin Microbiol. 1985;4:508.
33. Cendan I, KlapholzA, Talavera W. Pulmonary actinomycosis: a cause of endobronchial disease in a patient with AIDs. Chest 1993;103:1886–7
34. Jin SL, Lee HP, Kim JI, et al. A case of endobronchial actinomycosis. Korean J Intern Med. 2000;15:240–4.
35. Baek JH, Lee JH, Kim MS, Lee JC. Pulmonary actinomycosis associated with endobronchial vegetable foreign body. Korean J Thorac Cardiovasc Surg. 2014;47:566–8.
36. Kim TS, Han J, Koh WJ, et al. Endobronchial actinomycosis associated with broncholithiasis: CT findings for 9 patients. AJR Am J Roentgenol. 2005;185:347–53.
37. Godfrey AM, Diaz-Mandoza J, ray C, Simoff MJ. Endobronchial actinomycosis after airway stenting. J Bronchol Intervent Pulmonol 2012;19:315–8.
38. Ernst A, Rafeq S, Boiselle P, et al. Relapsing polychondritis and airway involvement. Chest. 2009;135:1024–30.

39. Staas BA, Utz JP, Michet CJ Jr. Relapsing polychondritis. Semin Respir Crit care Med. 2002;23:145–54.
40. McAdam LP, O'Hanlan MA, Bluestone R, et al. Relapsing polychondritis: prospective study of 23 patients and a review of the literature. Medicine. 1976;55:193–215.
41. Rafeq S, Trentham D, Ernst A. Pulmonary manifestations of relapsing polychondritis. Clin Chest Med. 2010;31:513–8.
42. Dunn TE, Specks U, Colby TV, et al. Tracheobronchial involvement in Wegener's granulomatosis. Am J Respir Crit Care Med 1995;151(2 pt 1):522–6.
43. Polychronopoulos VS, Prakash UBS, Goblin JM, Edell ES, Specks U. Airway involvement in Wegener's granulomatosis. Rheum Clin North Am. 2007;33:755–75.
44. Gluth MB, Shinners PA, Kasperbauer JL. Subglottic stenosis associated with Wegener's granulomatosis. Laryngoscope. 2003;113:1304–7.
45. Abdou NI, Kullman GJ, Hoffman GS, et al. Wegener's granulomatosis: survey of 701 patients in North America. Changes in outcome in the 1990s. J Rheumatol. 2002;29:309–16.
46. Taylor SD, Clayburgh DR, Rosenbaum JT, Schindler JS. Progression and management of Wegener's granulomatosis in the head and neck. Laryngoscope. 2012;122:1695–700.
47. Gilmore JD, Hawkins PN. Amyloidosis and the respiratory tract. Thorax. 1999;54:444–51.
48. Utz JP, Swensen SJ, Gertz MA. Pulmonary amyloidosis: the Mayo clinic experience from 1980 to 1993. Ann Intern Med. 1996;124:407–13.
49. O'Regan A, Fenlon HM, Beamis JF Jr, et al. Tracheobronchial amyloidosis. The Boston University experience from 1984 to 1999. Medicine (Baltimore). 2000;2000(79):69–79.
50. Ding L, Li W, Wang K, et al. Primary tracheobronchial amyloidosis in China: analysis of 64 cases and a review of literature. J Huazhong Univ Sci Technol (Med Sci). 2010;30:599–603.
51. Polychronopoulos VS, Prakash UBS. Airway involvement in sarcoidosis. Chest. 2009;136:1371–80.
52. Westcott JL, Noehren TH. Bronchial stenosis in chronic sarcoidosis. Chest. 1973;63:893–7.
53. Olsson T, Bjornstad-Pettersen H, Stjernberg NL. Bronchostenosis due to sarcoidosis. A cause of atelectasis and airway obstruction simulating pulmonary neoplasm and chronic obstructive pulmonary disease. Chest. 1979;75:663–6.
54. Brandstetter RD, Messina MS, Sprince NL, Grillo HC. Tracheal stenosis due to sarcoidosis. Chest. 1981;80:656.
55. Muller A, Brown KL, Teirstein AS. Stenosis of main bronchi mimicking fixed upper airway obstruction in sarcoidosis. Chest. 1985;88:244–8.
56. Rottoli P, Bargagli E, Chihichimo C, et al. Sarcoid with upper respiratory tract involvement. Respir Med. 2006;100:253–7.
57. Camus, P, Piard, F, Ashcroft, T, et al. The lung in inflammatory bowel disease. Medicine (Baltimore)1993;72:151–83.
58. Mahadeva R, Walsh G, Flower CD, et al. Clinical and radiological characteristics of lung disease in inflammatory bowel disease. Eur Respir J. 2000;15:41–8.
59. Black H, Mendoza M, Murin S. Thoracic manifestations of inflammatory bowel disease. Chest. 2007;131:524–32.
60. Kelley JH, Montgomery WW, Goodman ML, Mulvaney TJ. Upper airway obstruction associated with regional enteritis. Ann Otol. 1979;188:95–9.
61. Ulnick KM, Perkins J. Extraintestinal Crohn's disease: case report and review of literature. Ear Nose Throat J. 2001;80:97–100.
62. Lemann M, Messing B, D'Agay F. Crohn's disease with respiratory tract involvement. Gut. 1987;28:1669–72.
63. Lamblin C, Copin MC, Billaut C, et al. Acute respiratory failure due to tracheobronchial involvement in Crohn's disease. Eur Respir J. 1996;9:2176–8.
64. Shad JA, Sharief GQ. Tracheobronchitis as an initial presentation of ulcerative colitis. J Clin Gastroenterol. 2001;33:161–3.
65. Prakash U. Tracheobronchopathia osteochondroplastica. Semin Respir Crit Care Med. 2002;23:167–75.

66. Abu-Hijleh M, Lee D, Braman SS. Tracheobronchopathia osteochondroplastica: a rare large airway disorder. Lung. 2008;186:353–5.
67. Leske V, Lazor R, Coetmeur D, Crestani B, Chatte G, Cordier J-F. Tracheobronchopathia osteochondroplastica. A study of 41 patients. Medicine 2001;80:378–90.
68. Nienhuis DM, Prakash UBS, Edell ES. Tracheobronchopathia osteochondroplastica. Ann Otol Rhinol Laryngol. 1990;99:689–94.
69. Krustins E, Kravale Z, Buls A. Mounier-Kuhn syndrome or congenital tracheobronchomegaly: a literature review. Respir Med 2013;107:1822–8.
70. Simons M, Vremaroiu P, Andrei F. Mounier-Kuhn syndrome. J Bronchol Interv Pulmonol. 2014;21:145–9.
71. Woodring JH, Howard RS, Rehm SR. Congenital tracheobronchomegaly (Mounier Kuhn syndrome): a report of 10 cases and review of literature. J Thorac Imaging. 1991;6:1–10.
72. Seo JB, Song KS, Lee JS, et al. Broncholithiasis: review of the causes with radiologic-pathologic correlation. Radiographics. 2002;22:S199–213.
73. Kelly WA. Broncholithiasis: current concepts of an ancient disease. Postgrad Med. 1979;66:81–6.
74. Wynn GJ, Turkington PM, Drisscol BR. Anthracofibrosis, bronchial stenosis with overlying anthracotic mucosa: possibly a new occupational lung disorder: a series of seven cases from one UK hospital. Chest. 2008;134:1069–73.
75. Chung MP, Lee KS, Han J, et al. Bronchial stenosis due to anthracofibrosis. Chest. 1998;113:344–50.
76. Kim HY, Im JG, Goo JM, et al. Bronchial anthracofibrosis (inflammatory bronchial stenosis with anthracotic pigmentation): CT findings. AJR Am J Roentgenol. 2000;174:523–7.
77. Machuzak M, Santacruz JF, Gildea T, Murthy SC. Airway complications after lung transplant. Thorac Surg Clin. 2015;25:55–75.
78. Santacruz JF, Mehta AC. Airway complications and management after lung transplantation: ischemia, dehiscence and stenosis. Proc Am Thorac Soc. 2009;6:79–93.
79. Streitz JM Jr, Shapshay SM. Airway injury after tracheostomy and endotracheal intubation. Surg Clin North Am. 1991;71:1211–30.
80. Stauffer JL, Olson DE, Petty TL. Complications and consequences of endotracheal intubation and tracheostomy: a prospective study of 150 critically ill adult patients. Am J Med. 1981;70:65–76.
81. Norwood S, Vallina VL, Short K, saigusa M, Fernandez LG, McLarty JW. Incidence of tracheal stenosis and other late complications after percutaneous tracheostomy. Ann Surg 2000;232:233–41.
82. Murgu S, Colt H. Tracheobronchomalacia and excessive dynamic airway collapse. Clin Chest Med. 2013;34:527–55.
83. Feist JH, Johnson TH, Wilson RJ. Acquired tracheomalacia: etiology and differential diagnosis. Chest. 1975;68:340–5.
84. Carden KA, Boiselle PM, Waltz DA, Ernst A. Tracheomalacia and tracheobronchomalacia in children and adults: an in-depth review. Chest. 2005;127:984–1005.
85. Ikeda S, Hanawa T, Konishi T, Adachi M, Sawi S, Chiba W. Diagnosis, incidence, clinicopathology and surgical treatment of acquired tracheomalacia. Nihon Kyobu Shikkan Gakki Zasshi. 1992;30:1028–35.
86. Loring SH, O'Donnell CR, Feller-Kopman DJ, Ernst A. Central airway mechanics and flow limitation in acquired tracheobronchomalacia. Chest. 2007;131:1118–24.
87. Nuutinen J. Acquired tracheobronchomalacia. Eur J Respir Dis. 1982;63:380–7.
88. Samson IM, Rossoff LJ. Chronic lithoptysis with multiple bilateral broncholiths. Chest. 1997;112:563–5.
89. Bohadana A, Izbicki G, Kraman SS. Fundamentals of lung auscultation. N Engl J Med. 2014;370:744–51.
90. Miller RD, Hyatt RE. Obstructing lesions of the larynx and trachea: clinical and physiologic characteristics. Mayo Clin Proc. 1969;44:145–61.

91. Kryger M, Bode F, Antic R, Anthonisen N. Diagnosis of obstruction of upper and central airways. Am J Med. 1976;61:85–93.
92. Miller RW, Hyatt RE. Evaluation of obstructing lesions of the trachea and larynx by flow volume loops. Am Rev Respir Dis. 1973;108:475–81.
93. Campbell AH, Faulks LW. Expiratory airflow patterns in tracheobronchial collapse. Am Rev Respir Dis. 1965;92:781–91.
94. Majid A, Sosa AF, Ernst A, et al. Pulmonary function and flow volume loop patterns in patients with tracheobronchomalacia. Respir Care. 2013;58:1521–6.
95. Jayamanne DS, Epstein H, Goldring RM. Flow volume curve contour in COPD: correlation with pulmonary mechanics. Chest. 1980;77:749–57.
96. Anzueto A, Levine SM, Tillis WP, Calhoon JH, Bryan CL. Use of flow volume loop in the diagnosis of bronchial stenosis after single lung transplantation. Chest. 1994;105:934–6.
97. Gascoigne AD, Corris PA, Dark JH, Gibson GJ. The biphasic spirogram: a clue to unilateral narrowing of mainstem bronchus. Thorax. 1990;45:637–8.
98. Vincken WG, Cosio MG. Flow oscillations on the flow volume loop: clinical and physiological implications. Eur Respir J. 1989;2:543–9.
99. Sanders MH, Martin RJ, Pennock BE, Rogers RM. The detection of sleep apnea in the awake patient. The saw-tooth sign. JAMA. 1981;245:2414–8.
100. Vincken W, Cosio MG. Flow oscillations on the flow volume loop: a non-specific indicator of upper airway dysfunction. Bull Eur Physiopathol Respir. 1985;21:559–67.
101. Haponik EF, Meyers DA, Munster AM, et al. Acute upper airway injury in burn patients. Serial changes of flow volume curves and nasopharyngoscopy. Am Rev Respir Dis. 1987;135:360–6.
102. Schiffman PL. A saw-tooth pattern in Parkinson's disease. Chest. 1985;87:124–6.
103. Vincken W, Elleker G, Cosio MG. Detection of upper airway muscle involvement in neuromuscular disorders using the flow volume loop. Chest. 1986;90:52–7.
104. Garcia-Pachon E. Tracheobronchomalacia: a cause of flow oscillations on the flow volume loop. Chest. 2000;118:1519.
105. Nakajima A, Saraya T, Takata S, et al. The saw-tooth sign as a clinical clue for intra-thoracic central airway obstruction. BMC Research Notes. 2012;5:388–90.
106. Rendleman N, Quinn SF. The answer is blowing in wind: a pedunculated tumor with saw-tooth flow volume loop. J Laryngol Otol. 1998;112:973–5.
107. Guntupalli KK, Bandi V, Sirgi C, Pope C, Rios A, Eschenbacher W. Usefulness of flow volume loops in emergency centers and ICU settings. Chest. 1997;111:481–8.
108. Farmer W, Littner MR, Gee JBL. Assessment of therapy of upper airway obstruction. Arch Intern Med. 1977;137:309–12.
109. Vander Els NJ. Sorhage F, Bach AM, Straus DJ, White DA. Abnormal flow volume loops in patients with intrathoracic Hodgkin's disease. Chest. 2000;117:1256–61.
110. Miller MR, Pincock AC, Oates GD, Wilkinson R, Skene-Smith H. Upper airway obstruction due to goiter: detection, prevalence and results of surgical management. Q J Med. 1990;74 (274):177–88.
111. Modrykamien AM, Gudavalli R, McCarthy K, Liu X, Stoller JK. Detection of upper airway obstruction with spirometry results and flow volume loops: a comparison of quantitative and visual inspection criteria. Respir Care. 2009;54:474–9.
112. Andrade e Raposo L, Bugalho A, Marques Gomes MJ. Contribution of flow volume curves to the detection of central airway obstruction. J Bras Pneumol 2013;39:447–54.
113. Empey DW. Assessment of upper airway obstruction. BMJ. 1972;3:503–5.
114. Rotman HH, Liss HP, Weg JG. Diagnosis of upper airway obstruction by pulmonary function testing. Chest. 1975;68:796–9.
115. Pellegrino R, Viegi G, Brusasco V, et al. Interpretive strategies for lung function tests. Eur Respir J. 2005;26:948–68.
116. Brookes GB, Fairfax AJ. Chronic upper airway obstruction: value of flow volume loop examination in assessment and management. J Royal Soc Med. 1982;75:524–34.

117. Gelb AF, Tashkin DP, Epstein JD, Zamel N. Nd-YAG laser surgery for severe tracheal stenosis physiologically and clinically masked by severe diffuse obstructive pulmonary disease. Chest. 1987;91:166–70.
118. Handa H, Huang J, Murgu SD, et al. Assessment of central airway obstruction using impulse oscillometry before and after interventional bronchoscopy. Respir Care. 2014;59:231–40.
119. Dubois A, Brody A, Lewis D, Burgess BF Jr. Oscillation mechanics of lung and chest in man. J Appl Physiol. 1956;8:587–94.
120. Oostveen E, MacLeod D, Lorino H, et al. The forced oscillation technique in clinical practice: methodology, recommendations and future development. Eur Respir J. 2003;22:1026–41.
121. Smith SJ, Reinhold P, Goldman MD. Forced oscillation technique and impulse oscillometry. Eur Respir Mon. 2005;31:72–105.
122. Vicencio AG, Bent J, Tsirilakis K, Nandalike K, Veler H, Parikh S. management of severe tracheal stenosis using flexible bronchoscopy and impulse oscillometry. J Bronchol Intervent Pulmonol. 2010;17:162–4.
123. King GG. Cutting edge technologies in respiratory research: lung function testing. Respirology. 2011;16:883–90.
124. Horan T, Mateus S, Beraldo P, et al. Forced oscillation technique to evaluate tracheostenosis in patients with neurological injury. Chest. 2001;120:69–73.
125. van Narood JA, Wellens W, Clarysse I, Cauberghs M, Van de Woestijne K, Demedts M. Total respiratory resistance and reactance in patients with upper airway obstruction. Chest 1987;92:475-80.
126. Kang EY. Large airway diseases. J Thorac Imaging. 2011;26:249–62.
127. Boiselle PM. Multislice helical CT of the central airways. Radiol Clin North Am. 2003;41:561–74.
128. Boiselle PM, Reynolds KF, Ernst A. Multiplanar and three-dimensional imaging of the central airways with multidetector CT. AJR. 2002;179:301–8.
129. Grenier PA, Beigelman-Aubry C, Fetita C, Preteux F, Brauner MW, Lenoir S. New frontiers in CT imaging of airway disease. Eur Radiol. 2002;12:1022–44.
130. Lee KS, Boiselle PM. Update on multidetector computed tomography images of the airways. J Thorac Imaging. 2010;25:112–24.
131. LoCicero J III, Costello P, Campos CT, et al. Spiral CT with multiplanar and three-dimensional reconstructions accurately predicts tracheobronchial pathology. Ann Thorac Surg. 1996;62:811–7.
132. Lee KS, Lunn W, Feller-Kopman D, Ernst A, Hatabu H. Boiselle PM. Multislice CT evaluation of airway stents. J Thorac Imaging. 2005;20:81–8.
133. Fettetti GR, Kocier M, Calaque O, et al. Follow up after stent insertion in the tracheobronchial tree: role of helical computed tomography in comparison with flexible bromchoscopy. Eur Radiol. 2003;13:1172–8.
134. Dialani V, Ernst A, Sun M, et al. MDCT detection of airway stent complications: comparison with bronchoscopy. AJR Am J Roentgenol. 2008;191:1576–80.
135. Remy-Jardin M, Remy J, Artaud D, Fribourg M, Duhamel A. Volume rendering of the tracheobronchial tree: Clinical evaluation of bronchographic images. Radiology. 1998;208:761–70.
136. Hussein SRA. Role of virtual bronchoscopy in the evaluation of bronchial lesions: a pictorial essay. Curr Probl Diagn Radiol. 2013;42:33–9.
137. Haponik EF, Aquino SL, Vining DJ. Virtual bronchoscopy. Clin Chest Med. 1999;20:201–17.
138. Morshed K, Trojanowska A, Szymanski M, et al. Evaluation of tracheal stenosis: comparison between computed tomography virtual tracheobronchoscopy with multiplanar reformatting, flexible tracheobronchoscopy and intraoperative findings. Eur Arch Otorhinolaryngol. 2011;268:591–7.

139. Fleiter T, Merkle EM, Aschoff AJ, et al. Comparison of real time virtual and fiberoptic bronchoscopy in patients with bronchial carcinoma.: opportunities and limitations. AJR Am J Roentgenol. 1997;169:1591–5.
140. Finkelstein SE, Schrump DS, Nguyen DM, Hewitt SM, Kunst TF, Summers RM. Comparative evaluation of super high-resolution CT scan and virtual bronchoscopy for the detection of tracheobronchial malignancies. Chest. 2003;124:1834–40.
141. Allah MF, Hussein SRA, Al-Asmar ABH, et al. Role of virtual bronchoscopy in the evaluation of bronchial lesions. J Comput Assist Tomogr. 2012;36:94–9.
142. Asano F, Eberhardt R, Herth FJ. Virtual bronchoscopy navigationfor peripheral pulmonary lesions. Respiration. 2014;88:430–40.
143. De wever W, Vendecaveye V, Lanciotti S, Verschakelen JA. Multidetector CT-generated virtual bronchoscopy: an illustrated review of the potential clinical indications. Eur Respir J 2004;23:776–82.
144. Hoppe H, Dinkel HP, Walder B, von Allmen G, Gugger M, Vock P. Grading airway stenosis down to the segmental level using virtual bronchoscopy. Chest. 2004;125:704–11.
145. Gamsu G, Webb WR. Computed tomography of the trachea: normal and abnormal. AJR Am J Roentgenol. 1982;139:321–6.
146. Webb EM, Elicker BM, Webb R. Using CT to diagnose non-neoplastic tracheal abnormalities. Appearance of tracheal wall. AJR Am J Roentgenol. 2000;174:1315–21.
147. Stern EJ, Graham CM, Webb WR, Gamsu G. Normal trachea during forced expiration: dynamic CT measurements. Radiology. 1993;187:27–31.
148. Breatnach E, Abbott GC, Fraser RC. Dimensions of normal human trachea. AJR Am J Roentgenol. 1984;141:903–6.
149. Greene R, Lechner GL. Saber-sheath trachea: a clinical and functional study of marked coronal narrowing of intrathoracic trachea. Radiology. 1975;115:265–8.
150. Greene R. Saber-sheath trachea: relation to chronic obstructive pulmonary disease. AJR Am J Roentgenol. 1978;130:441–5.
151. Trigaux JP, Hermes G, Dubois P, et al. CT of saber-sheath trachea. Acta Radiol. 1994;35:247–50.
152. Ismail SA, Mehta AC. Saber-sheath trachea. J Bronchol. 2003;10:296–7.
153. Shin MS, Jackson RM, Ho KJ. Tracheobronchomegaly (Mounier Kuhn syndrome): CT diagnosis. AJR Am J Roentgenol. 1988;150:777–9.
154. Kim Y, Lee KS, Yoon JH, et al. Tuberculosis of the trachea and main bronchi: CT findings in 17 patients. AJR Am J Roentgenol. 1997;168:1051–6.
155. Moon WK, Im JG, Yeon KM, et al. Tuberculosis of central airways: CT findings of active and fibrotic disease. AJR Am J Roentgenol. 1997;169:649–53.
156. Choe K, Jeong HJ, Sohn HY. Tuberculous bronchial stenosis: CT findings in 28 cases. AJR Am J Roentgenol. 1990;155:971–6.
157. Franquet T, Muller NL, Oikonomou A, et al. Aspergillus infection of the airways: computed tomography and pathologic findings. J Comput Assist Tomogr. 2004;28:10–6.
158. Taouli B, Cadi M, Leblond V, Grenier PA. Invasive aspergillosis of mediastinum and left hilum. AJR Am J Roentgenol. 2004;183:1224–6.
159. Prince JS, Duhamel DR, Levine DL, Harrell JH, Friedman PJ. Non-neoplastic lesions of tracheobronchial wall:radiologic findings with bronchoscopic correlation. Radiographics. 2002;22:S215–30.
160. Miller A, Brown LK, Teirstein AS. Stenosis of main bronchi mimicking fixed upper airway obstruction in sarcoidosis. Chest. 1985;88:244–8.
161. Hennebicque AS, Nunes H, Brillet PY, et al. CT findings in severe thoracic sarcoidosis. Eur Radiol. 2005;15:23–30.
162. Bradstetter RD, Messina MS, Sprince NL, et al. Tracheal stenosis due to sarcoidosis. Chest. 1981;80:656.
163. Lenique F, Brauner MW, Grenier P, Battesti JP, Loiseau A, Valeyre D. CT assessment of bronchi in sarcoidosis: endoscopic and pathologic correlations. Radiology. 1995;194:419–23.

64 P. Jain and A.C. Mehta

164. Shad JA, Sharief GQ. Tracheobronchitis as an initial presentation of ulcerative colitis. J Clin Gastroenterol. 2001;33:161–3.
165. Asami T, Koyama S, Watanabe Y, et al. Tracheobronchitis in a patient with Crohn's disease. Intern Med. 2009;48:1475–8.
166. Kuzniar T, Sleiman C, Brugiere O, et al. Severe tracheobronchial stenosis in a patient with Crohn's disease. Eur Respir J. 2000;15:209–12.
167. Kinebuchi SI, Oohashi K, Takada T, et al. Tracheobronchitis associated with Crohn's disease improved on inhaled corticotherapy. Intern Med 2004;829–34.
168. Behar JV, Choi YW, Hartman TA, Allen NB, McAdams HP. Relapsing polychondritis affecting the lower respiratory tract. AJR Am J Roentgenol. 2002;178:173–7.
169. Lee KS, Ernst A, Trentham DE, et al. Relapsing polychondritis: prevalence of expiratory CT airway abnormalities. Radiology. 2006;240:565–73.
170. Zack JR, Rozenshtein A. Tracheobronchopathia osteochondroplastica: report of three cases. J Compu Assist Tomogr. 2002;26:33–6.
171. Mariotta S, Pallone S, Pedicelli G, Bisetti A. Spiral CT and endoscopic findings in a case of tracheobrochopathia osteochondroplastica. J Comput Assist Tomogr. 1997;21:418–20.
172. White BD, Kong A, Khoo E, Southcott AM. Computerized tomography diagnosis of tracheobronchopathia osteochondroplastica. Autralas Radiol. 2005;49:319–21.
173. Restrepo S, Pandit M, Villami MA, Rojas IC, Perez JM, Gascue A. Tracheobronchopathia osteochondroplastica: helical CT findings in 4 cases. J Thorac Imaging. 2004;19:112–6.
174. Georgiades CS, Neyman EG, Barish MA, Fishman EK. Amyloidosis: review and CT manifestations. Radiographics. 2004;24:405–16.
175. Kim HY, Im JG, Song KS, et al. Localized amyloidosis of the respiratory system: CT features. J Comput Assist Tomogr. 1999;23:627–31.
176. Pickford HA, Swensen SJ, Utz JP. Thoracic cross sectional imaging of amyloidosis. AJR Am J Roentgenol. 1997;168:351–5.
177. Crestani B, Monnier A, Kambouchner M, Battesti JP, Reynaud P, Valeyre D. Tracheobronchial amyloidosis with hilar lymphadenopathy associated with serum monoclonal immunoglobulin. Eur Respir J. 1993;6:1569–71.
178. Screaton NJ, Sivasothy P. Flower CD. Lockwood CM. Tracheal involvement in Wegener's granulomatosis: evaluation using spiral CT. Clin Radiol 1998;53:809–15.
179. Stein MG, Gamsu G, Webb WR, Stulbarg MS. Computed tomography of diffuse tracheal stenosis in Wegener's granulomatosis. J Coumpt Assist Tomogr. 1984;8:327–9.
180. Lee KS, Kim TS, Fugimoto K, et al. Thoracic manifestations of Wegener's granulomatosis: CT findings in 30 patients. Eur Radiol. 2003;13:43–51.
181. McCarthy MJ, Rosado-de-Christenson ML. Tumors of the trachea. J Thorac Imaging. 1995;10:180–98.
182. Kwak SH, Lee KS, Chung MJ, Jeong YJ, Kim GY, Know OJ. Adenoid cystic carcinoma of airways: helical CT and histopathological correlation. AJR Am J Roentgenol. 2004;183:277–81.
183. Spizarny DL, Shepard JA, McLoud TC, Grillo HC, Dedrick CG. CT of adenoid cystic carcinoma of the trachea. AJR Am J Roentgenol. 1986;146:1129–32.
184. Kim TS, Lee KS, Han J, et al. Mucoepidermoid carcinoma of the tracheobronchial tree: radiographic and CT findings in 12 patients. Radiology. 1999;212:643–8.
185. Jeung MY, Gasser B, Gangi A, et al. Bronchial carcinoid tumors of the thorax: spectrum of radiologic findings. Radiographics. 2002;22:351–65.
186. Ko JM, Jung JI, Park S, et al. Benign tumors of tracheobronchial tree: CT-pathologic correlations. AJR Am J Roentgenol. 2006;186:1304–13.
187. Mata JM, Caceres J, Ferrer J, Gomez E, Castaner F, Velayos A. Endobronchial lipoma: CT diagnosis. J Comput Assist Tomogr. 1991;15:750–1.
188. Gruden JF, Webb WR, Sides DM. Adult onset disseminated tracheobronchial papillomatosis: CT features. J Coumpt Assist Tomogr. 1994;18:640–2.
189. Kramer SS, Wehunt WD, Stocker JT, Kashima H. Pulmonary manifestations of juvenile laryngotracheal papillomatosis. AJR Am J Roengenol. 1985;144:687–94.

190. Yoon RG, Kim MY, Song JW, Chae EJ, Choi CM, Jang S. Primary endobronchial marginal zone B-cell lymphoma of bronchus associated lymphoid tissue: CT findings in 7 patients. Korean J Radiol. 2013;14:366–74.
191. McAdams HP, Palmer SM, Erasmus JJ, et al. Bronchial anastomotic complications in lung transplant recipients: virtual bronchoscopy for non-invasive assessment. Radiology. 1998;209:689–95.
192. Boiselle PM, Ernst A. Tracheal morphology in patients with tracheomalacia: prevalence of inspiratory lunate and expiratory frown shapes. J Thorac Imaging. 2006;21:190–6.
193. Lee KS, Sun MR, Ernst A, Feller-Kopman D, Majid A, Boiselle PM. Comparison of dynamic expiratory CT with bronchoscopy for diagnosing airway malacia: a pilot evaluation. Chest. 2007;131:758–64.
194. Ferretti GR, Jankowski A, Perrin MA, et al. Multi-detector CT evaluation in patients suspected of tracheobronchomalacia: comparison of end expiratory with dynamic expiratory volumetric acquisitions. Eur J Radiol. 2008;68:340–6.
195. Im JG, Chung JW, Han SK, Han MC, Kim CW. CT manifestations of tracheobronchial involvement in relapsing polychondritis. J Comput Assist Tomogr. 1988;12:792–3.
196. Lee KS, Ashiku SK, Ernst A, et al. Comparison of expiratory CT airway abnormalities before and after tracheoplasty surgery for tracheobronchomalacia. J Thorac Imaging. 2008;23:121–6.
197. Godoy MC, Saldana DA, Rao PP, et al. Multidetector CT evaluation of airway stents: what the radiologist should know. Radiographics. 2014;34:1793–806.
198. Yedururi S, Guillerman RP, Chung T, et al. Multimodality imaging of tracheobronchial disorders in children. Radiographics. 2008;28:e29.
199. Rimell FL, Shapiro AM, Meza MP, Goldman S, Hite S, Newman B. Magnetic resonance imaging of the pediatric airways. Arch Otolaryngol Head Neck Surg. 1997;123:999–1003.
200. Ciet P, Wielopolski P, Manniesing R, et al. Spirometer controlled cine-magnetic resonance imaging used to diagnose tracheobronchomalacia in pediatric patients. Eur Respir J. 2014;43:115–24.
201. Wang J, Takashima SS, Takayama F, et al. Tracheal invasion by thyroid carcinoma: prediction using MR imaging. AJR Am J Roengenol. 2001;177:929–36.
202. Freeman SJ, Harvey JE, Goddard PR. Demonstration of supranumerary tracheal bronchus by computed tomographic scanning and magnetic resonance imaging. Thorax. 1995;50:426–7.
203. Gilad R, Milillo P, Som PM. Severe diffuse systemic amyloidosis with involvement of pharynx, larynx, and trachea: CT and MRI findings. Am J Neuroradiol. 2007;28:1557–8.
204. Park KJ, Bergin CJ, Harrell J. MR findings of tracheal involvement in Wegener's granulomatosis. AJR Am J Roentgenol. 1998;171:524–5.
205. Rodriguez E, Soler R, Pombo F, Requejo I, Montero C. Fibrosing mediastinitis: CT and MR findings. Clin Radiol. 1998;53:907–10.
206. Hantous-Zannad S, Sebai L, Zidi A, et al. Tracheobronchopathia osteochondroplastica presenting as a respiratory insufficiency: diagnosis by bronchoscopy and MRI. Eur J Radiol 2003;113–6.
207. Park CM, Goo JM, Lee HF, et al. Tumors in the tracheobronchial tree: CT and FDG PET features. Radiographics. 2009;29:55–71.
208. Erasmus JJ, McAdams HP, Patz EF Jr, Coleman RE, Ahuja V, Goodman PC. Evaluation of primary pulmionary carcinoid tumors using FDG-PET. AJR Am J Roentgenol. 1998;170:1369–73.
209. Yamashita H, Takahashi H, Kubota K, et al. Utility of fluorodeoxyglucose positron emission tomography/computed tomography for early diagnosis and evaluation of disease activity of relapsing polychondritis: a case series and literature review. Rheumatology (Oxford). 2014;53:1482–90.
210. Wang J, Li S, Zeng Y, Chen P, Zhang N, Zhong N. 18 F-FDG PET/CT is a valuable tool for relapsing polychondritis diagnosis and therapeutic response monitoring. Ann Nucl Med. 2014;28:276–84.
211. Myer CM, O'Connor DM, Cotton RT. Proposed grading system for sub-glottic stenosis based on endotracheal tube sizes. Ann Otol Rhinol Laryngol. 1994;103:319–23.

212. Freitag L, Ernst A, Unger M, Kovitz K, Marquette CH. A proposed classification system of central airway stenosis. Eur Respir J. 2007;30:7–12.
213. Tremblay A, Coulter TD, Mehta AC. Modification of mucosal sparing technique using electrocautery and balloon dilation in endoscopic management of web-like benign airway stenosis. J Bronchol. 2003;10:268–71.
214. Murgu S, Colt H. Tracheobronchomalacia and excessive dynamic airway collapse. Clin Chest Med. 2013;34:527–55.
215. Murgu SD, Pecson J, Colt HG. Bronchoscopy during non-invasive ventilation: indications and technique. Respir Care. 2010;55:595–600.
216. Murgu SD. Pneumatic splinting for tracheobronchomalacia. J Bronchol Intervent Pulmonol. 2014;21:109–12.
217. Reidel M, Hauck RW, Stein HJ, et al. Preoperative bronchoscopic assessment of airway invasion by esophageal cancer. A prospective study. Chest. 1998;113:687–95.
218. Koike E, Yamashita H, Noguchi S, et al. Bronchoscopic diagnosis of thyroid cancer with laryngotracheal invasion. Arch Surg. 2011;136:1185–9.
219. Choi TK, Siu KF, Lam KH, Wong J. Bronchoscopy and carcinoma of the esophagus I. Findings of bronchoscopy in carcinoma of the esophagus. Am J Surg. 1984;147:757–9.
220. Oki M, Saka H. Thin bronchoscope for evaluating stenotic airways during stenting procedure. Respiration. 2011;82:509–14.
221. Schuurmans MM, Michaud GC, Diacon AH, Bolliger CT. Use of ultrathin bronchoscope in the assessment of central airway obstruction. Chest. 2003;124:735–9.
222. Kurimoto N, Murayama M, Yoshioka S, Nishisaka T, Inai K, Dohi K. Assessment of usefulness of endobronchial ultrasonography in determination of depth of tracheobronchial tumor invasion. Chest. 1999;115:1500–6.
223. Miyazu Y, Miyazawa T, Kurimoto N, Iwamoto Y, Kanoh K, Kohno N. Endobronchial ultrasonography in the assessment of centrally located early-stage lung cancer before photodynamic therapy. Am J Respir Crit Care Med. 2002;165:832–7.
224. Miyazawa T, Miyazu Y, Iwamoto Y, Ishida A, Kanoh K, Sumiyoshi H, Doi M, Kurimoto N. Stenting at the flow-limiting segment in tracheobronchial stenosis due to lung cancer. Am J Respir Crit Care Med. 2004;169:1096–102.
225. Herth F, Becker HD, LoCicero J 3rd, Ernst A. Endobronchial ultrasound in therapeutic bronchoscopy. Eur Respir J. 2002;20:118–21.
226. Herth F, Ernst A, Schultz M, Becker H. Endobronchial ultrasound reliably differentiates between airway infiltration and compression by tumor. Chest. 2003;123:458–62.
227. Wakamatsu T, Tsushima K, Yasuo M, et al. Usefulness of preoperative endobronchial ultrasound for airway invasion around the trachea: esophageal cancer and thyroid cancer. Respiration. 2006;73:651–7.
228. Nishimura Y, Osugi H, Inoue K, Takada N, Takamura M, Kinosita H. Bronchoscopic ultrasonography in diagnosis of tracheobronchial invasion of esophageal cancer. J Ultrasound Med. 2002;21:49–58.
229. Osugi H, Nishimura Y, Takemura M, et al. Bronchoscopic ultrasound for staging supracarinal esophageal squamous cell carcinoma: impact on outcome. World J Surg. 2003;27:590–4.
230. Murgu S, Kurimoto N, Colt H. Endobronchial ultrasound morphology of expiratory central airway collapse. Respiration. 2008;13:315–9.
231. Iwamoto Y, Miyazawa T, Kurimoto N, et al. Interventional bronchoscopy in the management of airway stenosis due to tracheobronchial tuberculosis. Chest. 2004;126:1344–52.
232. Miyazu Y, Miyazava T, Kurimoto N, et al. Endobronchial ultrasonography in the diagnosis and treatment of relapsing polychondritis with tracheobronchial malacia. Chest. 2003;124:2393–5.
233. Eksombatchai D, Boonsarngsuk V, Amornputtisathaporn N, Suwatanapongched T, Kurimoto N. Tracheobronchial involvement in relapsing polychondritis diagnosed on endobronchial ultrasound. Intern Med. 2013;52:801–5.

234. Irani S, Hofer M, Gaspert A, Bachmann LM, Russi EW, Boehler A. Endobronchial ultrasonography for the quantitative assessment of bronchial mural structures in lung transplant recipients. Chest. 2006;129:349–55.
235. Chambellan A, Turbie P, Nunes H, Brauner M, Battesti JP, Valeyre D. Endoluminal sarcoidosis of proximal bronchi in sarcoidosis. Bronchoscopy, function and evolution. Chest. 2005;127:427–81.
236. Hong G, Kim H. Clinical characteristics and treatment outcomes of patients with relapsing polychondritis with airway involvement. Clin Rheumatol. 2013;32:1329–35.
237. Solans-Laque R, Bosch-Gil JA, Canela M, Lorente J, Pallisa E, Vilardell-Tarres M. Clinical features and therapeutic management of subglottic stenosis in patients with Wegener's granulomatosis. Lupus. 2008;17:832–6.
238. Sahoo DH, Mehta AC. Active endobronchial Wegener's granulomatosis. J Bronchol. 2005;12:166–7.
239. Honing J, Gaissert HA, Verhagen AF, at al. Undertreatment of tracheal carcinoma: multidisciplinary audit of epidemiological data. Ann Surg Oncol 2009;16:246–53.
240. Wood DE. Management of malignant tracheobronchial obstruction. Surg Clin North Am. 2002;82:621–42.
241. Chao YK, Liu YH, Hsieh MJ, et al. Controlling difficult airway by rigid bronchoscope- an old but effective method. Interact CardioVasc Thorac Surg. 2005;4:175–9.
242. McGarvey JM, Pollock CV. Heliox in airway management. Emerg Med Clin N Am. 2008;26:905–20.
243. Skrinskas GJ, Hyland RH, Hutcheon MA. Using helium-oxygen mixtures in management of acute upper respiratory obstruction. Can Med Assoc J. 1983;128:555–8.
244. Curtis JL, Mahlmeister M, Fink JB, Lampe G, Matthay MA, Stulbarg MS. Helium-oxygen gas therapy. Use and availability for the emergency treatment of inoperable airway obstruction. Chest. 1986;90:455–7.
245. Khanlou H, Eiger G. Safety and efficacy of heliox as a treatment for upper airway obstruction due to radiation induced laryngeal dysfunction. Heart Lung. 2001;30:146–7.
246. Abu-Hijleh M, Lee D, Braman SS. Tracheobronchopathia osteochondroplastica: a rare large airway disorder. Lung. 2008;186:353–9.
247. Cerfolio RJ, Bryant AS, Maniscalco L. Rigid bronchoscopy and surgical resection for broncholithiasis and calcified mediastinal lymph nodes. J Thorac Cardiovasc Surg. 2008;136:186–90.
248. Capizzi SA, Betancourt E, Prakash UB. Tracheobronchial amyloidosis. Mayo Clin Proc. 2000;75:1148–52.
249. Nouraei SAR, Obholzer R, Ind PW, et al. Results of endoscopic surgery and intralesional steroid therapy for airway compromise due to tracheobronchial Wegener's granulomatosis. Thorax. 2008;63:49–52.
250. Ferguson GT, Benoist J. Nasal continuous positive airway pressure in the treatment of tracheobronchomalacia. Am Rev Respir Dis. 1993;147:457–61.
251. Shirit D, Kuchuk M, Zismanov V, Rahman NA, Amital A, Kramer MR. Bronchoscopic balloon dilation of tracheobronchial stenosis: long term follow-up. Eur J Cardiothorac Surg. 2010;38:198–202.
252. Wood DE, Liu YH, Vallieres E, et al. Airway stenting for malignant and benign tracheobronchial stenosis. Ann Thorac Surg. 2003;76:167–72.
253. Gaissert HA. Primary tracheal tumors. Chest Surg Clin North Am. 2003;13:247–53.
254. Ernst A, Simoff M, Ost D, Goldman Y, Herth FJF. Prospective risk-adjusted morbidity and mortality outcome analysis after therapeutic bronchoscopy procedures. Results of a multi-institutional outcome database. Chest 2008;134:514–9.
255. Monnier P, Mudry A, Stanzel F, et al. The use of the covered wallstent for the palliative treatment of inoperable tracheobronchial cancers. A prospective multicenter study. Chest. 1996;110:1161–8.
256. Ryu YJ, Kim H, Choi JC, Kwon YS, Kwon OJ. Use of silicone stents for the management of post-tuberculosis tracheobronchial stenosis. Eur Respir J. 2006;28:1029–35.

257. Damle SS, Mitchell JD. Surgery for tracheobronchomalacia. Semin Cardiothorac Vasc Anesth. 2012;16:203–8.
258. Dasgupta A, Dolmatch BL, Abi-Saleh WJ, et al. Self-expanding metallic airway stent insertion employing flexible bronchoscopy: preliminary results. Chest. 1998;114:106–9.
259. Freitag L, Darwiche K. Endoscopic treatment of tracheal stenosis. Thorac Surg Clin. 2014;24:27–40.
260. Saad PS, Murthy S, Krizmanich G, Mehta AC. Self expanding metal stents and flexible bronchoscopy. Chest. 2003;124:1993–9.
261. Gaissert HA, Grillo HC, Wright CD, Donahue DM, Wain JC, Mathisen DJ. Complications of benign tracheobronchial strictures by self expanding metal stents. J Thorac Cardiovasc Surg. 2003;126:744–7.
262. Lunn W, Feller-Kopman D, Wahidi M, et al. Endoscopic removal of metallic airway stents. Chest. 2005;127:2106–12.
263. Swanson KL, Edell ES, Praksh UBS, Brutinel WM, Midthun DE, Utz JP. Complications of metal stent therapy in benign airway obstruction. J Bronchol. 2007;14:90–4.
264. Datau H. Airway stenting for benign tracheal stenosis: what is really behind the choice of stents. Eur J Cardiothorac Surg. 2011;40:925–6.
265. Madden BP, Loke TK, Sheth AC. Do expandable metallic airway stents have a role in management of patients with benign tracheobronchial disease? Ann Thorac Surg. 2006;82:274–8.
266. Grillo HC, Mathisen DJ. Primary tracheal tumors: treatment and result. Ann Thorac Surg. 1990;49:69–77.
267. Gaissert HA, Grillo HC, Shadmehr MB, et al. Long-term survival after resection of primary adenoid cystic and squamous cell carcinoma of trachea and carina. Ann Thorac Surg. 2004;78:1889–97.
268. Fink G, Krelbaum T, Yellin A, et al. Pulmonary carcinoid. Presentation, diagnosis, and outcome in 141 cases in Israel and review of 640 patients from the literature. Chest. 2001;119:1647–51.
269. Detterbeck FC. Management of carcinoid tumors. Ann Thorac Surg. 2010;89:998–1005.
270. Stoelben E, Koryllos A, Beckers F, Ludwig C. Benign stenosis of the trachea. Thorac Surg Clin. 2014;24:59–65.
271. Olson EJ, Utz JP, Prakash UBS. Therapeutic bronchoscopy in broncholithiasis. Am J Respir Crit Care Med. 1999;160:766–70.
272. Faber LP, Jensik RJ, Chawla SK, Kittle CF. The surgical implications of broncholithiasis. J Thorac Cardiovasc Surg. 1975;70:779–89.
273. Li Y. Clinical manifestation and management of primary malignant tumors of the cervical trachea. Eur Arch Otorhinolaryngol. 2014;271:225–35.
274. Bugalho A. Management of subglottic stenosis and subglottic stenosis in systemic disease. In: Ernst A, Herth FJF, editors. Principles and practice of Interventional Pulmonology. New York: Springer Science; 2012. p. 409–20.
275. Acar T, et al. Computed tomography finding of tracheobronchial system disease: a pictorial essay. Jpn J Radiol. 2015;33:51–8.
276. Holland A. Der bronchoskopische zufallsbefund. Der Internist 2014;55(9):1039–44.
277. Sirajuddin A. Normal thoracic anatomy and common variants. In: Kanne JP, editor. Clinically oriented pulmonary imaging. New York: Humana Press; 2012. p. 1–17.
278. Barreiro TJ. Accessory cardiac bronchus. Lung. 2014;192(5):821–2.
279. Choi YK, et al. Bronchial anthracofibrosis: a potential false-positive finding on F-18 FDG PET. Ann Nucl Med. 2012;26:681–3.
280. Monnier P. Subglottic and tracheal stenosis. In: Remacle M, Eckel HE, editors. Surgery of Larynx and Trachea. Heidelberg: Springer; 2009. p. 137–58.
281. Hadique S, Jain P, Mehta AC. Therapeutic bronchoscopy for central airway obstruction. In: Mehta AC, Jain P, editors. Interventional bronchoscopy. New York: Humana Press; 2013. p. 143–76.

282. Hayden SJ. Imaging of airway disease. In: Kanne JP, editor. Clinically oriented pulmonary imaging. New York: Humana Press; 2012. p. 179–93.
283. Morshed K, et al. Evaluation of tracheal stenosis: comparison between computed tomography, virtual tracheobronchoscopy with multiplanar reformatting, flexible tracheofibroscopy and intra-operative findings. Eur Arch Otorhinolaryngol. 2011;268:591–7.
284. Sato M, et al. F-18 FDG PET/CT in relapsing polychondritis. Ann Nucl Med. 2010;24:687–90.
285. Wang J, et al. 18F-FDG PET/CT is a valuable tool for relapsing polychondritis diagnose and therapeutic response monitoring. Ann Nucl Med. 2014;28:276–84.
286. Anantham D. Management principles of nonmalignant airway obstruction. In: Ernst A, Herth FJF, editors. Principles and practice of Interventional Pulmonology. New York: Springer Science; 2012. p. 269–83.

Chapter 2
Sarcoidosis of the Upper and Lower Airways

Daniel A. Culver

Introduction

Sarcoidosis granulomas have a predilection for the submucosa of the entire respiratory tract. As a result, sarcoidosis may cause a variety of airway-based clinical syndromes, which can be the dominant clinical feature in some patients. Respiratory symptoms referable to airway disease are often similar to more common illnesses, such as rhinitis, sinusitis, and asthma, not infrequently leading to delayed diagnosis [1–4]. Moreover, the pathologic features of sarcoidosis can be confused with other inflammatory disorders, including granulomatosis with polyangiitis and tuberculosis [5].

Including patients with pulmonary function abnormalities, radiologic abnormalities, and symptoms, the reported prevalence of airway involvement in sarcoidosis ranges from 40 to 60 % [5]. Advanced parenchymal disease, especially fibrotic sarcoidosis, increases the risk of lower respiratory tract airway involvement [6], whereas the presence of lupus pernio is associated with a higher risk for sinonasal sarcoidosis [7]. When lower respiratory tract airways are affected, morbidity and mortality are both elevated [8]; upper respiratory tract involvement is strongly associated with a high risk for non-resolving sarcoidosis [9]. The frequency of involvement and the prognostic implications both imply that the presence of airway sarcoidosis should be actively sought and factored into management decisions when it is found.

D.A. Culver (✉)
Department of Pulmonary Medicine, Respiratory Institute,
Cleveland Clinic, 9500 Euclid Avenue, Desk A90, Cleveland, OH 44195, USA
e-mail: culverd@ccf.org

D.A. Culver
Department of Pathobiology, Lerner Research Institute,
Cleveland Clinic, 9500 Euclid Avenue, Desk A90, Cleveland, OH 44195, USA

© Springer International Publishing Switzerland 2016
A.C. Mehta et al. (eds.), *Diseases of the Central Airways*,
Respiratory Medicine, DOI 10.1007/978-3-319-29830-6_2

Upper Respiratory Tract

Presentation and Diagnosis

Sarcoidosis of the upper respiratory tract (SURT) occurs in 2–6 % of individuals with sarcoidosis [7, 10]. It occurs more commonly in black patients and in females [3, 11, 12]. Any structure from the nares to the vocal cords may be affected. The most commonly affected areas are the nasal mucosa and sinuses [7], but the larynx, epiglottis, pharynx, and oral mucosa may also be involved.

SURT typically presents with sinonasal congestion, crusting, nasal drainage, and variable degrees of hyposmia. Sometimes, sinonasal sarcoidosis may lead to sinus headache pain, epistaxis, watery eyes (from nasolacrimal duct obstruction), otitis media, and even destruction of nasal cartilage resulting in saddle nose deformity or septal perforation (Fig. 2.1). Glottic or supraglottic sarcoidosis symptoms may be due to exuberant granulomatous inflammation, or to strictures. Dyspnea, cough, stridor, obstructive sleep apnea, dysphagia, and dysphonia may be the presenting manifestations of laryngeal or pharyngeal sarcoidosis.

Nasal mucosal sarcoidosis is usually diagnosed by examination. Nodular pale white to yellow papular lesions, or exuberant inflammation with mucus crusting are the findings most typically observed with direct examination of the anterior nares, or by fiberoptic examination (Fig. 2.2) [4, 12]. Biopsy of the lesions should

Fig. 2.1 Collapse of anterior nasal cartilage from severe sinonasal sarcoidosis. There is also a substantial fleshy protuberance of the tip of the nose from granulomatous inflammation

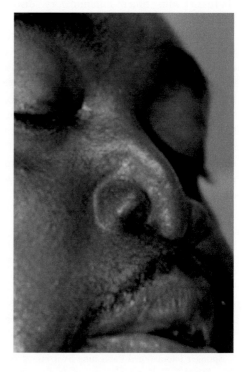

Fig. 2.2 Cobblestoning of
nasal mucosa. The nodular
lesions are typically pale
white yellow; there may be
associated hyperemia and
crusting [Courtesy of Martin
Citardi, MD.]

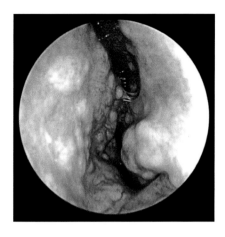

document predominantly well-formed non-necrotizing granulomas, with no evidence of infectious agents. Occasionally, the inflammatory lesions of granulomatosis with polyangiitis (GPA) may be difficult to distinguish from sarcoidosis [13]. Evidence of either disease outside of the upper respiratory tract is usually sufficient to confirm the diagnosis. In contradistinction to the well-formed discrete non-necrotizing granulomas of sarcoidosis, the "granulomas" of GPA show central geographic basophilic necrosis with palisading histiocytes and multinucleated giant cells and can be associated with vasculitis and neutrophilic microabscesses (Fig. 2.3a–c).

The prevalence of supraglottic and glottic involvement is approximately 1–2 % [3, 14]. It may occur in isolation, or in combination with sinonasal sarcoidosis. Fiberoptic examination findings include epiglottic thickening, masses, and granular infiltration of the aryepiglottic folds, false vocal cords, or surrounding tissues (Fig. 2.4a–b). Severe disease may lead to respiratory distress or respiratory failure, occasionally requiring tracheostomy [15]. Physical examination and inspection of the flow-volume curves are helpful adjunctive diagnostic tests when symptoms suggest the possibility of laryngeal sarcoidosis.

Management of Upper Respiratory Tract Sarcoidosis

The presence of SURT portends a low likelihood of spontaneous remission and also relative treatment resistance compared to many other organs [3, 16]. When the symptoms are relatively modest, topical therapy with corticosteroids and saline nasal washes may be adequate [12, 17, 18]. However, most patients with symptomatic SURT require systemic therapy [16]. In one center, emergence of SURT in patients with preexisting sarcoidosis led to a greater-than-four-fold escalation in the

Fig. 2.3 Well-formed
granulomas are typical in
sinonasal sarcoidosis (**a**),
where clustered histiocytes
are tightly arranged, and there
is no substantial necrosis. The
histiocytic inflammation seen
in granulomatosis with
polyangiitis, in contrast, is
usually less tightly organized
and may consist only of
clusters of multinucleated
giant cells with
microabscesses (**b**). Other
features (**c**) include clusters of
foamy histiocytes, and
histiocytes palisading
adjacent to basophilic
geographic necrosis [Courtesy
of Andrea Arrossi, MD.]

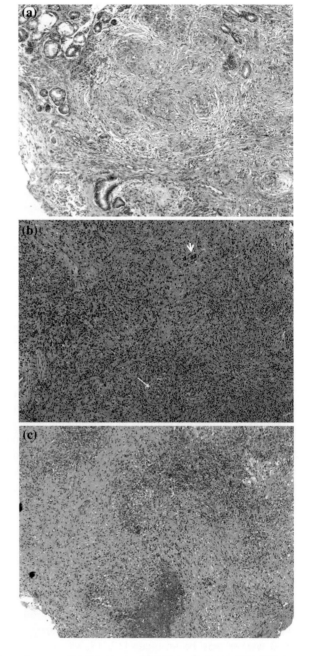

mean daily prednisone dose in an attempt to control the disease (4 mg/d to
18.6 mg/d) [3]. Despite the increased corticosteroid dose, intralesional steroid
injections, and surgical interventions, only 40 % of the patients had significant
symptomatic improvement [3].

(a)   **(b)**

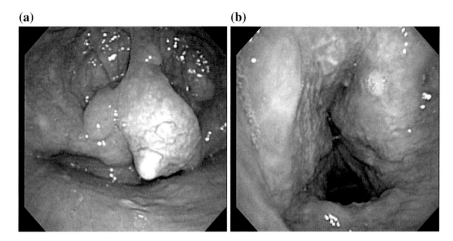

Fig. 2.4 Severe laryngeal sarcoidosis requiring debulking surgery. There is exuberant mass-like polypoid granulomatous inflammation of the epiglottis and aryepiglottic folds (**a**) leading to subtotal obstruction. The subglottic airway (**b**) is circumferentially infiltrated and narrowed by active granulomas and associated inflammation

Other immunosuppressive agents may be useful for SURT, but the data are sparse. In several series, the antimalarial agent hydroxychloroquine demonstrated modest efficacy, especially for milder cases [16, 19]. Cytotoxic agents, including methotrexate, azathioprine, and leflunomide were reportedly beneficial in small case series and case reports [13, 16, 19, 20]. Tumor necrosis factor antagonists, such as infliximab and adalimumab, are useful for treatment of sarcoidosis, but there are few data about their effectiveness for SURT. In a double-blind placebo-controlled trial of infliximab for pulmonary sarcoidosis, there was a trend ($p = 0.236$) for improvement of sinonasal sarcoidosis among the 7 patients who received infliximab, compared to four placebo-treated patients [21]. Obviously, this post hoc analysis was underpowered to provide meaningful information regarding infliximab for SURT.

Intralesional corticosteroid injections may be useful for isolated granulomatous masses. For sinonasal disease, their effectiveness appears to be relatively modest—in the series reported by Panselinas et al., only 2 of the 11 patients had improvement of symptoms at the end of the follow-up period [3]. For glottic and supraglottic lesions, several case reports have suggested that intralesional injections may be useful [18, 22–25]. Although intralesional injection may provide only temporary relief of severe airway obstruction, the resultant improvement of symptoms may allow sufficient time for slower-acting medications to effect longer term improvements [5]. Less commonly employed approaches to laryngeal sarcoidosis include laser ablation and external beam radiation [26, 27].

Sinus surgery may be necessary when there is severe sinus obstruction or suspected infection. Sinus surgery may provide temporary relief, but its benefits are usually not durable [3], and it may lead to nasal septal perforation and disease recurrence [7, 28]. It is usually reserved for severe SURT refractory to medical therapy, or when there is life-threatening upper airway obstruction.

Lower Respiratory Tract

Presentation and Diagnosis

Sarcoidosis can affect any part of the tracheobronchial tree. The manifestations may be subdivided according to whether they are mainly due to airway luminal (intrinsic) involvement, or to extraluminal (extrinsic) compression or distortion by sarcoidosis inflammation or fibrosis occurring in the peribronchial lung parenchyma. A second distinction may be drawn between those manifestations that are due to active granulomatous inflammation versus those due to fibrosis (Table 2.1). This section will be organized using this categorization, but it should be recognized that many patients have more than one mechanism responsible for symptoms and physiologic abnormalities. Obviously, lower respiratory tract sarcoidosis due to granulomatous inflammation may require inhaled or systemic immunosuppressive medications for treatment. The general principles for treatment of pulmonary sarcoidosis apply to these patients, but are beyond the scope of this chapter.

Lower respiratory tract sarcoidosis, regardless of the mechanism, commonly causes cough, wheezing or dyspnea. Although airway mucosa is often very friable, hemoptysis is rare and should prompt evaluation for other problems, such as mycetomas, infections, or concomitant malignancies [29]. Pulmonary function testing may demonstrate obstruction in 11–57 % of individuals with pulmonary sarcoidosis [10, 30, 31]. In African American cohorts, the prevalence of airflow limitation is even higher; in a study of 123 consecutive non-smoking patients, 63 % were found to have an FEV1/FVC ratio less than 0.75 [32]. On the other hand, obstruction appears to be unusual in Japanese patients—in one prospective study of 228 subjects, only 9 % exhibited reduced airflow [33]. One possible explanation for the higher frequency of airflow obstruction in African American patients may be a

Table 2.1 Mechanisms of tracheobronchial sarcoidosis

	Granulomatous	Non-granulomatous
Intrinsic	Granulomatous tracheobronchitis Hyper-reactive airways[a]	Endoluminal stenosis Bronchiectasis Hyper-reactive airways[a]
Extrinsic	Extraluminal inflammation (masses or bronchovascular bundle thickening) Lymph node enlargement	Bronchial distortion Traction bronchiectasis

[a]Contribution of granulomas to hyper-reactivity is unclear but associated with physiologic hyper-reactivity

higher granuloma density compared Caucasians [34, 35]. Measurements of small airway dysfunction, such as frequency dependence of dynamic compliance and closing volume to vital capacity ratio, confirm that airway disease occurs in more than 50 % of Scadding stage 1–2 patients and should be assessed when dyspnea is unexplained [36]. As a rule, however, obstruction tends to be more evident and more severe with advancing parenchymal lung involvement [33].

Intrinsic/Granulomatous

As mentioned previously, granulomas are very common in mucosal and submucosal airways. In up to 55 % of patients with pulmonary sarcoidosis, direct examination of the airways will reveal abnormalities [34]. Common features include erythema, edema, mucosal granularity, cobblestoning, and plaques (Fig. 2.5). The mucosa may be extremely friable, but overt hemoptysis is rare [29]. The endoluminal nodules seen in sarcoidosis are typically wax or pearly, whitish to yellowish, and when present in a non-contiguous distribution, resemble cobblestones. However, this appearance is not specific, so a biopsy is mandatory if the diagnosis has not been established previously.

Endobronchial forceps biopsy is a low-risk modality for securing histologic evidence of sarcoidosis. In patients with abnormal mucosa, the yield of directed endobronchial biopsy has ranged from 45 to 91 %, with most series in the 50–60 % range [37–41]. However, endobronchial biopsy may still be useful in suspected sarcoidosis when there is no visible mucosal abnormality, where performing 2–4 random mucosal biopsies results in 20–37 % sensitivity for granulomas [37, 39, 41]. In a retrospective review of 154 patients, the yield of endobronchial biopsy was 85 % for African American patients, versus 38 % for Caucasians [34]. These data

Fig. 2.5 Cobblestone appearance of tracheobronchial sarcoidosis at the main carina. The lesions tend to be more discrete in the trachea and mainstem bronchi and more like to coalesce into diffusely irregular mucosal inflammation in the lobar and segmental airways

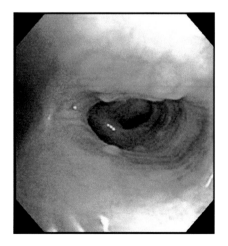

suggest that careful airway inspection and directed endobronchial biopsy is a useful part of bronchoscopic diagnosis, especially in African American patients.

Chest CT scan may be useful to identify patients with endobronchial involvement; in a series of 60 patients, CT scan revealed bronchial involvement in 65 % of the cases [42]. An additional CT feature that suggests small airway involvement is the presence of air trapping on expiratory scans. In one series, air trapping was found in 19 of 20 evaluated patients; its presence correlated with reduced mid-expiratory flow rate and increased residual volume, but not with other spirometric parameters [43]. It is unknown whether all air trapping in sarcoidosis is due to granulomatous inflammation or to other mechanisms.

Bronchial hyper-reactivity is common in sarcoidosis. It may be extremely difficult to distinguish from asthma, since extrinsic triggers like fumes, smoke, or pollen may precipitate exacerbations. As a result, misdiagnosis of asthma is not uncommon in sarcoidosis cohorts, resulting in delayed sarcoidosis diagnosis [44]. Bronchial provocation testing is abnormal in approximately 20 % of patients [45–47]. Bronchial hyper-reactivity appears to be more frequent patients with lower baseline FEV1 [46] and occurred solely in those with positive endobronchial biopsies in the study performed by Shorr et al. [45]. These observations raise the possibility that the presence of abnormal bronchial provocation responses may be due to intrinsic small airway disease with smaller baseline airway diameter, which could potentially lead to false-positive FEV1 declines. As further evidence that there may be no pathophysiologic association between asthma and sarcoidosis, a recent case–control study examined the likelihood of atopic eczema, asthma, or hay fever in a series of 225 sarcoidosis patients and 177 controls [48]. The prevalence of all three features was similar in sarcoidosis and control patients, raising the likelihood that the apparent relationship between asthma and sarcoidosis may be coincidental rather than pathologic.

Intrinsic/Non-granulomatous

Significant endoluminal stenosis is very rare, occurring in only 18 of 2500 (0.7 %) patients seen in a French institution from 1980 to 2000 [49]. Most of the lesions occur in the upper lobes or middle lobe and involve more than one lobar or segmental bronchus [49–51]. Occasionally, the stenosis may be diffuse [52]. Bronchoscopically, the lesions typically appear as webs or concentric narrowing by bland fibrotic tissue (Fig. 2.6a). However, in some patients, there may be a granulomatous component (Fig. 2.6b), so that endobronchial forceps biopsy and consideration of immunosuppressive therapy may be useful.

The presence of endoluminal stenosis may be suspected when there is cough, dyspnea, or wheezing; physical examination is extremely important as it may demonstrate focal prolongation of the expiratory phase or even wheezing. The flow-volume loop may likewise reveal variable emptying of large airways, sometimes visible as a notch on the expiratory limb. Endoluminal stenosis should be

(a)   (b)

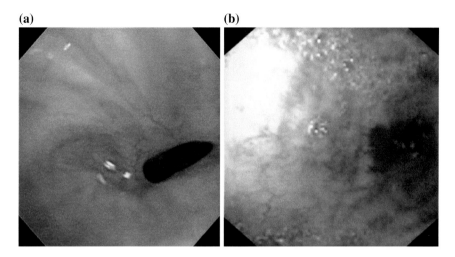

Fig. 2.6 Airway stenosis due to sarcoidosis. Isolated or multiple fibrotic webs may be found, usually in the segmental or subsegmental airways. **a** Depicts subtotal obstruction of the entire left lower lobe, with the anteromedial basal and lateral basal subsegments still visible. **b** There is extensive fibrogranulomatous proliferation at the level of the right mainstem bronchus leading to ventilation of the right lung through a pin-hole-size orifice

suspected in patients with dyspnea that is out of proportion to chest imaging findings, especially when airflow obstruction is present [53]. However, it may occur even in patients with normal pulmonary spirometry [49].

When active granulomatous disease is present, treatment should include immunosuppressive therapy, such as corticosteroids [49, 53]. In patients for whom immunosuppressive therapy is not helpful, mechanical dilatation via balloon bronchoplasty can be considered (Fig. 2.7). Bronchoplasty can be performed via rigid or flexible bronchoscopy [54, 55]. Repeat bronchoscopic evaluation is usually necessary since the stenosis may recur, requiring more than one session of dilatation before the airways remain fully patent. Although spirometry is often unchanged after bronchoplasty, it is not uncommon that dyspnea is alleviated [54]. For refractory cases, endobronchial stenting is an option, but it may lead to exuberant granulation tissue in sarcoidosis patients. Therefore, stenting should be reserved for as a last resort and performed only centers with substantial experience.

Extrinsic/Granulomatous

Sarcoidosis tends to involve the peribronchial lung parenchyma in the mid-to-upper lung zones. Sometimes, the sarcoidosis lesions coalesce in a perihilar distribution to form conglomerate inflammatory masses (Fig. 2.8). The perihilar conglomerate mass-like lesions are typically difficult to distinguish from enlarged lymph nodes

(a)   **(b)**

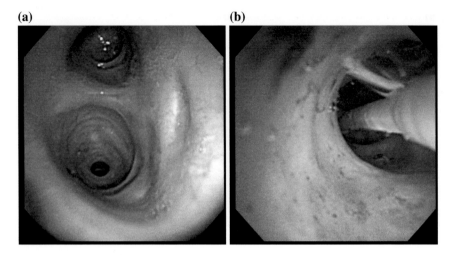

Fig. 2.7 Web-like stenosis of the airways (**a**) treated by advancing a balloon catheter into the obstructed segments (**b**) to perform bronchoplasty. The procedure requires that the operator is able to pass the catheter through the stenotic lesion. We routinely perform circumferential methylprednisolone injections at the level of the stenosis after dilatation [Courtesy of Thomas R. Gildea, MD.]

Fig. 2.8 Conglomerate perihilar inflammatory mass-like inflammation leading to compression of the right upper lobe, bronchus intermedius, and left lower lobe superior segment airways

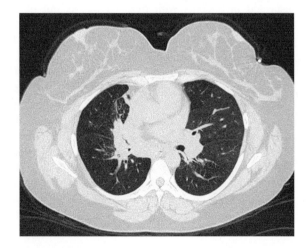

and usually occur in advanced or long-standing disease [56, 57]. Although the lesions may already have been treated with corticosteroids and other therapies, the emergence of flurodeoxyglucose positron emission tomography (FDG-PET) scanning has shown that many of these lesions previously thought to be fibrotic actually harbor active granulomatous inflammation [58]. The intensity of FDG uptake correlates positively with the magnitude of response to therapy [59]. Therefore, in patients with extrinsic airway compression from conglomerate parenchymal sarcoidosis, assessment of disease activity and trials of therapy should be attempted. In some patients, aggressive immunosuppressants, such as infliximab, are necessary to alleviate the impact on the airways [59].

Lymph node enlargement is a very rare cause of airway compression. In the French series of 2500 patients, only 2 patients had substantial main carina enlargement [49]. Lobar obstruction due to lymph node enlargement has been reported [60–62]. In a series of 42 patients with airflow obstruction, only one had obstruction solely due to compression from enlarged lymph nodes, but another 10 (36 %) had some contribution from lymph node enlargement [56]. Taken together, these data suggest that there are several granulomatous mechanisms of extrinsic airway obstruction in sarcoidosis; in the absence of failed treatment trials and negative FDG-PET scanning, the presumption should be that aggressive therapy has the potential to improve symptoms and physiologic indices.

Extrinsic/Non-granulomatous

Sequelae of granulomatous inflammation may lead to irreversible airflow obstruction when the airways get caught up in the peribronchial fibrotic response. The response may include parenchymal architectural distortion, leading to loss of airway patency, bullous disease, honeycombing, and traction bronchiectasis [57]. These radiologic features may all be present in Scadding stage IV chest radiographs and are all associated with physiologic and symptomatic airway obstruction [63]. The most common manifestation is bronchial distortion, which tends to occur in the mid-to-upper lung zones [56, 57] (Fig. 2.9).

Bronchiectasis from sarcoidosis can be localized, but it is usually diffuse. Diffuse cystic bronchiectasis occurs in two situations: due to traction from honeycombing or other parenchymal fibrosis, or from direct damage to the airways from granulomatous inflammation. In cases with localized bronchiectasis, long-standing endobronchial sarcoidosis or focal lymph node compression is usually the culprit [64]. Using chest CT, bronchiectasis has been found on 18–40 % of patients with a stage 4 chest radiograph [57, 65]. The rate of bronchiectasis may approach 100 % in patients who require lung transplantation [66].

Hemoptysis and substantial sputum production are unusual when bronchiectasis occurs in sarcoidosis, and their presence should prompt evaluation for other morbidities such as infections. However, in a minority of patients with bronchiectasis, the clinical course may be dominated by classical bronchiectasis features. In that situation, there may be a high rate of clubbing, crackles, and recurrent exacerbations requiring hospitalization [65]. Management of recurrent infectious exacerbations may be more useful than escalating corticosteroid doses. In a small series, the mortality rate in this situation was high (4 of 7) [65].

Fig. 2.9 Severe right upper lobe bronchus architectural distortion from parenchymal fibrosis. The airway is curved by the surrounding fibrotic process in a pattern that is nearly pathognomonic for sarcoidosis. Endoluminal irregularity is typically visible as well, as in this example

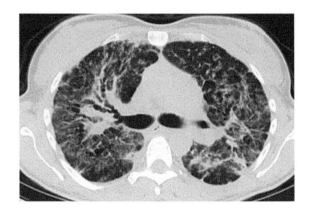

Conclusion

Airway involvement from sarcoidosis is common but under-recognized. Its presence implies a low likelihood of spontaneous remission and the need for more aggressive immunosuppression when treatment is indicated. Therefore, a treatment strategy that considers long-term tolerability and effectiveness should be initiated in those patients with significant airway disease. It is important to distinguish active granulomatous inflammation from fibrotic sequelae of sarcoidosis when formulating a treatment strategy, using imaging findings, response to therapeutic trials, biopsies, and FDG-PET scanning to assess activity.

References

1. Judson MA, et al. The diagnostic pathway to sarcoidosis. Chest. 2003;123(2):406–12.
2. Rodrigues MM, et al. Delayed diagnosis of sarcoidosis is common in Brazil. J Bras Pneumol. 2013;39(5):539–46.
3. Panselinas E, et al. Clinical manifestations, radiographic findings, treatment options, and outcome in sarcoidosis patients with upper respiratory tract involvement. South Med J. 2010;103(9):870–5.
4. Braun JJ, Gentine A, Pauli G. Sinonasal sarcoidosis: review and report of fifteen cases. Laryngoscope. 2004;114(11):1960–3.
5. Baughman RP, Lower EE, Tami T. Upper airway. 4: Sarcoidosis of the upper respiratory tract (SURT). Thorax. 2010;65(2):181–6.
6. Lavergne F, et al. Airway obstruction in bronchial sarcoidosis: outcome with treatment. Chest. 1999;116(5):1194–9.
7. Neville E, et al. Sarcoidosis of the upper respiratory tract and its association with lupus pernio. Thorax. 1976;31(6):660–4.
8. Viskum K, Vestbo J. Vital prognosis in intrathoracic sarcoidosis with special reference to pulmonary function and radiological stage. Eur Respir J. 1993;6(3):349–53.
9. Neville E, Walker AN, James DG. Prognostic factors predicting the outcome of sarcoidosis: an analysis of 818 patients. Q J Med. 1983;52(208):525–33.

10. Baughman RP, et al. Clinical characteristics of patients in a case control study of sarcoidosis. Am J Respir Crit Care Med. 2001;164(10 Pt 1):1885–9.
11. Reed J, et al. Clinical features of sarcoid rhinosinusitis. Am J Med. 2010;123(9):856–62.
12. Aloulah M, et al. Sinonasal manifestations of sarcoidosis: a single institution experience with 38 cases. Int Forum Allergy Rhinol. 2013;3(7):567–72.
13. Hasni SA, Gruber BL. Sarcoidosis presenting as necrotizing sinus destruction mimicking Wegener's granulomatosis. J Rheumatol. 2000;27(2):512–4.
14. Weiss JA. Sarcoidosis in otolaryngology. Report of eleven cases. Evaluation of blind biopsy as a diagnostic aid. Laryngoscope. 1960;70:1351–98.
15. Davis C, Girzadas DV Jr. Laryngeal sarcoidosis causing acute upper airway obstruction. Am J Emerg Med. 2008;26(1):114 e1–3.
16. Aubart FC, et al. Sinonasal involvement in sarcoidosis: a case-control study of 20 patients. Medicine (Baltimore). 2006;85(6):365–71.
17. Krespi YP, Kuriloff DB, Aner M. Sarcoidosis of the sinonasal tract: a new staging system. Otolaryngol Head Neck Surg. 1995;112(2):221–7.
18. Fergie N, Jones NS, Havlat MF. The nasal manifestations of sarcoidosis: a review and report of eight cases. J Laryngol Otol. 1999;113(10):893–8.
19. Zeitlin JF, et al. Nasal and sinus manifestations of sarcoidosis. Am J Rhinol. 2000;14(3):157–61.
20. Sahoo DH, et al. Effectiveness and safety of leflunomide for pulmonary and extrapulmonary sarcoidosis. Eur Respir J. 2011;38(5):1145–50.
21. Judson MA, et al. Efficacy of infliximab in extrapulmonary sarcoidosis: results from a randomised trial. Eur Respir J. 2008;31(6):1189–96.
22. Krespi YP, et al. Treatment of laryngeal sarcoidosis with intralesional steroid injection. Ann Otol Rhinol Laryngol. 1987;96(6):713–5.
23. Carasso B. Sarcoidosis of the larynx causing airway obstruction. Chest. 1974;65(6):693–5.
24. McKelvie P, et al. Sarcoidosis of the upper air passages. Br J Dis Chest. 1968;62(4):200–6.
25. Sakamoto M, Ishizawa M, Kitahara N. Polypoid type of laryngeal sarcoidosis–case report and review of the literature. Eur Arch Otorhinolaryngol. 2000;257(8):436–8.
26. Gerencer RZ, Keohane JD Jr, Russell L. Laryngeal sarcoidosis with airway obstruction. J Otolaryngol. 1998;27(2):90–3.
27. Fogel TD, et al. Radiotherapy in sarcoidosis of the larynx: case report and review of the literature. Laryngoscope. 1984;94(9):1223–5.
28. Marks SC, Goodman RS. Surgical management of nasal and sinus sarcoidosis. Otolaryngol Head Neck Surg. 1998;118(6):856–8.
29. Rubinstein I, et al. Hemoptysis in sarcoidosis. Eur J Respir Dis. 1985;66(4):302–5.
30. Harrison BD, et al. Airflow limitation in sarcoidosis–a study of pulmonary function in 107 patients with newly diagnosed disease. Respir Med. 1991;85(1):59–64.
31. Gibson GJ, et al. British Thoracic Society Sarcoidosis study: effects of long term corticosteroid treatment. Thorax. 1996;51(3):238–47.
32. Sharma OP, Johnson R. Airway obstruction in sarcoidosis. A study of 123 nonsmoking black American patients with sarcoidosis. Chest. 1988;94(2):343–6.
33. Handa T, et al. Clinical and radiographic indices associated with airflow limitation in patients with sarcoidosis. Chest. 2006;130(6):1851–6.
34. Torrington KG, Shorr AF, Parker JW. Endobronchial disease and racial differences in pulmonary sarcoidosis. Chest. 1997;111(3):619–22.
35. Burke RR, et al. Racial differences in sarcoidosis granuloma density. Lung. 2009;187(1):1–7.
36. Argyropoulou PK, Patakas DA, Louridas GE. Airway function in stage I and stage II pulmonary sarcoidosis. Respiration. 1984;46(1):17–25.
37. Shorr AF, Torrington KG, Hnatiuk OW. Endobronchial biopsy for sarcoidosis: a prospective study. Chest. 2001;120(1):109–14.
38. Bjermer L, et al. Endobronchial biopsy positive sarcoidosis: relation to bronchoalveolar lavage and course of disease. Respir Med. 1991;85(3):229–34.

39. Armstrong JR, et al. Endoscopic findings in sarcoidosis. Characteristics and correlations with radiographic staging and bronchial mucosal biopsy yield. Ann Otol Rhinol Laryngol. 1981; 90 (4 Pt 1):339–43.
40. Bilaceroglu S, et al. Combining transbronchial aspiration with endobronchial and transbronchial biopsy in sarcoidosis. Monaldi Arch Chest Dis. 1999;54(3):217–23.
41. Gupta D, et al. Endobronchial vis a vis transbronchial involvement on fiberoptic bronchoscopy in sarcoidosis. Sarcoidosis Vasc Diffuse Lung Dis. 2001;18(1):91–2.
42. Lenique F, et al. CT assessment of bronchi in sarcoidosis: endoscopic and pathologic correlations. Radiology. 1995;194(2):419–23.
43. Davies CW, et al. Air trapping in sarcoidosis on computed tomography: correlation with lung function. Clin Radiol. 2000;55(3):217–21.
44. Judson MA, et al. The diagnostic pathway to sarcoidosis. Chest. 2003;123(2):406–12.
45. Shorr AF, Torrington KG, Hnatiuk OW. Endobronchial involvement and airway hyperreactivity in patients with sarcoidosis. Chest. 2001;120(3):881–6.
46. Bechtel JJ, et al. Airway hyperreactivity in patients with sarcoidosis. Am Rev Respir Dis. 1981;124(6):759–61.
47. Marcias S, et al. Aspecific bronchial hyperreactivity in pulmonary sarcoidosis. Sarcoidosis. 1994;11(2):118–22.
48. Hajdarbegovic E, et al. Prevalence of atopic diseases in patients with sarcoidosis. Allergy Asthma Proc. 2014;35(4):e57–61.
49. Chambellan A, et al. Endoluminal stenosis of proximal bronchi in sarcoidosis: bronchoscopy, function, and evolution. Chest. 2005;127(2):472–81.
50. Westcott JL, Noehren TH. Bronchial stenosis in chronic sarcoidosis. Chest. 1973;63(6):893–7.
51. Olsson T, Bjornstad-Pettersen H, Stjernberg NL. Bronchostenosis due to sarcoidosis: a cause of atelectasis and airway obstruction simulating pulmonary neoplasm and chronic obstructive pulmonary disease. Chest. 1979;75(6):663–6.
52. Miller A, Brown LK, Teirstein AS. Stenosis of main bronchi mimicking fixed upper airway obstruction in sarcoidosis. Chest. 1985;88(2):244–8.
53. Stjernberg N, Thunell M. Pulmonary function in patients with endobronchial sarcoidosis. Acta Med Scand. 1984;215(2):121–6.
54. Fouty BW, et al. Dilatation of bronchial stenoses due to sarcoidosis using a flexible fiberoptic bronchoscope. Chest. 1994;106(3):677–80.
55. Brown KT, Yeoh CB, Saddekni S. Balloon dilatation of the left main bronchus in sarcoidosis. AJR Am J Roentgenol. 1988;150(3):553–4.
56. Naccache JM, et al. High-resolution computed tomographic imaging of airways in sarcoidosis patients with airflow obstruction. J Comput Assist Tomogr. 2008;32(6):905–12.
57. Abehsera M, et al. Sarcoidosis with pulmonary fibrosis: CT patterns and correlation with pulmonary function. AJR Am J Roentgenol. 2000;174(6):1751–7.
58. Mostard RL, et al. Severity of pulmonary involvement and (18)F-FDG PET activity in sarcoidosis. Respir Med. 2013;107(3):439–47.
59. Vorselaars AD, et al. Effectiveness of infliximab in refractory FDG PET-positive sarcoidosis. Eur Respir J. 2015;46(1):175–85.
60. Mendelson DS, et al. Bronchial compression: an unusual manifestation of sarcoidosis. J Comput Assist Tomogr. 1983;7(5):892–4.
61. Arkless HA, Chodoff RJ. Middle lobe syndrome due to sarcoidosis. Dis Chest. 1956; 30(3):351–3.
62. Abramowicz MJ, et al. Tumour-like presentation of pulmonary sarcoidosis. Eur Respir J. 1992;5(10):1286–7.
63. Remy-Jardin M, et al. Pulmonary sarcoidosis: role of CT in the evaluation of disease activity and functional impairment and in prognosis assessment. Radiology. 1994;191(3):675–80.
64. Udwadia ZF, et al. Bronchoscopic and bronchographic findings in 12 patients with sarcoidosis and severe or progressive airways obstruction. Thorax. 1990;45(4):272–5.

65. Lewis MM, et al. Clinical bronchiectasis complicating pulmonary sarcoidosis: case series of seven patients. Sarcoidosis Vasc Diffuse Lung Dis. 2002;19(2):154–9.
66. Xu L, Kligerman S, Burke A. End-stage Sarcoid Lung Disease Is Distinct From Usual Interstitial Pneumonia. Am J Surg Pathol. 2013;37(4):593–600.

Chapter 3
Airway Complications of Inflammatory Bowel Disease

Shekhar Ghamande and Prasoon Jain

Introduction

Most physicians are aware of extra-intestinal manifestations of inflammatory bowel disease (IBD). Over the course of disease, extra-intestinal manifestations occur in 20–40 % of IBD patients [1]. The most common extra-intestinal manifestations include arthritis, ankylosing spondylitis, pyoderma gangrenosa, erythema nodosum, sclerosing cholangitis, episcleritis, uveitis, pancreatitis, thyroiditis, and pericarditis. These extra-intestinal manifestations tend to correlate with the extent of ulcerative colitis, and as many as 25 % of the patients have more than one extra-intestinal manifestations [2]. Furthermore, the probability of these manifestations increases with the duration of IBD [3]. Over past several decades, there is an increasing recognition of involvement of pulmonary system in patients with IBD. These include involvement of upper and central airways, small airways, pulmonary parenchyma, pulmonary vasculature, and pleura. Unfortunately, high-quality studies addressing pulmonary complications of IBD are lacking, and the majority of information on this subject comes from small series or case reports. Due to low incidence, the lack of general awareness and absence of any established criteria to associate pulmonary manifestations with underlying IBD, the appropriate diagnosis, and therapies are often delayed. To make the matter more difficult, many of the drugs used for the treatment of IBD have important pulmonary complications that

S. Ghamande (✉) · P. Jain
Pulmonary and Critical Care, Louis A Johnson VA Medical Center,
Clarksburg, WV, 26301, USA
e-mail: sghamande@sw.org

P. Jain
e-mail: prasoonjain.md@gmail.com

S. Ghamande
Texas A&M University, College Station, TX, USA

© Springer International Publishing Switzerland 2016
A.C. Mehta et al. (eds.), *Diseases of the Central Airways,*
Respiratory Medicine, DOI 10.1007/978-3-319-29830-6_3

are difficult to differentiate from the pulmonary abnormalities inherently associated with the underlying disease process.

In this chapter, we discuss the clinical presentation, diagnosis, and treatment airway diseases associated with IBD. We also discuss the emerging views on the possible association of IBD with other common airway diseases such as chronic obstructive pulmonary disease (COPD) and asthma. We provide practical suggestions to recognize and treat airway complications of IBD in a timely fashion.

Historical Background

Early studies looking into extra-intestinal manifestations did not recognize the association of IBD with pulmonary manifestations [4, 5]. Kraft and associates in 1976 were first to identify the pulmonary involvement in IBD in 6 patients [6]. All patients in this series presented with chronic productive cough with 4 of 6 patients having findings consistent with bronchiectasis and 5 of 6 patients having airflow obstruction on pulmonary function tests (PFTs). Overt pulmonary symptoms first developed following procto-colectomy in 2 patients in this series. Several subsequent reports have confirmed such association with most notable contribution coming from a detailed account of 33 patients with a variety of pulmonary complications in patients with both ulcerative colitis (UC) and Crohn's disease (CD) [7].

Incidence

IBD is a common gastrointestinal disease. In an analysis of 9 million health insurance claims, the prevalence of CD and UC in adults was 201 (95 % CI, 197–204) and 238 (95 % CI, 234–241) per 100,000, respectively [8]. The incidence of pulmonary complications in IBD remains unknown. In fact, many epidemiological studies have failed to recognize any such association [1–3]. For example, in an earlier study, no respiratory complications were reported in 624 patients with IBD [4]. Another study looking into extra-intestinal manifestations found no instance of pulmonary disease among 700 patients with IBD [9]. The evidence for respiratory complications of IBD mostly comes from case reports and short series. For example, in one study, PFTs and high-resolution chest computed tomography (HRCT) were performed in 17 patients with IBD. Obstructive, restrictive, or combined defect was found in 11 (65 %) and abnormalities on HRCT were detected in 16 (94 %) patients [10]. In another study of 39 patients with IBD, PFT abnormalities were present in 56 % and HRCT abnormalities were detected in 64 % of patients [11]. A somewhat lower prevalence of abnormalities was reported in a prospective study of 95 IBD patients in which PFT was abnormal in 28.5 % and HRCT was abnormal in 22 % of patients [12]. Generally, the incidence of clinical symptoms was lower than PFT abnormalities, and HRCT changes in these studies. Overall review of these clinical reports leaves little doubt regarding an association between IBD and pulmonary involvement. Most likely, prior studies failed to identify these complications due to non-specific nature of respiratory symptoms and clinical presentation in IBD. Population studies looking into survival and cause-specific mortality further support an association between IBD and lung disease. Several of these studies have shown higher than expected mortality from COPD [13–15], asthma, pulmonary embolism, and pneumonia [16] in patients with IBD.

There is a strong evidence for subclinical pulmonary involvement in IBD. Non-specific respiratory symptoms are common in patients with IBD. In a case–control study, a nearly threefold increase in prevalence of dyspnea and sputum production was found in IBD patients as compared with control subjects [17]. Abnormalities on PFTs have been found in as many as 50 % of patients with IBD [18]. Notably, many authors have reported PFT abnormalities in patients free of any respiratory symptom, suggesting presence of a latent pulmonary involvement in IBD [19–21]. Non-specific bronchial hyperresponsiveness has been reported in as many as 71 % of children with CD in the absence of any pulmonary symptoms [22]. In addition to altered pulmonary functions, abnormal findings on HRCT are found in many asymptomatic patients with IBD. For example, in one study, HRCT showed abnormal findings such as air trapping, peripheral reticular opacities, and bronchiectasis in 19 of 36 (53 %) patients. Eight of 19 (42 %) patients with abnormal HRCT findings had no respiratory symptom [19]. In a prospective study, HRCT was performed in 95 patients with IBD. Abnormalities were detected in 21 (22 %) patients. A majority of patients with abnormal HRCT findings in this study had no respiratory symptoms [12]. A further evidence of subclinical pulmonary involvement comes from studies in which bronchoalveolar lavage (BAL) was performed. In one such study, BAL was performed in 18 patients with CD [23]. All patients included in this study were free of any symptoms. Lymphocytic alveolitis was detected in 11 (61 %) subjects. Other studies have also demonstrated similar findings [24]. Taken together, these data leave little doubt that pulmonary involvement is common in IBD but is often overlooked because many such patients have a latent disease that is difficult to detect in a routine clinical setting. Even in symptomatic patients, non-specific presentation, confounding effect of tobacco use, non-availability of a reliable test, and a general lack of awareness among clinicians about such association contribute to underdiagnosis of pulmonary complications in IBD.

Pathophysiology

IBD is the end result of a complicated interaction between environmental, genetic, microbial factors, and abnormal immune response [25]. Smoking is clearly associated with increased risk of CD [26]. Epidemiologic studies suggest a link between air pollution and risk of IBD [27]. There is evidence for an association between the reduced biodiversity and other changes in intestinal microbiome and IBD [28, 29]. A variety of defects in innate as well as adaptive immune response have been reported in IBD. Increasing body of data supports an important role of altered innate immunity in response to intestinal bacterial antigens in IBD, mediated by pattern recognition receptors (PRRs) expressed by cells involved in innate immunity. The nucleotide-binding oligomerization domain containing protein-2 (NOD2) in the cytoplasm and the Toll-like receptor (TLR) on the cell membrane are two important PRR families associated with mucosal immunity [30, 31]. NOD2 recognizes peptidoglycan in bacterial cell wall. An alteration in the function of NOD2 receptor due to a frameshift mutation is shown to be associated with increased risk of CD [32]. Such mutation results in a stronger TLR-2 response, disruption of epithelial barrier, and increased Th-1 response, all contributing to the pathophysiology of CD [33].

It cannot go unnoticed that nearly all of the factors associated with pathogenesis of IBD mentioned above have also been associated with a variety of lung diseases, including COPD. Smoking and air pollution are the leading causes of respiratory morbidity. An increasing number of studies are reporting association between altered lung microbiome and chronic lung diseases such as COPD, asthma, idiopathic pulmonary fibrosis, and bronchiectasis [34–36]. Several studies have also established an important role of altered innate immunity in pathogenesis of COPD [37]. For example, NOD2 single nucleotide polymorphism has been described in COPD and is shown to be associated with reduced lung function in COPD [38]. In this regard, it is also interesting to note the similarities between the organ-specific and systemic inflammatory process in COPD and IBD. In both diseases, there is noticeable dysfunction of epithelial mucosal barrier. Smoking is the main cause of the breakdown of respiratory epithelium in COPD [39]. A similar epithelial barrier dysfunction is also a key feature in IBD, although it is unclear whether the epithelial dysfunction is the cause or the effect of the disease [40]. The loss of epithelial barrier may initiate an intestinal inflammatory response and promote increased bacterial translocation. Whether intestinal epithelium barrier dysfunction in IBD is related in any way to the epithelium barrier dysfunction in airway diseases in IBD is unknown.

Based on aforementioned discussion, convincing similarities can be drawn between the nature and origins of inflammation in IBD and lung diseases such as COPD. However, any such discussion provides no information on how pulmonary system without any direct anatomical connection gets involved with the inflammatory cascades that originates in the gastrointestinal tract in IBD [41].

Both of these organ systems evolve from the primitive foregut during human development [42, 43]. Despite an anatomic separation during subsequent development, gastrointestinal and pulmonary organ systems continue to share many similarities at a structural and organizational level. Both organ systems have similar mucosal epithelial barrier, protective mucus layer, submucosal loose connective tissue, and mucosa-associated lymphoid tissue (MALT). It is very likely that both these organ systems share similar antigens due to a common embryonic ancestry. The presence of a shared antigen between these organ systems provides the likely link that allows cross talk between the inflammatory responses that originates in the gastrointestinal tract and goes on to involve pulmonary system [41]. Aberrant homing of the gut-derived lymphocytes is shown to occur in liver, synovial, and ocular tissues, possibly contributing to systemic manifestations [44]. It is interesting to speculate whether a similar homing of gut-derived lymphocytes also occurs in the lung tissues of IBD patients with pulmonary complications. Such mechanism might explain the onset of active pulmonary disease for the first time after colectomy in some patients with IBD [45]. Additional factors may include soluble mediators of inflammation and TLR4 gene variations causing exaggerated lung and intestinal mucosal immune response to lipopolysaccharide antigens from gut bacteria in patients with IBD [46].

Pulmonary Disorders in IBD

Pulmonary manifestations of IBD are summarized in Table 3.1. Pulmonary diseases in IBD involving airways, lung parenchyma, pulmonary vasculature, and pleura are extensively reviewed elsewhere [47–49]. Unfortunately, most clinical reports on this subject are cross-sectional and retrospective and are limited to a handful of cases. Therefore, the details on clinical course and natural history of the pulmonary complications are not readily available. The largest series was reported by Camus and associates who reviewed 33 patients with various pulmonary manifestations of IBD [7]. The male-to-female distribution was roughly 1:2, and the age at the diagnosis varied from 17 to 80 years. Majority of patients were non-smokers. Pulmonary complications were airway diseases in 20 cases, interstitial lung diseases in 10 patients, necrobiotic lung nodules in 2 cases, and serositis in 1 case. The onset of pulmonary complications varied widely in relation to the underlying IBD. Most commonly, the pulmonary disease was identified after the diagnosis of IBD was already established, although some patients experienced pulmonary symptoms before or at the time of IBD diagnosis. In another series of 10 patients, Higenbottam and associates reported predominantly airway involvement in 6 patients and lung parenchymal involvement in 4 patients [50]. A similar pattern of predominant central airway involvement has also been reported by others [51].

In recent years, data have emerged to suggest a higher than expected burden of asthma and COPD in IBD. In subsequent sections, we briefly discuss this emerging information but mainly focus on the involvement of central airways with IBD.

Asthma and IBD

Epidemiological studies suggest higher than expected incidence of asthma in IBD compared to the control subjects. For instance, in a large population-based study from Manitoba, the prevalence ratio of asthma was 1.66 (95 % CI 1.46–1.88) in UC and 1.43 (95 % CI 1.26–1.62) in CD [52]. In another study, an increased prevalence of UC (OR 2.81, 1.15–6.9) but not of CD was found in patients with asthma [53]. D'Arienzo and associates reported a higher prevalence (42.2 %) of allergic disease including asthma in 45 subjects with UC compared to 13.5 % prevalence among 37 healthy controls. There was a family history of allergic diseases in 48.9 % of

Table 3.1 Pulmonary manifestations of inflammatory bowel disease

Large airway diseases
• Subglottic stenosis
• Tracheobronchitis
• Bronchitis
• Bronchiectasis
Small airway disease
• Bronchiolitis
• Bronchiolitis obliterans
• Diffuse panbronchiolitis
Interstitial lung disease
• Bronchiolitis obliterans with organizing pneumonia
• Non-specific interstitial pneumonia
• Desquamative interstitial pneumonia
• Eosinophilic pneumonia
• Fibrosing alveolitis
• Sarcoidosis
Pulmonary vascular disease
• Pulmonary thromboembolism
• Pulmonary vasculitis
Pleural disease
• Pleural effusion
• Pleuro-pericarditis
• Pleural thickening
• Pneumothorax
• Colo-pleural fistula
Drug induced lung disease
• Sulfasalazine
• Azathioprine
• Methotrexate
• Biological agents
Miscellaneous
• Laryngeal involvement
• Lymphocytic alveolitis
• Necrobiotic pulmonary nodules

patients with UC and 16.2 % of healthy controls. Skin prick tests were almost twice as likely to be positive in UC patients as in control subjects [54].

Studies have shown a high incidence of bronchial hyperresponsiveness (BHR) in patients with IBD. In one such study, BHR was detected with methacholine challenge testing in 45 % of IBD patients without pulmonary symptoms compared to 17 % of healthy controls [55]. Others have reported a similar increase in prevalence of BHR among patients with CD [56]. Higher sputum eosinophil count and eosinophilic cationic protein levels have also been detected among IBD patients compared to healthy controls in absence of respiratory symptoms [57, 58]. High levels of serum IgE have also been reported in patients with IBD [59]. However, not all studies have reached similar conclusions in this regard. Some studies have not found an increased incidence of allergic disorders in IBD. For example, one study found no correlation between atopy and IBD [60]. Further, Ceyhan and associates did not find significant BHR or elevated IgE, even though there were more respiratory and allergic symptoms in patients with IBD compared to control subjects [61]. Another recent study has reported a low prevalence of BHR and respiratory involvement in children with IBD [62].

Notwithstanding, the overall evidence does suggest a higher than expected incidence of asthma and allergic disorders among patients with IBD. Apparently, this association is an underappreciated extra-intestinal manifestation of IBD. More work is needed to understand the full clinical implications of this association between asthma and other allergic disorders and IBD. Particularly, troubling in this context is a report of higher than expected asthma mortality among patients with IBD [63]. Future studies are needed to address this issue and to determine whether the natural course of asthma differs in any way among patients with or without IBD.

COPD and IBD

Smoking is a common risk factor for both COPD and CD. It is therefore not surprising that there is suggestion of an epidemiologic association between COPD and IBD. For example, in a Swedish population-based cohort study, Ekbom and associates demonstrated an increased risk of UC (HR 1.83; 95 % CI 1.61–2.09) and CD (HR 2.72; 95 % CI 2.33–3.18) in patients with COPD. Furthermore, the first-degree relatives of COPD patients had an increased risk of CD (HR 1.25; 95 % CI 1.09–1.43) but not of UC (HR 1.09; 95 % CI 0.96–1.23) [13]. Moreover, COPD contributes to mortality risk in patients with CD but not UC. In a Danish cohort, mortality in IBD was assessed over a 30 year period. The risk of mortality from respiratory disease was high in the first year of diagnosis of CD (HR 3.10, 2.4–4) and declined slightly but remained elevated even after 10 years (HR 2.32, 1.96–2.74) [14]. As in asthma, it is unclear how clinical course of COPD is different in patients with or without underlying IBD.

Central Airway Disorders in IBD

Central airway is the most common site of respiratory involvement in IBD [7, 10]. In a review of 155 patients from 55 case series, large airway disease accounted for 39 % of respiratory involvement in IBD [64]. In one series, the prevalence of IBD was significantly higher (Odds ratio 4.26, 95 % CI 1.48–11.71) than expected among patients with airway disease in a respiratory clinic [53]. Airway disease typically follows several years of intestinal manifestations. However, in some case, pulmonary involvement precedes bowel disease, most notably in younger patients [7, 65, 66]. As is true for other manifestations, airway involvement becomes clinically manifest for the first time months to years after colectomy in some patients [7, 45, 67]. Airway disease occurs usually in UC with a female preponderance and an average age of onset in the fifth decade. Other extraintestinal manifestations including ocular, arthritic, dermatological, and hepatic are concurrently found in up to 40 % of cases [7, 10, 64].

Upper airway disease with IBD has been described in several case reports. The site of inflammation in many of these cases has included the vocal cords, subglottic region, and tracheobronchial tree. Isolated involvement of larynx is uncommon [68, 69]. It is more usual to have a generalized tracheobronchitis with laryngeal and subglottic involvement [70]. The patients usually present with progressive hoarseness, cough, and dyspnea often mistaken for asthma or chronic bronchitis for months to years before the correct diagnosis is identified [7, 67, 71–76]. There are several reports of a more dramatic presentation with severe respiratory distress and stridor [7, 71, 72, 77]. Acute respiratory failure requiring immediate intubation and mechanical ventilation due to severe tracheobronchitis has been described in a handful of case reports [78, 79]. Sometimes, urgent bronchoscopic interventions have been needed to alleviate airway narrowing in these patients [73, 80]. Persistent airway inflammation has led to large airway stenosis in some cases [7, 67, 75]. Obstructive defect on PFTs with abnormalities in flow volume loop may provide a clue to correct underlying diagnosis [71, 72, 81]. Bronchoscopy confirms the diagnosis and provides useful information on the severity and extent of central airway involvement. There is considerable resolution after the treatment with systemic steroids.

Bronchiectasis is the most common airway manifestation of IBD. It accounts for 66 % of airway complications in patients with IBD [64]. 6 of 15 patients reported by Camus and associates had clinical and radiological evidence of bronchiectasis [7]. In a study of 17 patients with IBD, 13 (76 %) patients had evidence of bronchiectasis on HRCT [10]. These results were similar to those reported in an earlier series in which 5 of 7 IBD patients with chronic cough and sputum production had evidence of bronchiectasis on chest computed tomography (CT) [82]. Bronchiectasis is reported to occur more commonly in UC than in CD. The respiratory symptoms usually develop months to years after onset of gastrointestinal symptoms. The usual symptoms are chronic cough and copious sputum production. Early to mid-inspiratory coarse crackles can be appreciated on auscultation of lung fields [83]. Periodic exacerbation of symptoms is reported by many patients, needing repeated courses of antibiotics. Hemoptysis is uncommon but is occasionally reported [84]. Interestingly, there are several reports of chronic bronchitis and bronchial suppuration without any prior tobacco use in IBD. Many such patients were described before availability of HRCT [65]. It is plausible that some of the patients thought to have bronchitis or bronchial suppuration in earlier reports had underlying bronchiectasis that could not be detected with the available imaging modalities. In this regard, it is important to point out that bronchiectasis is the most common radiologic abnormality on HRCT in IBD and several patients with this finding have minimal or no pulmonary symptoms [10, 12].

As discussed above, several patients have developed large airway complications for the first time after undergoing colectomy for IBD [7, 45, 85]. For example, 8 of 10 patients in a series developed bronchiectasis 2 weeks to 30 years after undergoing colectomy for IBD [45]. Similarly, 9 of 15 patients with large airway disease reported by Camus and associates had undergone prior colectomy [7]. It is suggested that a reduction in immunomodulating drugs after colectomy for IBD may unmask an underlying airway disease in some of these patients [45].

PFTs may reveal airflow obstruction, but normal results do not exclude the diagnosis [82]. A HRCT is indicated when bronchiectasis is suspected in patients with IBD. Dilatation of bronchi is most prominent in both lower lobes. A routine bronchoscopy is not helpful in bronchiectasis. Many patients with IBD-associated bronchiectasis have experienced a dramatic improvement in symptoms after institution of systemic corticosteroids [65, 82]. Such response is not typical for bronchiectasis unrelated to IBD. Use of inhaled corticosteroids has also led to resolution of symptoms in some of these cases [7, 50].

Small airways are also involved in some patients with IBD. Radiological studies using HRCT have shown suggestion of small airway disease in 33–52 % of patients [10, 19]. In many instances, the CT findings suggest simultaneous involvement of both large and small airways with the disease process. In other cases, small airway involvement is associated with interstitial changes in the lung. Small airway involvement appears to be more common in CD than in UC. Cough and dyspnea are the usual complaints, although many patients have no symptoms. Symptomatic disease tends to present earlier and in younger patients compared to large airway disease. It can precede bowel involvement and pose a diagnostic dilemma [66, 80, 86–89]. PFTs can be normal, but the reported changes include obstructive defect, restrictive defect, or a combined defect. No correlation has been detected between HRCT abnormalities and PFTs [19]. Small airway dysfunction is observed in some patients in the absence of any abnormality on standard PFTs. For example, Tzanakis and associates assessed small airway function using method based on density dependence of flow in 30 patients with IBD. The forced vital capacity (FVC), forced expiratory volume in 1 s (FEV1), FEV1/FVC ratio, or total lung capacity were similar in both groups of patients [90]. Small airway dysfunction was identified in patients with untreated disease and active UC treated with mesalamine but not in those treated with steroids, possibly reflecting beneficial effects of steroids on small airway disease [91]. Optimal therapy is not defined for small airway disease in IBD. However, several patients have experienced improvement or resolution of symptoms with oral or inhaled corticosteroids [7, 89, 91].

Pulmonary Function Tests

PFTs are indicated in IBD patients suspected to have respiratory complications. Pulmonary function abnormalities can be detected not only in symptomatic but also in many asymptomatic patients with subclinical involvement of respiratory system. The prevalence of PFT abnormalities in IBD has varied from 6 to 58 % in different case series [11, 12, 19, 21, 24, 90, 92–95]. This heterogeneity may be related to difference in disease activity, severity of lung disease, use of corticosteroids, and inclusion of smokers in the patient groups. In a vast majority of studies, the most common abnormality is a small but statistically significant reduction in DLCO [11, 12, 19, 24, 90, 93, 94]. Mild obstructive, restrictive, or combined defects have been reported, but many other studies have failed to show any major abnormality in FEV1, FEV1/FVC ratio, and mid-expiratory flow rates in the patients with IBD [19, 24, 90]. Air trapping or hyperinflation possibly due to small airway dysfunction has been reported in a few studies [19, 24, 94]. The correlation of PFT abnormalities with the degree of disease activity was demonstrated in a majority of the studies with a drop in DLCO being the most frequent abnormality. However, longitudinal data on this are too scant to draw any firm conclusions. In the pediatric CD of 26 patients, Munck et al. [20] reported a decrease in DLCO only with active disease. But more recently in a larger study, Peradzynska et al. [62] did not find any significant PFT abnormalities in 50 patients with pediatric IBD compared to controls and furthermore there was no correlation of PFTs with disease activity.

Airflow obstruction is readily detectable in IBD patients with predominant involvement of central airways. Untreated tracheobronchitis may lead to central airway stenosis with flattening of inspiratory and expiratory components of flow volume loop [71, 72]. Treatment with systemic corticosteroids leads to improvement or resolution of pulmonary function defects as well as flow volume loop abnormalities [71, 72]. An improvement in PFTs and flow volume loop provides an easy and noninvasive objective parameter to assess the response to corticosteroid therapy in patients with central airway obstruction.

Exhaled Nitric Oxide

A simple tool to detect early and asymptomatic airway involvement and to monitor airway inflammation is highly desired in IBD. Unfortunately, clinical evaluation, chest radiograph, and routine pulmonary function testing are inadequate for this purpose. Exhaled nitric oxide (FeNO) has been used to monitor airway inflammation and steroid responsiveness in bronchial asthma [96]. Recent data suggest a potential role of FeNO in early detection of airway involvement in IBD. Elevation in FeNO is shown to correlate with the CD activity index suggesting the presence of subclinical pulmonary involvement [97, 98]. Most useful data in this regard come from a study from Turkey in which FeNO was measured in 33 patients with IBD and was compared with 25 matched controls [99]. Pulmonary involvement could be established in 15 patients on the basis of detailed clinical evaluation, PFTs, bronchoscopy, and HRCT. Bronchiectasis and large airway obstruction were diagnosed in 12 of 15 (80 %) IBD patients with pulmonary involvement. The levels of FeNO were higher in patients with pulmonary involvement (FeNO 32 ± 20 ppb) than in those without pulmonary involvement (24 ± 8 ppb) and healthy controls (14 ± 8 ppb). Higher FeNO levels were not associated with symptoms, abnormalities on PFT, or disease activity. Sensitivity and specificity analyses failed to identify a cutoff value for the diagnostic FeNO levels. With these encouraging results, further work is needed to establish the role of FeNO in medical assessment of IBD patients with respiratory complications. Most important initial step in this regard is to establish a cutoff level of FeNO with an adequate sensitivity, specificity, and predictive value to identify presence or absence of airway involvement in IBD.

Imaging Studies

Most patients with IBD have a normal chest radiographs irrespective of respiratory symptoms [7, 53, 100]. In an occasional patient with central airway disease, narrowing of tracheal air column can be appreciated on plain chest radiograph [71]. Soft tissue swelling of upper airways is sometimes encountered with involvement of hypopharynx, larynx, and upper trachea [101]. Chest radiograph has low sensitivity for detecting bronchiectasis, but the reported findings include bronchial wall thickening, tramline pattern, and dilated bronchi in advanced cases [7, 83].

Chest CT is a useful radiological investigation in IBD patients suspected to have respiratory tract involvement. In tracheobronchitis, CT findings include irregularity of airway mucosa, concentric thickening of airway wall, narrowing, and large airway stenosis [67, 77, 79]. Similar findings have also been shown on magnetic resonance imaging (MRI) in some reports [51, 71, 73]. In the absence of comparative studies, it is unclear whether MRI is better than CT for this purpose, but at least in one case, thickening of airway wall and stenosis were seen on MRI but not on CT [73]. In one report, an increased activity was noted over the posterior wall of trachea on 2-deoxy-2[^{18}F] fluoro-D-glucose positron emission tomography (^{18}F-FDG PET) scan that resolved with systemic steroids in 3 months [102]. The authors propose PET scan to have a possible value in noninvasive assessment of tracheobronchial involvement with IBD, but it is difficult to draw any conclusion on the basis of a single case report.

HRCT should be performed in IBD patients suspected to have bronchiectasis [7]. In addition to cylindrical or cystic bronchiectasis changes, HRCT may also reveal bronchial wall thickening, mucus plugging, and airway stenosis [51]. Evidence of associated small airway involvement is not unusual on HRCT in patients with bronchiectasis [7, 10, 12, 19], as suggested by the presence of air trapping, centrilobular nodules, and tree-in-bud appearance. Additional findings on HRCT may include ground glass changes, reticular changes, parenchymal bands, and cystic changes [10–12].

Bronchoscopy

Bronchoscopy should be performed without delay in IBD patients with suspected central airway involvement. Examination in patients with tracheobronchial involvement usually shows diffuse erythematous, inflamed, edematous, and friable mucosa with scattered white mucosal plaques and nodular changes [7, 50, 66, 73, 75, 80, 82, 103] (Fig. 3.1). Purulent secretions may be found in some cases. In some instances, stripes of tracheal cartilage and longitudinal mucosal folds of the membranous portion of trachea cannot be appreciated on bronchoscopic inspection [81]. Narrowing of trachea and bronchi is seen in more advanced cases [7, 67, 75]. Web-like obstruction of lobar bronchi has also been reported [73]. In some patients, the disease process is most pronounced in subglottic trachea [71], but it is more usual to find a generalized involvement of trachea and main-stem bronchi with the disease process [75, 77]. In one report, endobronchial ultrasound showed circumferential thickening of the mucosa with preservation of tracheobronchial cartilage [104]. The ability of endobronchial ultrasound to identify sparing of cartilage may be helpful in differentiating IBD-associated tracheobronchitis from disorders such as relapsing polychondritis.

The abnormal bronchoscopic findings usually resolve with corticosteroid therapy in 1–3 months [70, 75, 78, 81, 103–105]. Development of stenosis in the areas of circumferential inflammation is a concern and requires airway monitoring [67]. Fortunately, only a minority of patients develop this complication with early

Fig. 3.1 Inflammatory and nodular endobronchial changes causing partial obstruction of right middle lobe bronchus in a patient with inflammatory bowel disease

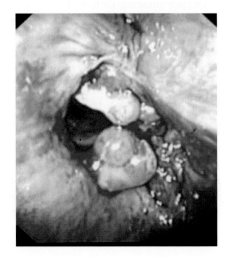

detection and appropriate treatment. The need for a repeat bronchoscopy must be assessed on a case-by-case basis.

Bronchoscopy has a more limited role in patients with IBD-associated bronchiectasis. Bronchoscopy may be normal [82] or may show mucosal erythema, purulent secretions, and extensive dilatation of distal bronchi [7, 51, 85]. BAL shows increased cellularity with neutrophilic predominance [7]. Isolation of pathogens may be helpful in appropriate selection of anti-microbial agents in selected patients.

Similarly, bronchoscopy has no major role in assessment of other respiratory diseases associated with IBD. Histological diagnosis of small airway disease and other pathologies affecting lung parenchyma cannot be established on bronchoscopic lung biopsies. The role of bronchoscopy in these patients is largely limited to exclusion of an underlying infectious etiology.

Pathology

Endobronchial biopsies in IBD patients with tracheobronchial disease reveal mucosal and submucosal inflammation. The epithelial lining is ulcerated sometimes with squamous metaplasia [76, 78, 105]. Lymphocytes and plasma cells are the predominant infiltrating cells along with a few neutrophils and red cells [7]. Loosely formed granuloma may be found in some cases [70, 77, 103]. On forceps biopsies, the cartilage cannot be sampled, but in surgical specimens, underlying cartilage is entirely spared [104]. Many of the histological changes resolve with corticosteroid administration within 1–3 months [75]. Minimal fibrotic changes and non-specific inflammation of little clinical significance may persist in some cases [70, 78].

Pathologic confirmation of small airway involvement requires surgical lung biopsy. Histopathologic findings in these patients include bronchiolitis, peribronchial granuloma, concentric small airway fibrosis, and panbronchiolitis [12, 64]. Surgical biopsy is not essential in every case, and the decision to perform invasive biopsy should be preceded by a careful risk–benefit analysis.

Treatment

Corticosteroids are the mainstay for treatment of airway complications associated with IBD [7, 106]. Systemic corticosteroids must be started without delay in IBD patients found to have involvement of central airways to avoid development of fixed and irreversible airway narrowing. Currently, the dose and duration of therapy with systemic corticosteroids are not defined as there are no controlled studies addressing this issue. Based on numerous case reports and our own experience, it is reasonable to initiate therapy with oral prednisone at a starting dose of 40–60 mg per day. We recommend reducing dose by 10 mg/day every two weeks till a stable dose of 10 mg/day is reached and maintaining patient on this dose for next 4–6 months. Higher doses of intravenous corticosteroids may be required in patients who develop respiratory failure due to critical airway stenosis and severe subglottic stenosis. Several such patients have experienced a rapid clinical improvement and resolution of airway pathology with high-dose steroids.

There are isolated reports of successful outcome with anti-tumor necrosis factor treatment in respiratory complications of IBD. In the first report, a patient with severe airway involvement responded well to infliximab therapy after failure of systemic corticosteroids to control the disease process [77]. In second report, infliximab therapy successfully controlled disease process in a patient with bron-chiolitis obliterans with organizing pneumonia associated with CD who could not tolerate systemic corticosteroids [107]. While further data are clearly needed to clarify the usefulness of infliximab for these patients, these two reports provide some reassurance to clinicians looking for an alternative therapy for patients not responding to corticosteroids.

It is reasonable to initiate inhaled corticosteroids in addition to systemic steroids for their local anti-inflammatory action. We recommend the use of inhaled corti-costeroids for an extended period after withdrawal of systemic steroids. Some patients with mild to moderate large airway disease have shown adequate response to high-dose inhaled corticosteroids alone without needing systemic therapy. A close clinical follow-up to monitor the disease process is essential in such patients.

There is no established role of interventional bronchoscopy procedures in the management of airway complications in IBD patients. Some patients refractory to oral steroids have received direct instillation of methylprednisolone in right and main-stem bronchi every 2–3 days [7]. In the absence of controlled trials, this approach cannot be recommended for routine care of these patients. Other inter-ventional procedures such as laser photocoagulation [7, 106], balloon dilation [80], and tissue ablation with microdebrider [73] have been employed for the treatment of critical airway narrowing, but the indications for such procedures are poorly defined. Attempted balloon dilation was complicated by airway perforation and death in one reported case [80].

Patients with bronchiectasis seem to respond well to systemic and inhaled cor-ticosteroids [7, 65, 82]. Such rapid response to steroids is unusual with other causes of non-cystic fibrosis bronchiectasis. This observation has led some investigators to speculate that an immunological mechanism may have a more dominant role in IBD-related bronchiectasis than in idiopathic bronchiectasis where infection seems to play a more important role [85]. Although some patients with small airway disease have responded to inhaled steroids [7, 91], oral steroids seem more effective and are preferred over inhaled steroids for initial therapy [87, 89]. More work is needed to identify the most effective treatment approach in these patients.

Conclusion

Involvement of central airways in IBD is well documented in the literature but is underappreciated in clinical practice. The airway complications of IBD include laryngeal inflammation, tracheobronchitis, bronchiectasis, and small airway disease. Clinical presentation varies from chronic cough and sputum production to acute respiratory failure needing intubation and mechanical ventilation. Many patients develop respiratory complications months to years after undergoing colectomy for IBD. A high index of suspicion is needed for early recognition of airway disease associated with IBD. PFTs may be normal or may reveal airflow obstruction and abnormalities in flow volume loop. Chest radiograph is usually unremarkable. CT is the imaging modality of choice. The main finding on CT is diffuse thickening of airway wall. HRCT should be performed for the assessment of patient suspected to have IBD-associated bronchiectasis and small airway disease. Bronchoscopy provides important diagnostic information and should be performed without any delay in patients suspected to have central airway involvement with IBD. Systemic steroids should be initiated as soon as the diagnosis is established. Inhaled steroids are also effective in mild disease. The majority of patients experience resolution of symptoms and airway pathology with corticosteroid therapy. There is no established role of interventional bronchoscopy procedures. A careful clinical follow-up supplemented by PFTs, radiological imaging, and in selected cases, bronchoscopy is essential for optimal outcome. There is emerging role of exhaled nitric oxide monitoring for this purpose.

References

1. Bernstein CN, Blanchard JF, Rawsthorne P, Yu N. The prevalence of extraintestinal diseases in inflammatory bowel disease: a population-based study. Am J Gastroenterol. 2001;96:1116–22.
2. Monsén U, Sorstad J, Hellers G, Johansson C. Extracolonic diagnoses in ulcerative colitis: an epidemiological study. Am J Gastroenterol. 1990;85:711–6.
3. Veloso FT, Carvalho J, Magro F. Immune-related systemic manifestations of inflammatory bowel disease. A prospective study of 792 patients. J Clin Gastroenterol. 1996;23:29–34.
4. Edwards FC, Truelove SC. The course and prognosis of ulcerative colitis III. complications. Gut. 1964;5:1–22.
5. Rogers BH, Clark LM, Kirsner JB. The epidemiologic and demographic characteristics of inflammatory bowel disease: an analysis of a computerized file of 1400 patients. J Chronic Dis. 1971;24:743–73.
6. Kraft SC, Earle RH, Roesler M, Esterly JR. Unexplained bronchopulmonary disease with inflammatory bowel disease. Arch Intern Med. 1976;136:454–9.
7. Camus P, Piard F, Ashcroft T, et al. The lung in inflammatory bowel disease. Medicine (Baltimore). 1993;72:151–83.
8. Kappelman MD, Rifas-Shiman SL, Kleinman K, et al. The prevalence and geographic distribution of Crohn's disease and ulcerative colitis in the United States. Clin Gastroenterol Hepatol. 2007;5:1424–9.

9. Greenstein AJ, Janowitz HD, Sachar DB. The extra-intestinal complications of crohn's disease and ulcerative colitis: a study of 700 patients. Medicine. 1976;55:401–12.
10. Mahadeva R, Walsh G, Flower CD, et al. Clinical and radiological characteristics of lung disease in inflammatory bowel disease. Eur Respir J. 2000;15:41–8.
11. Yilmaz A, Yilmaz Demirci N, Hoşgün D, Uner E, Erdoğan Y, Gökçek A, Cağlar A. Pulmonary involvement in inflammatory bowel disease. World J Gastroenterol. 2010;16:4952–7.
12. Desai D, Patil S, Udwadia Z, Maheshwari S, Abraham P, Joshi A. Pulmonary manifestations in inflammatory bowel disease: a prospective study. Indian J Gastroenterol. 2011;30:225–8.
13. Ekbom A, Brandt L, Granath F, Lofdahl CG, Egesten A. Increased risk of both ulcerative colitis and Crohn's disease in a population suffering from COPD. Lung. 2008;186:167–72.
14. Jess T, Frisch M, Simonsen J. Trends in overall and cause-specific mortality among patients with inflammatory bowel disease from 1982 to 2010. Clin Gastroenterol Hepatol. 2013;11:43–8.
15. Duricova D, Pedersen N, Elkjaer M, Gamborg M, Munkholm P, Jess T. Overall and cause specific mortality in Crohn's disease: a meta-analysis of population based studies. Inflamm Bowel Dis. 2010;16:347–53.
16. Winthers KV, Jess T, Langholz E, Munkholm P, Binder V. Survival and cause specific mortality in ulcerative colitis: follow-up of a population-based cohort in Copenhagen county. Gastroenterology. 2003;125:1576–82.
17. Birring SS, Morgan AJ, Prudon B, et al. Respiratory symptoms in patients with treated hypothyroidism and inflammatory bowel disease. Thorax. 2003;58:533–6.
18. Heatley RV, Prokipchuk EJ, Gauldie J, Sieniewicz DJ, Bienenstock J. Pulmonary function abnormalities in patients with inflammatory bowel disease. Q J Med. 1982;203:241–50.
19. Songür N, Songür Y, Tüzün M, Dogan I, Tüzün D, Ensari A, Hekimoglu B. Pulmonary function tests and high-resolution CT in the detection of pulmonary involvement in inflammatory bowel disease. J Clin Gastroenterol. 2003;37:292–8.
20. Munck A, Murciano D, Pariente R, Cezard JP, Navarro J. Latent pulmonary function abnormalities in children with Crohn's disease. Eur Respir J. 1995;8:377–80.
21. Dierkes-Globisch A, Mohr H-H. Pulmonary function abnormalities in respiratory asymptomatic patients with inflammatory bowel disease. Eur J Intern Med. 2002;13:385–8.
22. Mansi A, Cucchiara S, Greco L, Sarnelli P, Pisanti C, Franco MT, Santamaria F. Bronchial hyperresponsiveness in children and adolescents with Crohn's disease. Am J Respir Crit Care Med. 2000;161:1051–4.
23. Wallert B, Colombel JF, Tonnel AB, et al. Evidence of lymphocyte alveolitis in Crohn's disease. Chest. 1985;87:363–7.
24. Bonniere P, Wallaert B, Cortot A, Marchandise X, Riou Y, Tonnel AB, Colombel JF, Voisin C, Paris JC. Latent pulmonary involvement in Crohn's disease: biological, functional, bronchoalveolar lavage and scintigraphic studies. Gut. 1986;27:919–25.
25. Zhang YZ, Li YY. Inflammatory bowel disease: pathogenesis. World J Gastroenterol. 2014;20:91–9.
26. Birrenbach T, Bocker U. Inflammatory bowel disease and smoking: a review of epidemiology, pathophysiology and therapeutic implications. Inflamm Bowel Dis. 2004;10:848–59.
27. Kaplan GG, Hubbard J, Korzenik J, et al. The inflammatory bowel disease and ambient air pollution: a novel association. Am J Gastroenterol. 2010;105:2412–9.
28. Eckburg PB, Bik EM, Bernstein CN, et al. Diversity of human intestinal microbial flora. Science. 2005;308:1635–8.
29. Joossens M, Huys G, Cnockaert M, et al. Dysbiosis of the fecal microbiota in patients with Crohn's disease and their unaffected relatives. Gut. 2011;60:631–7.
30. Eckmann L, Karin M. NOD2 and Crohn's disease: loss or gain of function? Immunity. 2005;22:661–7.
31. Bauer S, Muller T, Hamm S. Pattern recognition by Toll-like receptors. Adv Exp Med Biol. 2009;653:15–34.

32. Ogura Y, Bonen DK, Inohara N, et al. A framshift mutation in NOD2 associated with susceptibility to Crohn's disease. Nature. 2001;411:603–6.
33. Strober W, Kitani A, Fuss I, Asano N, Watanabe T. The molecular basis of NOD2 susceptibility mutations in Crohn's disease. Mucosal Immunol. 2008;1(Suppl 1):S5–9.
34. Beck JM, Young VB, Huffinagle GB. The microbiome of lung. Transl Res. 2012;160: 258–66.
35. Haung YJ, Lynch SV. The emerging relationship between the airway microbiota and chronic respiratory disease: clinical implications. Expert Rev Respir Med. 2011;6:809–21.
36. Molyneaux PL, Cox MJ, Willis-Owens SA, et al. The role of bacteria in pathogenesis and progression of idiopathic pulmonary fibrosis. Am J Respir Crit Care Med. 2014;190:906–13.
37. Brusselle GG, Joos GF, Bracke KR. New insight into the immunology of chronic obstructive pulmonary disease. Lancet. 2011;378:1015–26.
38. Kinose D, Ogawa E, Hirota T, et al. A NOD2 gene polymorphism is associated with the prevalence and severity of chronic obstructive pulmonary disease in a Japanese population. Respirology. 2012;17:164–7.
39. Shaykhiev R, Otaki F, Bonsu P, Dang DT, Teater M, Strulovici-Barel Y, et al. Cigarette smoking reprograms apical junctional complex molecular architecture in the human airway epithelium in vivo. Cell Mol Life Sci. 2011;68:877–92.
40. McGuckin MA, Eri R, Simms LA, Florin TH, Radford-Smith G. Intestinal barrier dysfunction in inflammatory bowel disease. Inflamm Bowel Dis. 2009;15:100–13.
41. Wang H, Liu JS, Peng SH, et al. Gut-lung crosstalk in pulmonary involvement with inflammatory bowel diseases. World J Gastroenterol. 2013;19:6794–804.
42. Shu W, Lu MM, Zhang Y, Tucker PW, Zhou D, Morrisey EE. Foxp2 and Foxp1 cooperatively regulate lung and esophagus development. Development. 2007;134:1991–2000.
43. Ramalho-Santos M, Melton DA, McMahon AP. Hedgehog signals regulate multiple aspects of gastrointestinal development. Development. 2000;127:2763–72.
44. Salmi M, Jalkanen S. Lymphocyte horning to the gut: attraction, adhesion, and commitment. Immunol Rev. 2005;206:100–13.
45. Kelly MG, Frizelle FA, Thornley PT, Beckert L, Epton M, Lynch AC. Inflammatory bowel disease and the lung: is there a link between surgery and bronchiectasis? Int J Colorectal Dis. 2006;21:754–7.
46. Keely S, Talley NJ, Hansbro PM. Pulmonary-intestinal cross-talk in mucosal inflammatory disease. Mucosal Immunol. 2012;5:7–18.
47. Storch I, Sachar D, Katz S. Pulmonary manifestations of inflammatory bowel disease. Inflamm Bowel Dis. 2003;9:104–15.
48. Lu DG, Ji XQ, Liu X, Li HJ, Zhang CQ. Pulmonary manifestations of Crohn's disease. World J Gatroenterol. 2014;20:133–41.
49. Casella G, Villanacci V, Di Bella C, Antonelli E, Baldini V, Bassotti G. Pulmonary diseases associated with inflammatory bowel diseases. J Crohn's Colitis. 2010;4:384–9.
50. Higenbottom T, Cochrane GM, Clark TJ. Bronchial disease in ulcerative colitis. Thorax. 1980;35:581–5.
51. Garg K, Lynch DA, Newell JD. Inflammatory airways disease in ulcerative colitis: CT and high resolution CT features. J Thorac Imaging. 1993;8:159–63.
52. Bernstein CN, Wajda A, Blanchard JF. The clustering of other chronic inflammatory diseases in inflammatory bowel disease: a population-based study. Gastroenterology. 2005;129: 827–36.
53. Raj AA, Birring SS, Green R, Grant A, de Caestecker J, Pavord ID. Prevalence of inflammatory bowel disease in patients with airways disease. Respir Med. 2008;102:780–5.
54. D'Arienzo A, Manguso F, Scarpa R, et al. Ulcerative colitis, seronegative spondyloarthropathies and allergic diseases: the search for a link. Scand J Gastroenterol. 2002;37:1156–63.

55. Louis E, Louis R, Drion V, Bonnet V, Lamproye A, Radermecker M, Belaiche J. Increased frequency of bronchial hyperresponsiveness in patients with inflammatory bowel disease. Allergy. 1995;50:729–33.
56. Bartholo RM, Zaltman C, Elia C, et al. Bronchial hyperresponsiveness and analysis of induced sputum cells in Crohn's disease. Braz J Med Biol Res. 2005;38:197–203.
57. Louis E, Louis R, Shute J, et al. Bronchial eosinophilic infiltration in Crohn's disease in the absence of pulmonary disease. Clin Exp Allergy. 1999;29:660–6.
58. Fireman E, Masarwy F, Groisman G, et al. Induced sputum eosinophilia in ulcerative colitis patients: the lung as a mirror image of intestine? Respir Med. 2009;103:1025–32.
59. Levo Y, Shalit M, Wolner S, Fich A. Serum IgE levels in patients with inflammatory bowel disease. Ann Allergy. 1986;56:85–7.
60. Troncone R, Merrett TG, Ferguson A. Prevalence of atopy is unrelated to presence of inflammatory bowel disease. Clin Allergy. 1988;18:111–7.
61. Ceyhan BB, Karakurt S, Cevik H, Sungur M. Bronchial hyperreactivity and allergic status in inflammatory bowel disease. Respiration. 2003;70:60–6.
62. Peradzyńska J, Krenke K, Lange J, et al. Low prevalence of pulmonary involvement in children with inflammatory bowel disease. Respir Med. 2012;106:1048–54.
63. Persson PG, Bernell O, Leijonmarck CE, Farahmand BY, Hellers G, Ahlbom A. Survival and cause specific mortality in inflammatory bowel disease: a population based cohort study. Gastroenterology. 1996;110:1339–45.
64. Black H, Mendoza M, Murin S. Thoracic manifestations of inflammatory bowel disease. Chest. 2007;131:524–32.
65. Butland RJ, Cole P, Citron KM, et al. Chronic bronchial suppuration and inflammatory bowel disease. Q J Med. 1981;50(197):63–75.
66. Desai SJ, Gephardt GN, Stoller JK. Diffuse panbronchiolitis preceding ulcerative colitis. Chest. 1989;95:1342–4.
67. Kuzniar T, Sleiman C, Brugiere O, et al. Severe tracheobronchial stenosis in a patient with Crohn's disease. Eur Respir J. 2000;15:209–12.
68. Kelley JH, Montgomery WW, Goodman ML, Mulvaney TJ. Upper airway obstruction associated with regional enteritis. Ann Otol. 1979;188:95–9.
69. Ulnick KM, Perkins J. Extraintestinal Crohn's disease: case report and review of literature. Ear Nose Throat J. 2001;80:97–100.
70. Lemann M, Messing B, D'Agay F. Crohn's disease with respiratory tract involvement. Gut. 1987;28:1669–72.
71. Rickli, H, Fretz, C, Hoffman, M, et al. Severe inflammatory upper airway stenosis in ulcerative colitis. Eur Respir J. 1994;7:1899–902.
72. Janssen WJ, Bierig LN, Beuther DA, et al. Stridor in a 47-year-old man with inflammatory bowel disease. Chest. 2006;129:1100–6.
73. Plataki M, Tzortzaki E, Lambiri I, Giannikaki E, Ernst A, Siafakas NM. Severe airway stenosis associated with Crohn's disease: case report. BMC Pulm Med. 2006;6:7.
74. Ahmed KA, Thompson JW, Joyner RE, Stocks RMS. Airway obstruction secondary to tracheobronchial involvement of asymptomatic undiagnosed Crohn's disease in a pediatric patient. Int J Pediatr Otorhinolaryngol. 2006;69:1003–5.
75. Henry MT, Davidson LA, Cooke NJ. Tracheobronchial involvement with Crohn's disease. Eur J Gastroenterol Hepatol. 2001;13:1495–7.
76. Iwama T, Higuchi T, Imajo M, Akagawa S, Matsubara O, Mishima Y. Tracheobronchitis as a complication of Crohn's disease—a case report. Jpn J Surg. 1991;21:454–7.
77. Kirkcaldy J, Lim WS, Jones A, Pointon K. Stridor in Crohn's disease and use of infliximab. Chest. 2006;130:579–81.
78. Lamblin C, Copin MC, Billaut C, et al. Acute respiratory failure due to tracheobronchial involvement in Crohn's disease. Eur Respir J. 1996;9:2176–8.
79. Shad JA, Sharief GQ. Tracheobronchitis as an initial presentation of ulcerative colitis. J Clin Gastroenterol. 2001;33:161–3.

80. Wilcox P, Miller R, Miller G, et al. Airway involvement in ulcerative colitis. Chest. 1987;92:18–22.
81. Kinebuchi SI, Oohashi K, Takada T, et al. Tracheobronchitis associated with Crohn's disease improved on inhaled corticotherapy. Intern Med. 2004;43:829–34.
82. Spira A, Grossman R, Balter M. Large airway disease associated with inflammatory bowel disease. Chest. 1998;113:1723–6.
83. Moles KW, Varghese G, Hayes JR. Pulmonary involvement in ulcerative colitis. Br J Dis Chest. 1988;82:79–83.
84. Gibb WR, Dhillon DP, Zilkha KJ, Cole PJ. Bronchiectasis with ulcerative colitis and myelopathy. Thorax. 1987;42:155–6.
85. Eaton TE, Lambie N, Well AU. Bronchiectasis following colectomy for Crohn's disease. Thorax. 1998;53:529–31.
86. Ward H, Fisher KL, Waghray R, et al. Constrictive bronchiolitis and ulcerative colitis. Can Respir J. 1999;6:197–200.
87. Hilling, GA, Robertson, DA, Chalmers, AH, et al. Unusual pulmonary complication of ulcerative colitis with a rapid response to corticosteroids: case report. Gut. 1994;35:847–8.
88. Veloso FT, Rodrigues H, Aguiar MM. Bronchiolitis obliterans in ulcerative colitis. J Clin Gastroenterol. 1994;1:339–41.
89. Vandenplas O, Casel S, Delos M, et al. Granulomatous bronchiolitis associated with Crohn's disease. Am J Respir Crit Care Med. 1998;158:1676–9.
90. Tzanakis N, Bouros D, Samiou M, Panagou P, Mouzas J, Manousos O, Siafakas N. Lung function in patients with inflammatory bowel disease. Respir Med. 1998;92:516–22.
91. Trow TK, Morris DG, Miller CR, Homer RJ. Granulomatous bronchiolitis of Crohn's disease successfully treated with inhaled budesonide. Thorax. 2009;64:546–7.
92. Mohamed-Hussein AA, Mohamed NA, Ibrahim ME. Changes in pulmonary function in patients with ulcerative colitis. Respir Med. 2007;101:977–82.
93. Herrlinger KR, Noftz MK, Dalhoff K, Ludwig D, Stange EF, Fellermann K. Alterations in pulmonary function in inflammatory bowel disease are frequent and persist during remission. Am J Gastroenterol. 2002;97:377–81.
94. Douglas JG, McDonald CF, Leslie MJ, Gillon J, Crompton GK, McHardy GJ. Respiratory impairment in inflammatory bowel disease: does it vary with disease activity? Respir Med. 1989;83:389–94.
95. Tunc B, Filik L, Bilgic F, Arda K, Ulker A. Pulmonary function tests, high-resolution computed tomography findings and inflammatory bowel disease. Acta Gastroenterol Belg. 2006;69:255–60.
96. Dweik RA, Boggs PB, Erzurum SC, Irvin CG, Leigh MW, Lundberg JO, American Thoracic Society Committee on Interpretation of Exhaled Nitric Oxide Levels (FENO) for Clinical Applications. An official ATS clinical practice guideline: interpretation of exhaled nitric oxide levels (FENO) for clinical applications. Am J Respir Crit Care Med. 2012;184:602–15.
97. Malerba M, Ragnoli B, Buffoli L, et al. Exhaled nitric oxide as a marker of lung involvement in Crohn's disease. Int J Immunopathol Pharmacol. 2011;24:1119–24.
98. Quenon L, Hindryckx P, De Vos M, et al. Hand-held fractional exhaled nitric oxide measurements as a non-invasive indicator of systemic inflammation in Crohn's disease. J Crohns Colitis. 2013;7:644–8.
99. Ozyilmaz E, Yildirim B, Erbas G, et al. Value of fractional exhaled nitric oxide (FENO) for the diagnosis of pulmonary involvement due to inflammatory bowel disease. Inflamm Bowel Dis. 2010;16:670–6.
100. Hoffmann RM, Kruis W. Rare extraintestinal manifestations of inflammatory bowel disease. Inflamm Bowel Dis. 2004;10:140–7.
101. Ulrich R, Goldberg R, Line WS. Crohn's disease: a rare cause of upper airway obstruction. J Emerg Med. 2000;19:331–2.
102. Jouan Y, Venel Y, Lioger B, et al. Tracheal involvement in ulcerative colitis: clinical presentation and potential interest of 2-deoxy-2[F-18]fluoro-D-glucose positron emission tomography (F-18-FDG PET) for the management. Ann Nucl Med. 2012;26:830–4.

103. Asami T, Koyama S, Watanabe Y, et al. Tracheobronchitis in a patient with Crohn's disease. Intern Med. 2009;48:1475–8.
104. Nakamura M, Inoue T, Ishida A, Miyazu YM, Kurimoto N, Miyazawa T. Endobronchial ultrasonography and magnetic resonance imaging in tracheobronchial stenosis from ulcerative colitis. J Bronchology Interv Pulmonol. 2011;18:84–7.
105. Bayraktaroglu S, Basoglu O, Ceylan N, Aydin A, Tuncel S, Savas R. A rare extraintestinal manifestation of ulcerative colitis: tracheobronchitis associated with ulcerative colitis. J Crohn's Colitis. 2010;4:679–82.
106. Camus P, Colby TV. The lung in inflammatory bowel disease. Eur Respir K. 2000;15:5–10.
107. Alrashid AI, Brown RD, Mihalov ML, et al. Crohn's disease involving the lung, resolution with infliximab. Dig Dis Sci. 2001;46:1736–9.

Chapter 4
Airway Involvement in Granulomatosis with Polyangiitis

Sonali Sethi, Nirosshan Thiruchelvam and Kristin B. Highland

Introduction

Wegener's granulomatosis, now referred to as granulomatosis with polyangiitis (GPA), is a multisystem disease characterized by necrotizing vasculitis and granuloma formation that affects primarily the upper and lower respiratory tracts and kidneys. It typically presents as sinusitis, pulmonary infiltrates, and glomerulonephritis [1]. Unlike pulmonary parenchymal involvement, the tracheobronchial disease manifestations are less well recognized by physicians. These extra-parenchymal pulmonary manifestations include involvement of the oral cavity, larynx, and trachea. Airway involvement is found in 15–55 % of patients, and disease activity in the airway poorly correlates with proteinase-3 (PR3) antineutrophil cytoplasm antibody (PR3-ANCA) [2–4]. The evaluation and diagnosis of a patient with suspected tracheobronchial GPA requires a combination of clinical assessment, serologic testing, sinus and chest imaging, pulmonary function tests, bronchoscopy, and tissue biopsy. The diagnosis is established when serologic and histopathologic evidence of vasculitis and granulomatous inflammation is present in a patient with a compatible clinical presentation. For those patients who remain symptomatic despite appropriate medical management, endoscopic management is an option. Early recognition and treatment of airway involvement can prevent untoward effects of improper therapy. In this chapter, we discuss the clinical, radiological, and bronchoscopic findings in patients with central airway involvement with GPA. We also outline the principles of treatment in these challenging patients.

S. Sethi (✉) · K.B. Highland
Respiratory Institute, Cleveland Clinic, 9500 Euclid Avenue, Cleveland, OH 44195, USA
e-mail: sethis@ccf.org

N. Thiruchelvam
Department of Pulmonary Medicine, Respiratory Institute, Cleveland Clinic Foundation, Cleveland, OH, USA

© Springer International Publishing Switzerland 2016
A.C. Mehta et al. (eds.), *Diseases of the Central Airways*,
Respiratory Medicine, DOI 10.1007/978-3-319-29830-6_4

Historical Background

GPA was initially described by Klinger in 1931 as a variant of polyarteritis nodosa, and then in greater detail as a separate entity by Wegener in two different articles in 1936 and 1939 [5–7]. The term Wegener's granulomatosis was then introduced into the English literature by Drs. Godman and Churg in [8]. There has been a subsequent shift from honorific eponyms to disease-descriptive or etiology-based nomenclature by the American College of Rheumatology, the Society of Nephrology, and the European league against Rheumatism, and the term GPA is now preferred as this terminology is based on pathology, rather than historical reference. The change in nomenclature was also catalyzed by the fact that Dr. Friedrich Wegener was a member of the Nazi party before and during World War II [9].

Incidence

The incidence of GPA in the adult population ranges from 3 to 14 cases/million/year, and several studies have indicated a worrisome increase in annual incidence [10–14]. A Swedish study during the period of 1975–2001 showed increasing incidence of GPA among adults, before antineutrophil cytoplasmic antibody (ANCA) testing was introduced [12]. Another population study from Southern Alberta during 1993–2009 demonstrated a steep increase in annual incidence among children from 2.75 cases/million/year to 6.39 cases/million/year over the study period [13]. Likewise, GPA prevalence in Norwich County in the UK doubled during the period 1990–2005 [14]. Whether the increasing GPA incidence reflects new environmental influences, changing classification, or increased awareness is a matter of uncertainty. Keeping the caveat in mind that the time elapsed since introduction of routine ANCA testing is still short, there are some indications that the rising GPA incidence has not leveled off in the post-ANCA era [12, 15, 16]. GPA remains rare in childhood, and peak incidence is in the 65–70-year-old group [11]. There is no gender-specific incidence of GPA [16], but it is more common in Caucasians compared with other races [11].

GPA decreases with decreasing latitude, both north and south of the equator, and is more common in the North of Europe compared with the South [16]. A similar observation was demonstrated in the southern hemisphere within the country of New Zealand [17]. The incidence of the limited form of GPA is 5 % of all GPA, 46 % of whom are ANCA-positive, and typically presents as saddle nose deformity, bony destruction of sinuses, subglottic stenosis, or visual loss due to orbital granuloma [18].

Etiology

GPA is a multisystem disease of unknown etiology, characterized by granulomata of the respiratory tract and a systemic necrotizing vasculitis. It usually starts in the respiratory tract and in the majority of patients progresses to systemic disease with ANCA directed against PR3-ANCA. Current epidemiological evidence indicates that GPA develops as a result of complex gene–environment interactions. The initiating event is a combination of environment (i.e., infectious agents and/or toxins) and individual risk factors, such as genetic background and epigenetic regulation.

Antineutrophil cytoplasmic antibodies are IgG-class autoantibodies directed against molecules located in the granules of neutrophils and the lysosomes of monocytes. Specifically, the target antigens of ANCAs are PR3 and myeloperoxidase (MPO). Positivity for PR3-ANCA or MPO-ANCA is highly specific for ANCA-associated vasculitis (AAV). PR3-ANCAs are more common in GPA, whereas MPO-ANCAs are more common in microscopic polyangiitis [19, 20]. The PR3-ANCA (also called c-ANCA or classic ANCA) has a cytoplasmic staining pattern and is seen in 75–90 % of patients with GPA. Although more common in microscopic polyangiitis, MPO-ANCA is observed in approximately 5–20 % of patients with GPA [21].

The importance of genetic contribution to the pathogenesis of GPA has been identified by many recent studies. An antibody response against PR3 may be a central pathogenic feature of PR3-ANCA-associated vasculitis. A genome-wide association study (GWAS) of 1233 patients with AAV and 5884 control subjects in the UK found both major histocompatibility complex (MHC) and non-MHC associations. This study was then replicated with a cohort of 1454 Northern European AAV patients and 1666 control subjects. Combined analysis of the discovery and replication cohorts showed that four single-nucleotide polymorphisms (SNPs) exceeded the significance threshold for association. Three of these SNPs were associated with the MHC; the most significant association was within the gene encoding HLA-DPB1. The fourth SNP was the *SERPINA1* locus, which previously has been associated with alpha-one antitrypsin deficiency (α_1AT). Alpha-one antitrypsin is a serine protease inhibitor, and PR3 is one of its substrates. Deficiency in the production of the α_1AT has been shown to be substantially overrepresented in patients with GPA [22, 23].

Environmental triggers are also implicated in the pathogenesis of GPA. They are hypothesized to break self-tolerance by molecular mimicry, unveiling of self-epitopes, bystander damage, and/or determinant molecular spreading. The pathogen *Staphylococcus aureus* (*S. aureus*) specifically has been associated with AAV. In GPA, chronic nasal carriage of *S. aureus* is a risk factor for relapse, and prophylactic treatment with co-trimoxazole reduces relapses of GPA by 60 % [24, 25]. High-intensity exposure to silica, propylthiouracil, and levamisole-contaminated cocaine has also been shown to be associated with the onset of AAV [26–28].

The nature of these risk factors and pathogenic mechanisms involved, however, is only just beginning to be understood.

The pathogenic interactions at the molecular level between ANCAs and their target antigens, neutrophils, neutrophil extracellular traps (NETs), T cells, B cells, and vascular endothelial cells are intimately involved in the pathogenesis of GPA. Clinical data and in vitro experimentation suggest that the initiating antigen(s) stimulates antigen-presenting cells to activate T cells. T cells are then stimulated to activate B cells, and downstream these B cells to increase the production of ANCAs by plasma cells. ANCAs bind and activate neutrophils, which then adhere to endothelial cells within small vessels. Each immune cell subsequently releases proinflammatory cytokines in response to activation signals, which leads to additional neutrophil recruitment and activation [25, 29]. Neutrophil activation leads to the release of proteolytic granule enzymes (including PR3 and MPO) and resultant vascular injury [20]. Vessel wall destruction then leads to perivascular hemorrhage and extravasation of macrophages and neutrophils.

Clinical Features

Clinical features of GPA include persistent pneumonitis with bilateral nodular and cavitary infiltrates, chronic sinusitis, mucosal ulcerations of the nasopharynx, renal disease, skin rashes, muscle pains, articular involvement, mononeuritis, or polyneuritis and fever.

With regard to pulmonary manifestations, patients with GPA have either upper airway or pulmonary involvement with the majority of patients having both (Table 4.1). Most patients with active GPA present with nasal crusting (69 %), chronic rhinosinusitis symptoms (61 %), nasal obstruction (58 %), and serosanguinous nasal discharge (52 %) [30]. With regard to the lung parenchyma, the most frequent findings of GPA are pulmonary nodules, ground glass opacities and patches of consolidation, diffuse alveolar hemorrhage, and lung masses with organizing pneumonia [31]. Other abnormalities include airway involvement with subglottic, tracheal, and bronchial stenosis. Subglottic stenosis occurs in an estimated 8.5–23 % of patients with GPA, and GPA accounts for 45 % of patients who present with subglottic stenosis [32, 33]. Patients with GPA are more likely to present with grade 1 subglottic stenosis, and higher grades are seen in non-GPA patients. Clinical features are further outlined in detail in the bronchoscopy section.

Laboratory Investigations

The clinical presentation and exam findings are essential pieces of the puzzle in the diagnosis of GPA. Because of the wide ranges in both disease severity and involvement (i.e., systemic or localized), it is not uncommon for these patients to go

Table 4.1 Pulmonary manifestations of GPA—patients have either upper airway or pulmonary involvement with the majority of patients having both

Upper respiratory tract			
Nasal disease	Sinus disease	Ear disease	Oropharynx
Nasal crusting	Sinus pain	Serous otitis	Gingivitis
Chronic rhinosinusitis	Sinus mucoceles	Hearing loss	Ulceration and hemorrhage
Mucosal ulceration			
Nasal septal perforation			
Saddle nose deformity			
Lower respiratory tract			
Epiglottis	Glottis and larynx	Tracheal disease	Bronchial disease
Ulceration and hemorrhage	Ulceration and hemorrhage	Subglottic stenosis— simple or complex	Bronchial ulceration
Edema	Edema	Tracheal stenosis	Bronchial stenosis
Granuloma	Granuloma	Tracheoesophageal fistulae	Bronchomalacia
	Nodules and masses	Tracheomalacia	Cobblestone mucosa
	Vocal cord involvement	Cartilaginous deformities	Polyps and pseudopolyps
	Stenosis		Submucosal tunnels
			Nodule and masses (pseudotumor)
			Mucosal edema and erythema

undiagnosed or be misdiagnosed at the time of initial presentation. It is important that the patients' presentation, history, and physical exam findings are recognized and correctly correlated in order to proceed with a workup that will yield the correct diagnosis.

The differential diagnosis of GPA is broad and includes eosinophilic granulomatosis with polyangiitis (EGPA) also known as Churg–Strauss Syndrome, microscopic polyangiitis (MPA), sarcoidosis, rheumatoid arthritis, and infection (fungal and mycobacterial).

According to the Chapel Hill Consensus Conference (CHCC), GPA, MPA, and EGPA were distinguished from other systemic small vessels vasculitis by the absence of immune deposits. In clinical practice, patients are classified as having GPA if they have destruction in their upper respiratory tract and/or nodules and cavities in the lower respiratory tract, and/or have granulomatosis on biopsy of any organ. Thus, patients who have nasal disease and necrotizing vasculitis on biopsy, but no evidence of granulomatosis, would be classified as having MPA [34]. While the specificity of c-ANCA has been reported to be as high as 98 %, the sensitivity of c-ANCA varies with disease activity: 90 % (active systemic), 80 % (localized), and 30 % (remission) [35]. Although PR3-ANCA antibodies are highly suggestive of GPA, their presence is not sufficient for a definitive diagnosis. It has been reported that MPO-ANCA is the primary antibody present in approximately 5–20 % of patients with GPA, and there are some cases of GPA in which no ANCA antibodies are present [36, 37]. Because serum concentrations of ANCA are only weakly associated with disease activity, it is not recommended that ANCA is used as a biomarker of disease activity [35].

The gold standard for the diagnosis of GPA remains a tissue biopsy of diseased tissue showing a triad of vasculitis, necrosis, and granulomatous inflammation. Histologically, the classic description is that of a necrotizing vasculitis with granulomatous inflammation consisting of multinucleated giant cells and palisading histiocytes. Tissue biopsy is usually obtained from the skin or kidney. If the pulmonary system is involved, lung biopsies are the most reliable for histological diagnosis. Nasal biopsies are associated with more false-negative results than either lung or renal biopsy due to the small amount of tissue that can be removed. Lung biopsy most often requires open or thoracoscopic lung biopsy. In a small number of cases (<10 %), sufficient tissue for diagnosis can be obtained by transbronchial biopsy. A positive lung biopsy precludes the need for a kidney biopsy in many cases; a renal biopsy may be indicated in patients who are diagnosed by lung biopsy and have severe or rapid worsening of renal dysfunction since the presence of active vasculitis in the kidney should be confirmed by histology [36, 37].

All specimens or biopsies taken should also be cultured to rule out infectious causes of granulomatous inflammation (e.g. fungal, TB). All patients who are suspected of having GPA should have a urinalysis obtained to assess for renal involvement, including microscopic analysis of urinary sediment in order to determine the presence of hematuria and proteinuria. Other tests that may be appropriate in the workup for GPA include the following: antinuclear antibody (ANA), complement levels (C3 and C4), cryoglobulins, hepatitis serology, human immunodeficiency virus (HIV) screening, liver functions tests, sinus films, basic metabolic panel, erythrocyte sedimentation rate (ESR), C-reactive protein (CRP), autoimmune panel, and a venereal disease research laboratory test (VDRL) or rapid plasma regain test (RPR) to screen for syphilis and blood cultures. Cultures for *S. aureus* should also be obtained, because in GPA, its chronic nasal carriage is a potential risk factor for relapse [24].

Imaging

A majority of patients with GPA will have an abnormal chest radiograph which reveals cavitary nodules, lobar or segmental atelectasis, patchy or diffuse infiltrates or pleural opacities, and/or lymphadenopathy. The most commonly reported chest radiograph findings are nodules which may be single or multiple and range in diameter [38]. Because chest radiographs are non-specific, computed tomography (CT) scan is the preferred imaging modality for evaluating patients with GPA. Sinus CT scans disclose mucosal thickening in the nasal cavity and paranasal sinuses in 61 and 75 %, respectively. Other findings include bony destruction of the paranasal sinuses (54 %), bony destruction of the nasal cavity (57 %), bony thickening of the paranasal sinuses (18 %), and subtotal sinus opacification (25 %) [39].

Chest CT may disclose lesions not seen on chest radiograph in 43–63 % of the patients and is usually performed without contrast because of underlying renal insufficiency. Common CT findings (Figs. 4.1, 4.2, and 4.3) include multiple pulmonary nodules (58 %) and patchy or diffuse ground glass or consolidative opacities (67 %). Pulmonary nodules tend to be bronchocentric or subpleural and peripheral. They are generally less than 10 in number and range in size from a few millimeters to 10 cm. Approximately 20–50 % of nodules are cavitary.

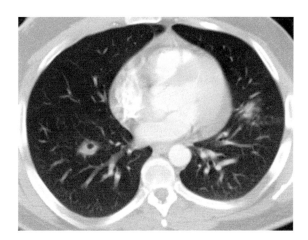

Fig. 4.1 CT imaging with cavitary nodules commonly seen in GPA

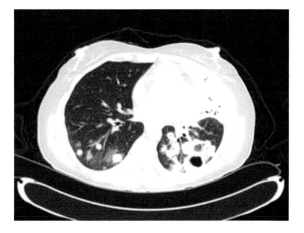

Fig. 4.2 CT image showing multiple pulmonary nodules of different sizes in a patient with GPA

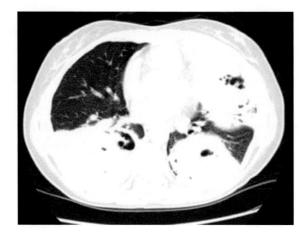

Fig. 4.3 Multiple large cavitary GPA masses may reach up to 10 cm in size

Consolidation and ground glass opacities can present as peribronchial consolidation, focal consolidations with or without cavitation, parenchymal bands, peripheral consolidation areas mimicking pulmonary infarctions, and diffuse and bilateral ground glass opacity areas corresponding to alveolar hemorrhage [40] (Fig. 4.4). Chest CT imaging can also have other findings that may suggest the diagnosis of vasculitis, including feeding vessels leading to nodules and cavities, wedge-shaped lesions suggestive of pulmonary microinfarction, or unsuspected tracheal or bronchial stenosis. Less often, CT imaging may reveal pleural disease (5–20 %) and mediastinal lymphadenopathy [41].

Although airway involvement occurs in approximately 50 % of patients with GPA, these findings are less frequently appreciated radiographically. Large airway

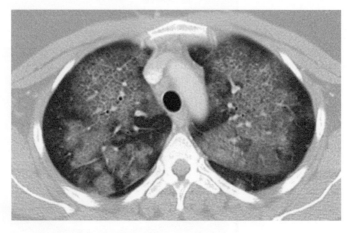

Fig. 4.4 CT image with bilateral ground glass opacities corresponding to alveolar hemorrhage in GPA

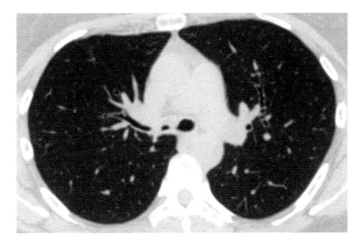

Fig. 4.5 CT image showing right main-stem bronchial stenosis. Fifty percentage of patients with GPA have airway involvement which can be seen radiographically

involvement may consist of focal or elongated segments of stenosis (Fig. 4.5). Other findings include calcifications and thickening of the tracheal rings [42]. Bronchial abnormalities, including bronchiectasis and peribronchial thickening of the small airways, have been reported in 40 % of cases and are best visualized with high-resolution CT scanning [43].

Creating two- and three-dimensional reconstructions from CT imaging may further assist in defining the degree and extent of stenosis by providing thin-section, high-spatial resolution images of the airway (Fig. 4.6). Magnetic resonance imaging

Fig. 4.6 Two- and three-dimensional reconstructions from CT imaging may assist in further defining the degree and extent of stenosis. Notice right main-stem and right upper lobe bronchial stenosis

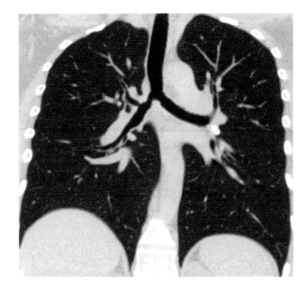

(MRI) of the trachea has also been used in assessing the degree of airway involvement in GPA. MRI of the upper airways may demonstrate diffuse thickening of tracheobronchial submucosal tissues and luminal narrowing.

Pulmonary Function Tests

Pulmonary function testing is an integral part of a comprehensive approach to the diagnosis and management of GPA. However, pulmonary function and flow-volume tracings are not uniformly abnormal in all patients with GPA, and their severity depends on the extent of compromise of the airway lumen. The most frequent abnormality seen is airflow obstruction with reduced lung volumes and diffusing capacity for carbon monoxide (DLCO). The DLCO may be markedly increased in the presence of active alveolar hemorrhage. Narrowing or stenosis of tracheal or bronchial airways typically reveals flattening of the inspiratory and expiratory flow-volume tracings. Lung functions frequently improve following treatment, although the DLCO may not return to normal. Patients who receive treatment or have had interventional procedures should have flow-volume tracings obtained both before and after treatment.

Bronchoscopy

Tracheobronchial manifestations of GPA may appear for the first time after remission has been achieved with appropriate immunosuppressive therapy, and it does not necessarily indicate failure of therapy. Therefore, bronchoscopy with visualization of the airways remains the major diagnostic procedure in the evaluation, diagnosis, and management of airway disease in GPA. It is the most important diagnostic procedure in the assessment of location and degree of airway involvement below the vocal cords and is a therapeutic tool to restore the functional airway patency.

Bronchoscopy is also used for diagnostic tissue sampling. Endobronchial bronchoscopic biopsy can confirm inflammation in 50 % of cases, revealing either vasculitis, necrosis, microabscesses, or giant cells [2]. Therefore, if suspicious mucosal abnormalities are detected, adequate tissue samples should be obtained for histologic documentation. However, non-diagnostic bronchoscopic biopsies are not unusual even when obtained from abnormal appearing areas.

Subglottic Stenosis

The subglottic region is particularly susceptible to narrowing secondary to laryngopharyngeal reflux, limited blood supply, and turbulent airflow. Subglottic stenosis occurs in 8.5–23 % of GPA patients and occurs independently of systemic GPA activity. It is the most frequent airway manifestation of GPA and may be the initial presenting feature in 1–6 % of patients [44]. Subglottic inflammation is a common feature at the time of active disease. At the time of bronchoscopy, erythematous, edematous, and friable mucosa and ulcerations may be seen with lesions typically being circumferential (Fig. 4.7). The vocal cords may or may not be involved (Fig. 4.8). With or without the treatment, fibrotic scarring may occur during the resolution of inflammation; however, early treatment may limit the degree of scar severity and airway lumen compromise. Isolated subglottic stenosis (Fig. 4.9) is observed in approximately 50 % of patients with strictures. Patients present with cough, dyspnea, and stridor. Stridor is usually a sign of severe laryngeal or tracheal obstruction, signaling more than 70 % airway lumen narrowing [45]. For those patients who remain symptomatic despite appropriate medical management, endoscopic management is an option with topical

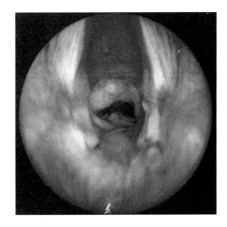

Fig. 4.7 Bronchoscopic image showing subglottic inflammation. Subglottic inflammation is a common feature at the time of active disease

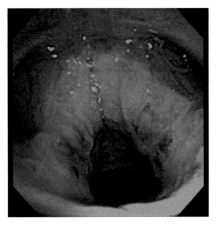

Fig. 4.8 Bronchoscopic image showing vocal cord involvement in GPA

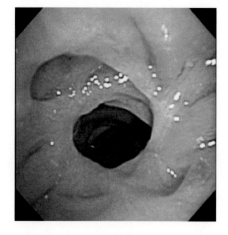

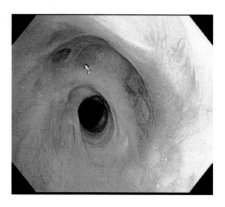

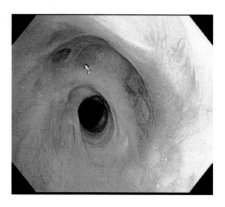

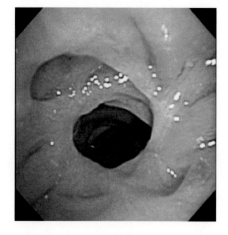

Fig. 4.9 Bronchoscopic image showing subglottic stenosis due to GPA. Fibrotic scarring during resolution of inflammation leads to subglottic stenosis. Isolated subglottic stenosis is observed in approximately 50 % of patients with strictures due to GPA

corticosteroids, laser incisions or resection, serial dilatations, and local mitomycin-C application. Patients often require multiple mechanical dilations and other therapy to restore airway patency. Overall, 10-year survival is 75 %.

Web Stenosis (Tracheobronchial Stenosis)

Similar inflammatory processes that occur in the subglottic region can occur at any level in the tracheobronchial tree. Web stenosis results from scarring secondary to acute inflammation and is usually unresponsive to immunosuppression (Figure 4.10). These stenotic regions can be simple and localized or complex with luminal distortion. Most of the web stenoses are eccentric or circumferential, and the mucosa in the stenotic segment is thickened. In active disease, the stenotic area may exhibit erythematous and edematous mucosa with the formation of ulceration and pseudomembranes. Bronchial inflammation and stenosis are less frequent than subglottic disease and is almost always associated with disease activity elsewhere. Isolated bronchial stenosis however has been described.

Fig. 4.10 Bronchoscopic image showing tracheal cicatricial stenosis, which results from scarring secondary to acute inflammation and is usually unresponsive to immunosuppression. These stenotic regions can be simple and localized or complex with luminal distortion

Mucosal Abnormalities

Mucosal abnormalities can be seen anywhere in the tracheobronchial tree. They may either be isolated lesions or are patchy in distribution. The most common mucosal abnormalities include inflammation with edema or erythema (Fig. 4.11), thickening, granularity or cobblestone changes of the mucosal surface (Fig. 4.12), shallow mucosal ulcers (Figs. 4.13 and 4.14), mucosal plaques (Fig. 4.15), hypertrophic tissue (Fig. 4.16), diverticula, and the formation of submucosal tunnels in the trachea and main-stem bronchi (Fig. 4.17). While cobblestoning is a marker for active inflammation, submucosal bridges result from excessive mucosal pseudomembrane formation which incorporates into the normal mucosa by epithelization. There may also be crusting secondary to purulent secretions and excessive mucous production (Fig. 4.18).

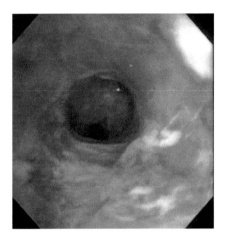

Fig. 4.11 Bronchoscopic image showing mucosal surface inflammation with erythema and friable mucosa in GPA

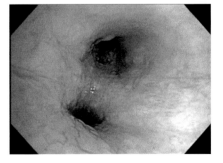

Fig. 4.12 Bronchoscopic image showing mucosal surface inflammation with cobblestone changes. Cobblestoning is a marker for active inflammation

Fig. 4.13 Bronchoscopic
image showing shallow
superficial mucosal ulcer in
GPA

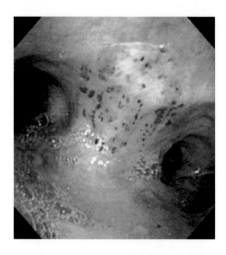

Fig. 4.14 Another
bronchoscopic image
showing mucosal ulceration
in a patient with GPA.
Ulcerations may be secondary
to GPA or to a superimposed
infection. All such ulcers
should be biopsied

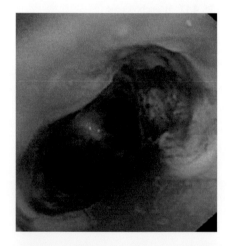

Fig. 4.15 Bronchoscopic
image of a mucosal plaque in
GPA

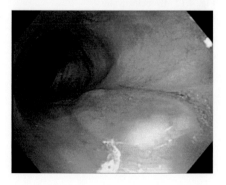

Fig. 4.16 Bronchoscopic image of mucosal abnormalities secondary to inflammation with hypertrophic tissue in GPA

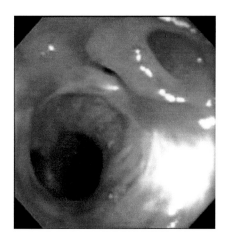

Fig. 4.17 Bronchoscopic image showing submucosal bridges resulting from mucosal pseudomembrane formation which incorporates into the normal mucosa by epithelization

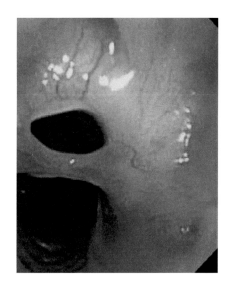

Fig. 4.18 Tracheal crusting secondary to purulent secretions and excessive mucous production in a patient with GPA

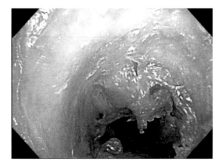

Masses and Polyps

Tracheal or bronchial mass lesions or inflammatory pseudotumors may develop in either the trachea or bronchi. These lesions mimic malignancy and therefore should be biopsied to establish GPA as the etiology. Of note, these lesions may ulcerate and cause hemoptysis [46]. Inflammatory pseudotumors may either present at the time of initial diagnosis of GPA or at the time of relapse and are generally a reflection of active disease.

Other Airway Abnormalities

GPA occasionally leads to tracheomalacia or bronchomalacia. Other airway abnormalities include acquired tracheoesophageal fistula, right middle lobe syndrome, and destruction of cartilage (Fig. 4.19).

Pathology

The gold standard for the diagnosis of GPA remains a tissue biopsy of diseased tissue showing a triad of vasculitis, necrosis, and granulomatous inflammation. Tissue biopsy is usually obtained from the skin or kidney; however, if the pulmonary system is involved, lung biopsies are reliable for a histological diagnosis.

Bronchoscopic tissue sampling of tracheobronchial luminal abnormalities reveals typical histologic features of GPA only in the minority of cases. However, endobronchial biopsies are useful for excluding other diseases such as endobronchial malignancy or sarcoidosis. Endobronchial biopsies typically reveal

Fig. 4.19 Acquired bronchomalacia of the bronchus intermedius secondary to the destruction of cartilage in GPA

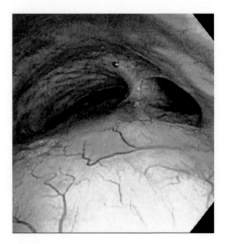

granulation tissue or non-specific inflammation including vasculitis, necrosis, microabscesses, or giant cells. Biopsy specimens from the subglottic region generally demonstrate only fibrosis and inflammation without the evidence of vasculitis.

The main indication for lung biopsy is the evaluation of single or multiple pulmonary nodules. Generally, transbronchial biopsies are too small for making a definitive diagnosis of GPA, and sufficient tissue for diagnosis is only obtained in 10 % of cases. Therefore, the gold standard continues to be a surgical lung biopsy. Microscopically, transmural infiltration of blood vessels with inflammatory cells is noted, associated with granulomatous inflammation in the surrounding tissue. Necrosis of the vessel walls and/or necrosis of inflammatory cells within the vessel walls may be visible [47].

The granulomatous inflammation of GPA is characterized by palisading histiocytes that are oriented with their long axis perpendicular to the necrotic center [48]. Non-caseating granulomas may be present, but are not prominent. In general, the inflammatory changes associated with GPA are angiocentric, although a rare bronchocentric variant has been described [38]. The infiltrating inflammatory cells include neutrophils, lymphocytes, multinucleated giant cells, and eosinophils, but eosinophils are generally not abundant. Special stains and cultures should be considered to exclude the presence of infections that can produce granulomas, vasculitis, or necrosis.

Bronchoalveolar lavage should be performed in patients with diffuse parenchymal opacities on chest imaging to identify alveolar hemorrhage and to obtain samples for microbiologic and cytologic analysis. Hemosiderin-laden macrophages are often identified on Prussian blue staining of cells from the BAL fluid.

Because inflammatory lesions secondary to infection often mimic GPA, endobronchial biopsies should be performed in all cases to rule out concomitant infection such a cryptococcus or mycobacteria.

Treatment/Prognosis

The goals of treatment in GPA are to improve survival and quality of life while preventing organ failure. This is done through the induction of remission followed by maintenance therapy and often requires a collaborative effort coordinated by a rheumatologist. Untreated GPA is rapidly fatal with median survival of less than 5 months [49]. Predictors of relapse include female gender, African American ethnicity, presentation with severe kidney disease, upper respiratory or pulmonary involvement, and persistent serologic positivity [50–52].

With glucocorticoids alone, death occurs within 1 year from either infection and/or uncontrolled disease [53, 54]. The first successful treatment regimen involved induction with a combination of oral cyclophosphamide and glucocorticoids [1, 55]. Provided that leukopenia was avoided, this regimen resulted in 91 %

improvement, 75 % remission, 80 % survival, and only 50 % relapse. Unfortunately, 42 % of patients develop drug toxicity [56]. Monthly pulse cyclophosphamide has been shown to have similar efficacy in regard to survival, induction of remission and relapse rate with less risk of infection, leukopenia, and bladder toxicity [57]. Methotrexate has also been shown to be similar to cyclophosphamide at six months in inducing remission in patients with mild disease. However, the patients on methotrexate took longer to achieve remission and had a higher relapse rate, although less drug toxicity [58]. Most recently, rituximab was found to be non-inferior to cyclophosphamide followed by azathioprine for complete remission at 6, 12, and 18 months with a more favorable safety profile [59].

Azathioprine and methotrexate have been used for maintenance therapy allowing for limited exposure to cyclophosphamide although despite maintenance therapy, relapse can occur in as many as 15 % of patients [60, 61]. Leflunomide recently was shown to be somewhat more efficacious than methotrexate for maintenance of remission [62]. Maintenance studies for rituximab are ongoing.

Finally, in a study of patients who had achieved remission, there was 82 % relapse rate in patients randomized to placebo versus 60 % relapse rate in patients randomized to trimethoprim–sulfamethoxazole. Occurrence of upper airway disease was reduced, although there was no difference in major organ relapses [24]. Prophylaxis with trimethoprim–sulfamethoxazole is also key in preventing pneumocystis pneumonia, a common complication of immunosuppressive therapy used to treat GPA.

Bronchoscopic Treatment

Fibrotic scarring stenosis found in GPA does not generally respond to immunosuppressive therapy, and therefore, bronchoscopic treatment is a good alternative. Options for the treatment of stenosis include intralesional injection of corticosteroids, laser or electrosurgical incisions or resection, serial dilations, balloon dilation, and local mitomycin-C application. Patients often require multiple mechanical dilations and other therapy to restore airway patency. Therefore, when endoscopically managing benign disease in the airway, it is important to be cognizant of a therapeutic plan that requires a combination of modalities and the potential need for future therapies. Morphologically, weblike stenosis can be managed by repeated endoscopic dilation; however, complex stenosis may be best treated by stent implantation or surgery in experienced hands with close follow-up required. One should keep in mind that these therapies should be limited so not to perpetuate further inflammation and should therefore only be performed by experienced physicians.

Instrumentation

The basic instrumentation has not changed significantly over time with the continued use of rigid laryngoscopes and bronchoscopes with dilators, and flexible fiberoptic bronchoscopes. The rigid bronchoscope is a stainless-steel tube that ranges in diameter from 8 cm to 14 mm and in length from 27 to 40 cm. It allows for the simultaneous delivery of oxygen and anesthetic agents, as well as the passage of large instruments, while maintaining a generous view of the trachea. The distal end of the rigid bronchoscope is beveled and can be used as a coring device allowing for blunt dilation of stenotic areas and stenting open of the airway during the procedure. In addition, it allows for a series of various sized dilators to pass through a larger size rigid scope. It may allow for gentle dilation of the stricture without damage to normal mucosa.

Intraluminal Steroids

Intralesional corticosteroid injections have potentially shown benefit in GPA, and their use may reduce the need for systemic therapy. Methylprednisolone acetate dosed at 40 mg/ml may be injected directly into multiple areas of the stenotic segments or areas of inflammation just underneath the mucosa using a 25-g sclerotherapy injection needle (Fig. 4.20).

Balloon Dilation

Focal circumferential strictures are endoscopically best managed by balloon dilation of the airway. Balloonplasty of the stenotic airway is safe, rapid, and effective. Balloon dilation is particularly effective when the fibrotic stenosis is not accompanied by cartilage destruction. Airway balloons may be inserted through the working channel of the flexible bronchoscope or through a rigid bronchoscope. The stricture should be seated in the middle of the expanding balloon, and as the balloon expands, the energy is transmitted to the area of least resistance. The balloon should

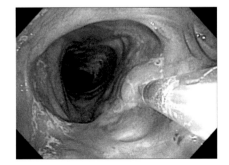

Fig. 4.20 Corticosteroid injections with methylprednisolone acetate dosed at 40 mg/ml being injected in areas of inflammation just underneath the mucosa using a 25-g sclerotherapy injection needle

Fig. 4.21 Circumferential
strictures are endoscopically
managed with balloonplasty.
The stricture should be seated
in the middle of the
expanding balloon

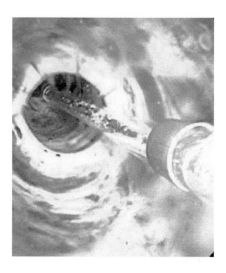

be inflated in increments with frequent deflation to observe progress and potential
airway injury [63] (Fig. 4.21). Apnea is required during the periods of balloon
inflation, and some desaturation may occur, limiting the inflation time. Potential
complications include perforation, wall injury or rupture, bleeding, pneumothorax,
bronchospasm, mediastinitis, chest pain, and recurrent stenosis.

Laser

Endoscopic laser techniques rely on laser–tissue interactions based on biologic,
chemical, or thermal reactions. They have sufficient power to vaporize tissue and
produce an excellent coagulation effect. Knowledge of tissue effects in specific
settings is important since inappropriate laser settings or resection techniques can
enhance laser-related adverse effects and alter local anatomy. Factors found to be
associated with poor results or failure include circumferential strictures longer than
1 cm in vertical dimension, tracheomalacia, posterior laryngeal inlet scarring with
arytenoids fixation, and a previous history of severe bacterial infection associated
with tracheostomy [64]. It should be recognized that some experts believe that
tissue damage and coagulation necrosis caused by laser therapy promotes fibrosis,
scarring, and granulation tissue which consequently leads to restenosis.

CO_2 *laser*: Based on laser–tissue interactions, the CO_2 laser is the preferred laser
for treating benign stenosis. There is no scatter and no deep penetration; therefore,
the risk for collateral mucosal damage or airway perforation is lower. The CO_2 laser
is used in the ultrapulse mode with a fluence of 150 mJ/cm^2 at a frequency of 10 Hz
to avoid heat diffusion into surrounding tissues and charring [65]. It is an excellent
cutting tool with an almost scalpel-like precision.

KTP laser: Compared with the CO_2 laser, KTP laser tissue penetration is significantly deeper and caution must be taken to avoid airway perforation.

Nd:YAG laser: This laser is best used in conjunction with dilation to release the tension of the stricture by performing radial incision in the stenotic tissues. Nd: YAG has greater depth of penetration compared to CO_2 and, hence, should at all times be directed parallel to the tracheal wall, skimming the surface of the target tissue to avoid damage to the underlying cartilage rings. There are experts, including our group who believe that this should not be used as treatment since it could cause more scarring and complicate further options for open surgical interventions [66].

Electrosurgery Knife/Blade

In an attempt to reduce local injury caused by laser therapy, an electrosurgery knife can be used in the endoscopic management of weblike benign airway stenosis [67]. It works by contact and can easily cut through the tracheal or bronchial wall and cartilage with radial incisions. Macroscopically, a clean cut is observed in the tissue. The use of an electrosurgery knife instead of laser results in several advantages; cost of equipment for electrosurgery is cheaper; it offers more precise and limited tissue vaporization.

Mitomycin

Mitomycin is an antibiotic that was isolated from the bacteria Streptomyces caespitosus in 1956. Its C-form is an alkylating agent that inhibits deoxyribonucleic acid synthesis. It was first used as an anticancer drug. It has been used to reduce scarring in the treatment of benign airway stenosis. There are a number of studies that show mitomycin-C's inhibitory effects in modulating the mediators and proteins involved in scar formation, reducing fibroblast density, reducing wound contracture and fibrosis, and improving airway patency [68]. It is usually placed on a cottonoid pledget typically with a concentration of 0.4 mg/ml and topically applied to the area of scar. The length of application varies from two to three repeat applications of two minutes each. The use and dose of mitomycin-C are debated with multiple studies having both positive and negative outcomes. Although the contribution of its activity is difficult to quantify in the success of treatment of stenosis, no side effects have been identified.

Summary

GPA is characterized by granulomatous inflammation and necrotizing vasculitis, affecting mainly small arteries, arterioles, capillaries, and venules of the upper and lower respiratory tract and kidneys. The involvement of the airways is one of the major characteristics of GPA and occurs in 15–55 % of patients. Airway involvement can be part of a multisystem disease, an isolated presentation, or a chronic complication of progressive disease or disease in remission. Symptoms include cough, stridor, wheezing, hemoptysis, and dyspnea. GPA can cause alterations in any segment of the airway including inflammation, ulceration, tracheobronchomalacia, formation of pseudomembranes, mucosal tunneling, endobronchial masses, and simple or complex airway stenosis. Therapeutic options for airway involvement caused by GPA include pharmacologic, bronchoscopic interventions, and surgery.

References

1. Fauci AS, Haynes BF, et al. Wegener's granulomatosis: prospective clinical and therapeutic experience with 85 patients for 21 years. Ann Intern Med. 1983;98:76–85.
2. Daum TE, Specks U, et al. Tracheobronchial involvement in Wegener's granulomatosis. Am J Respir Crit Care Med. 1995;151:522–6.
3. Gluth MB, Shinners PA, Kasperbauer JL. Subglottic stenosis associated with Wegener's granulomatosis. Laryngoscope. 2003;113(8):1304–7.
4. Cordier JF, Valeyre D, et al. Pulmonary Wegener's granulomatosis: a clinical and imaging study of 77 cases. Chest. 1990;97(4):906–12.
5. Klinger H. Grenzformen der Periarteriitis Nodosa. Frankf Z Pathol. 1931;42:455–80.
6. Wegener F. Ueber generalisierte septische Gefasserkrankungen. Verh Deut Pathol Ges. 1936;29:202–10.
7. Wegener F. Ueber eine eigenartige rhinogene Granulomatose mit besonderer Beteiligung des Arteriensystems und der Nieren. Beitr Pathol Anat. 1939;102:30–68.
8. Godman GC, Churg J. Wegener's granulomatosis: pathology and review of the literature. Arch Pathol. 1954;58:533–53.
9. Falk RJ, Jennette JC. ANCA disease: where is this field going? J Am Soc Nephrol. 2010;21 (745):52.
10. Watts RA, Scott DG, Lane SE. Epidemiology of Wegener's granulomatosis, microscopic polyangiitis, and Churg-Strauss syndrome. Cleve Clin J Med. 2002;69 Suppl 2:SII84–6.
11. Lane SE, Watts R, Scott DG. Epidemiology of systemic vasculitis. Curr Rheumatol Rep. 2005;7(4):270–5.
12. Knight A, Ekbom A, Brandt L, et al. Increasing incidence of Wegener's granulomatosis in Sweden, 1975–2001. J Rheumatol. 2006;33(10):2060–3.
13. Grisaru S, Yuen GW, Miettunen PM, et al. Incidence of Wegener's granulomatosis in children. J Rheumatol. 2010;37(2):440–2.
14. Watts RA, Al-Taiar A, Scott DG, et al. Prevalence and incidence of Wegener's granulomatosis in the UK general practice research database. Arthritis Rheum. 2009;61(10):1412–6.
15. Koldingsnes W, Nossent H. Epidemiology of Wegener's granulomatosis in northern Norway. Arthritis Rheum. 2000;43(11):2481–7.
16. Gibelin A, Maldini C, Mahr A. Epidemiology and etiology of Wegener granulomatosis, microscopic polyangiitis, churg-strauss syndrome and goodpasture syndrome: vasculitides with frequent lung involvement. Semin Respir Crit Care Med. 2011;32(3):264–73.
17. O'Donnell JL, Stevanovic VR, Frampton C, et al. Wegener's granulomatosis in New Zealand: evidence for a latitude-dependent incidence gradient. Intern Med J. 2007;37(4):242–6.
18. Holle JU, Gross WL, Holl-Ulrich K, et al. Prospective long-term follow-up of patients with localised Wegener's granulomatosis: does it occur as persistent disease stage? Ann Rheum Dis. 2010;69(11):1934–39.

19. Csernok E, Moosig F, Gross WL. Pathways to ANCA production: from differentiation of dendritic cells by proteinase 3 to B lymphocyte maturation in Wegener's granuloma. Clin Rev Allergy Immunol. 2008;34:300–6.
20. Gómez-Puerta JA, Bosch X. Anti-neutrophil cytoplasmic antibody pathogenesis in small-vessel vasculitis. Am J Pathol. 2009;175(5):1790–8.
21. Langford C. Vasculitis. J Allergy Clin Immunol. 2010;125(2):S216–25.
22. Lyons PA, Rayner TF, Trivedi S, et al. Genetically distinct subsets within ANCA-associated vasculitis. N Engl J Med. 2012;367(3):214–23.
23. Mahr AD, Edberg JC, Stone JH et al., for the Wegener's Granulomatosis Genetic Respiratory Research Group. Alpha$_1$-antitrypsin deficiency—related alleles Z and S and the risk of Wegener's granulomatosis. Arthritis Rheum. 2010;62(12):3760–67.
24. Stegeman CA, Tervaert JW, Sluiter WJ. Association of chronic nasal carriage of Staphylococcus aureus and higher relapse rates in Wegener granulomatosis. Ann Intern Med. 1994;120(1):12–7.
25. Kallenberg CGM. Pathogenesis of PR3-ANCA associated vasculitis. J Autoimmun. 2008;30:29–36.
26. Hogan SL, Cooper GS, Savitz DA, et al. Association of silica exposure with anti-neutrophil cytoplasmic autoantibody small-vessel vasculitis: a population-based, case-control study. Clin J Am Soc Nephrol. 2007;2(2):290–9.
27. Zhang AH, Chen M, Gao Y, Zhao MH, Wang HY. Inhibition of oxidation activity of myeloperoxidase (MPO) by propylthiouracil (PTU) and anti-MPO antibodies from patients with PTU-induced vasculitis. Clin Immunol. 2007;122(2):187–93.
28. Gross RL, Brucker J, Bache-Altuntas A, et al. A novel cutaneous vasculitis syndrome induced by levamisole-contaminated cocaine. Clin Rheumatol. 2011;30(10):1385–92.
29. Flint J, Morgan MD, Savage CO. Pathogenesis of ANCA-associated vasculitis. Rheum Dis Clin North Am. 2010;36(3):463–77.
30. Hseu AF, Benninger MS, Haffey TM, et al. Subglottic stenosis: a ten-year review of treatment outcomes. Laryngoscope. 2014;124(3):736–41.
31. Gómez-Gómez A, Martínez-Martínez MU, Cuevas-Orta E et al. Pulmonary manifestations of granulomatosis with polyangiitis. Reumatol Clin. 2014;10(5):288–93.
32. Lebovics RS, Hoffman GS, Leavitt RY, et al. The management of subglottic stenosis in patients with Wegener's granulomatosis. Laryngoscope. 1992;102(12 Pt 1):1341–5.
33. Cannady SB, Batra PS, Koening C, et al. Sinonasal Wegener granulomatosis: a single institution experience with 120 cases. Laryngoscope. 2009;119:757–61.
34. Jennette JC, Falk RJ, Andrassy K, et al. Nomenclature of systemic vasculitides. Proposal of an international consensus conference. Arthritis Rheum. 1994;37:187.
35. Finkielman JD, Lee AS, Hummel AM, et al. ANCA are detectable in nearly all patients with active severe Wegener's granulomatosis. Am J Med. 2007;120(643):e9.
36. Falk RJ, Jennette JC. ANCA small-vessel vasculitis. J Am Soc Nephrol. 1997;8:314.
37. Hagen EC, Daha MR, Hermans J, et al. Diagnostic value of standardized assays for anti-neutrophil cytoplasmic antibodies in idiopathic systemic vasculitis. EC/BCR project for ANCA assay standardization. Kidney Int. 1998;53:753.
38. Katzenstein AL, Locke WK. Solitary lung lesions in Wegener's granulomatosis. Pathologic findings and clinical significance in 25 cases. Am J Surg Pathol. 1995;19:545.
39. Lohrmann C, Uhl M, Warnatz K, et al. Sinonasal computed tomography in patients with Wegener's granulomatosis. J Comput Assist Tomogr. 2006;30:122.
40. Cordier JF, Valeyre D, Guillevin L, et al. Pulmonary Wegener's granulomatosis. A clinical and imaging study of 77 cases. Chest. 1990;97:906.
41. Hoffman GS, Kerr GS, Leavitt RY, et al. Wegener granulomatosis: an analysis of 158 patients. Ann Int Med. 1992;116(6):488–98.
42. Sheehan RE, Flint JD, Muller NL. Computed tomography features of the thoracic manifestations of Wegener granulomatosis. J Thorac Imaging. 2003;18(1):34–41.
43. Papiris SA, Manoussakis MN, Drosos AA, et al. Imaging of thoracic Wegener's granulomatosis: the computed tomographic appearance. Am J Med. 1992;93(5):529–36.

44. Hernandez-Rodriguez J, Hoffman GS, Koening CL. Surical interventionas and local therpay for Wegener's granulomatosis. Curr Opin Rheumatol. 2010;22:29–36.
45. Murgu S, Colt HG. Morphometric bronchoscopy in adults with central airway obstruction: case illustrations and review of the literature. Laryngoscope. 2009;119:1318–24.
46. Daum TE, Specks U, Colby TV, et al. Tracheobronchial involvement in Wegener's granulomatosis. Am J Respir Crit Care Med 1995;151(2 Pt1):522–26.
47. Mark EJ, Flieder DB, Matsubara O. Treated Wegener's granulomatosis: distinctive pathological findings in the lungs of 20 patients and what they tell us about the natural history of the disease. Hum Pathol. 1997;28(4):450.
48. Yousem SA. Wegener's granulomatosis. In: Churg AM, Myers JL, Tazelaar HD, Wright JL, editors. Thurlbeck's pathology of the lung, 3rd eds. New York: Thieme; 2005. p. 371.
49. Walton EW. Giant-cell granuloma of the respiratory tract (Wegener's Granulomatosis). Br Med J. 1958;2:265–80.
50. Slot MC, Tervaert JW, Boomsma MM, Stegeman CA. Positive classic antineutrophil cytoplasmic antibody (c-ANCA) titer at switch to azathioprine therapy associated with relapse in proteinase 3-related vasculitis. Arthritis Rheum. 2004;14:269–73.
51. Sanders JSF, Huitma MG, Kallenberg CGM, Stegeman CA. Prediction of relapses in PR3-ANCA-associated vasculitis by assessing responses of ANCA titres to treatment. Rheumatol. 2006;45:724–9.
52. Hogan SL, Falk RJ, Chin H, Cai J, Jennette CE, Jennette JC, Nachman PH. Predictors of relapse and treatment resistance in antineutrophil cytoplasmic antibody-associated small-vessel vasculitis. Ann Intern Med. 2005;143:621–31.
53. Hollander D, Manning RT. The use of alkylating agents in the treatment of Wegener's granulomatosis. Ann Int Med. 1967;67:393–8.
54. Hoffman G. Wegener's granulomatosis. Curr Opin Rheumatol. 1983;5:11–7.
55. Fauci AS, Wolff SM. Wegener's granulomatosis: studies in eighteen patients and a review of the literature. Medicine. 1973;52:535–61.
56. Hoffman GS, Kerr GS, Leavitt RY, Hallahan CW, Lebovics RS, Travis WD, Rottem M, Fauci AS. Wegener's granulomatosis: an analysis of 158 patients. Ann Intern Med. 1992;116:488–98.
57. de Groot K, Adu D, Savage CO, EUVAS (European Vasculitis Study Group). The value of pulse cyclophosphamide in ANCA-associated vasculitis: meta-analysis and critical review. Nephrol Dial Transplant. 2001;16:2018–27.
58. de Groot K, Rasmussen N, Bacon PA, Tervaert JW, Feighery C, Gregorini G, Gross WL, Luqmani R, Jayne DR. Randomized trial of cyclophosphamide versus methotrexate for induction of remission in early systemic antineutrophil cytoplasmic antibody-associated vasculitis. Arthritis Rheum. 2005;52:2461–9.
59. Stone JH, Merkel PA, Spiera R, Seo P, Langford CA, Hoffman GS, et al. Rituximab versus cyclophosphamide for ANCA-associated vasculitis. New Engl J Med. 2010;363(221–3):2.
60. Jayne D, Rasmussen N, Adrassy K, Bacon P, Tervaert JW, Dadoniene J, et al. A randomized trial of maintenance therapy for vasculitis associated with antineutrophil cytoplasmic autoantibodies. New Engl J Med. 2003;349:36–44.
61. Langford CA, Talar-Williams C, Barron KS, Sneller MC. A staged approach to the treatment of Wegener's granulomatosis: induction of remission with glucocorticoids and daily cyclophosphamide switching to methotrexate for remission maintenance. Arthritis Rheum. 1999;42:2666–73.
62. Metzler C, Miehle N, Manger K, Iking-Konert C, de Groot K, Hellmich B, et al. Elevated relapse rate under oral methotrexate versus leflunomide for maintenance of remission in Wegener's granulomatosis. Rheumatology. 2007;46:1087–91.
63. McArdle JR, Gildea TR, Mehta AC. Balloon bronchoplasty: its indications, benefits, and complications. J Bronchol. 2005;12(2):123–7.
64. Simpson GT, Strong MS, Healy GB, et al. Predictive factors of success or failure in the endoscopic management of laryngeal and tracheal stenosis. Ann Otol Rhinol Laryngol. 1982;91:384–8.

65. Monnier P, George M, Monod ME, et al. The role of the CO_2 laser in the management of laryngotracheal stenosis: a survey of 100 cases. Eur Arch Otorhinolaryngol. 2005;262:602–8.
66. Mehta AC, Lee FY, Cordasco EM, et al. Concentric tracheal and subglottic stenosis-management using the Nd-YAG laser for mucosal sparing followed by gentle dilation. Chest. 1993;104(3):673–7.
67. Tremblay A, Coulter T, Mehta AC. Modification of a mucosal-sparing technique using electrocautery and balloon dilation in the endoscopic management of web-like benign airway stenosis. J Bronchol. 2003;10(4):268–71.
68. Perepelitsyn I, Shapshay SM. Endoscopic treatment of laryngeal and tracheal stenosis—has mitomycin improved outcome? Otolaryngol Head Neck Surg. 2004;131:16–20.

Chapter 5
Tracheobronchomalacia and Excessive Dynamic Airway Collapse

Erik Folch

Introduction

Tracheobronchomalacia is the weakness of the tracheal or bronchial walls and supporting cartilages with the resultant collapsibility of central airways. If left untreated, it leads to significant morbidity, healthcare utilization with frequent emergency room visits, and limitations in quality of life. Given its diverse symptom profile and heterogeneous population, it is frequently mislabeled as difficult to treat asthma, chronic bronchitis, and other respiratory conditions.

The significant overlap with other respiratory conditions and the presence of comorbidities makes diagnosis and management of tracheobronchomalacia complicated, and is better suited for high-volume centers with multidisciplinary teams that include interventional pulmonologists, thoracic surgeons, and thoracic radiologists. In this chapter, the definitions, classification, clinical and radiologic evaluation, and therapeutic interventions such as airway stent trial and tracheoplasty are discussed.

Definition

Strictly speaking, TBM is weakness of the tracheal or bronchial walls and supporting cartilages in a diffuse or segmental distribution. This loss of structural integrity of the cartilaginous structure of the airway leads to a shape and functional

E. Folch (✉)
Division of Thoracic Surgery and Interventional Pulmonology,
Beth Israel Deaconess Medical Center, Harvard Medical School,
185 Pilgrim Road, Deaconess 201, Boston, MA 02215, USA
e-mail: efolch@bidmc.harvard.edu

© Springer International Publishing Switzerland 2016
A.C. Mehta et al. (eds.), *Diseases of the Central Airways*,
Respiratory Medicine, DOI 10.1007/978-3-319-29830-6_5

compromise during the respiratory cycle. This flaccidity of the airway is usually most apparent during coughing or forced expiration.

In an attempt to define TBM, we should separate it from its close resembling condition: excessive dynamic airway collapse (EDAC), which is the dynamic invagination of the posterior membrane and resultant obstruction of the central airway lumen. Unfortunately, TBM and EDAC can coexist in the same patient and respond to the same treatments. These patients can have both incompetence of the cartilaginous scaffold and posterior membrane invagination [1].

The behavior of the normal airway wall during the respiratory cycle changes due to weakness of the cartilaginous structure. In the normal airway, during inspiration, the tracheobronchial lumen increases in size as the relaxed posterior membrane bulges outward due to increased transmural pressure as pleural pressure becomes increasingly negative. During exhalation, the posterior membrane bulges inward causing narrowing of the tracheobronchial lumen. During forced exhalation, tension in the smooth muscle opposes exaggerated invagination of the posterior membrane and stabilizes the airway structure against excessive narrowing. The normal tracheobronchial lumen decreases approximately 10 % to 30 % with expiration or coughing because of normal invagination of the posterior membranous tracheal wall [2].

Although the exact prevalence of TBM is currently unknown, 12 % of patients with respiratory diseases who undergo fiber-optic bronchoscopy are estimated to have TBM [3]. Approximately 23 % of patients with COPD on fiber-optic bronchoscopy and 69 % of patients with cystic fibrosis on chest CT are reported to have TBM [4]. In a retrospective study of full-inspiratory and end-expiratory CT scans in 1071 patients with emphysema, approximately 10 % of men and 17 % of women had more than 50 % reduction in cross-sectional tracheal luminal area at end-expiration [5]. Thus, there is a clear association between TBM and chronic respiratory diseases such as emphysema [6]. Interestingly, if 50 % or greater narrowing of the airway lumen is used as a cutoff to define TBM, as many as 55 to 78 % of healthy volunteers were found to have TBM [7]. For this reason, many experts consider 90 % obstruction as a more appropriate cutoff point to define those patients who warrant treatment [5].

Etiology

In TBM, there is a decrease in the ratio of cartilage to soft tissues. In normal individuals, this ratio is 5:1, while in TBM it is 2:1. In excessive dynamic airway collapse, there is atrophy and decrease in the number of longitudinal elastic fibers of the posterior membrane [8].

The underlying causes of TBM can be divided into primary and secondary (Table 5.1). Primary TBM is associated with congenital deficiency of the cartilage. Acquired TBM is caused by trauma, COPD, chronic cough, infection, or connective tissue diseases (i.e., relapsing polychondritis). Focal areas of malacia can also be

Table 5.1 Causes of TBM

Primary
Genetic
Idiopathic
Tracheobronchomegaly or Mounier-Kuhn syndrome
Secondary
Secondary to trauma
• Post-intubation
• Post-tracheostomy
• Thoracic trauma
• Post-lung transplant
Emphysema
Chronic bronchitis
Chronic inflammation
• Relapsing polychondritis
External compression of the trachea
• Benign tumors
• Malignant tumors
• Cysts
• Abscess
• Aortic aneurysm
• Vascular rings

caused by aberrant vessels compressing the airway, large goiters, mediastinal masses, and aortic aneurysms or be idiopathic.

Classification

Clinically, TBM can be classified as primary or secondary. Primary TBM is either congenital or idiopathic. Secondary TBM may be related to post-traumatic, chronic infection, chronic inflammation, and chronic external compression.

Although there is no consensus with regard to severity, TBM has been classified as mild (70–79 %), moderate (80–89 %), and severe (more than 90 %) collapse of airway lumen [9].

As mentioned before, many experts only consider clinically significant TBM with more than 90 % airway obstruction in order to have higher specificity and prevent overdiagnosis. Two radiologic studies have demonstrated that as many as 73–78 % of normal individuals will have some degree of dynamic collapse of the airway during exhalation. For these reasons, the 50 % threshold is not considered clinically meaningful [10].

With regard to shape during airway collapse, TBM can be described as crescent shape, saber-sheath, circumferential, and excessive dynamic airway collapse. As previously mentioned, it can involve the trachea (22 %), bronchi (15 %), or both (63 %) in a diffuse or focal distribution [8].

Murgu et al. [9] described a classification based on functional class, etiology, morphology, origin, and severity of TBM. However, this classification has not been adopted in routine clinical practice or extensively used in the published literature.

Clinical Manifestations

The clinical manifestations of TBM are variable. Patients can be asymptomatic, present with dyspnea, cough, mucostasis, wheezing, stridor, or failure to wean and extubate. Although it is not pathognomonic, the presence of a barking (or "seal-like") cough frequently alerts the clinician to the possibility of TBM. Patients with TBM will frequently have recurrent pulmonary infections with difficulty expectorating sputum. On occasion, these cough spells will result in syncope. Although none of these symptoms are specific to TBM, failure to respond to customary treatments should prompt the consideration of structural reasons such as TBM or tracheal stenosis. The patients may also reproduce the symptoms when they perform Valsalva maneuvers and become recumbent, or with forced exhalation and cough. This adds a new layer of complexity to their pulmonary function testing and interpretation. On occasion, they describe a series of cough episodes that seem to be reiterated and intensified. So the more they cough, the higher the need to keep coughing. This is both debilitating and uncomfortable.

Differential Diagnosis

The differential diagnosis of TBM includes chronic bronchitis, emphysema, asthma, bronchiectasis, and chronic cough due to other causes. Other conditions that can mimic TBM or coexist include congestive heart failure, bronchiectasis, cystic fibrosis, obesity hypoventilation syndrome, recurrent low-grade aspiration, vocal cord dysfunction, and chronic gastroesophageal reflux disease (GERD). A meticulous diagnostic workup will allow the clinician to either rule out those conditions or at least address them appropriately and assign the remaining symptoms to TBM or excessive dynamic collapse of the posterior wall. Frequently clinicians will describe it as a "disproportionate range of symptoms" for the underlying lung disease.

The use of a standardized protocol in patients with suspected TBM that includes diagnostic procedures and optimization of these conditions is very effective to minimize overdiagnosis. At our center, patients with TBM undergo an extensive array of tests that include pulmonary function tests (PFTs), inspiratory and expiratory airway CT, GERD evaluation (impedance testing, manometry), laryngoscopy for vocal cord dysfunction, and evaluation for sleep apnea (with questionnaires and polysomnogram).

Diagnostic Interventions

In order to establish the diagnosis of TBM, the clinician may use dynamic airway computed tomography. This technology is widely available, and the radiologist should be alerted of the clinical suspicion for TBM so that they can perform inspiratory and expiratory imaging. The radiologic studies frequently reveal dilation of the conducting airways during inspiration with premature collapse during exhalation. The expiratory or exhalation part of the CT is remarkably different from the inspiratory images (Fig. 5.1).

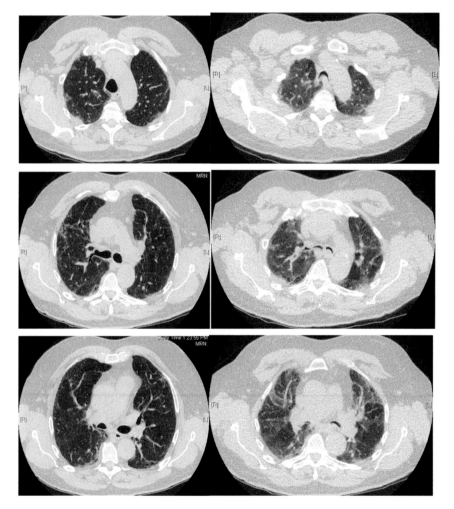

Fig. 5.1 Dynamic computed tomography of the chest on inspiration and full expiration demonstrating diffuse severe TBM involving the mid-trachea, distal trachea, and main-stem bronchi. The lung parenchyma demonstrates a significant air trapping

Lee et al. [11] have described the use of the collapsibility index resulting from the measurement of the cross-sectional area (CSA) of the airway during inspiration and expiration (Collapsibility index = CSA end inspiration − CSA dynamic exhalation/CSA end inspiration × 100).

The dynamic flexible bronchoscopy is the gold standard for the diagnosis of TBM [1, 9]. During bronchoscopy, the clinician encounters bowing of the cartilage wall as well as excessive invagination of the posterior wall of the trachea and bronchi to the point where the bronchoscope cannot be advanced any further.

Although the evaluation of TBM can be done with rigid or flexible broncho-scope, in practice, the flexible bronchoscope is the instrument of choice as it allows the patient to breathe spontaneously and follow commands to perform deep breathing and forced exhalation. It is important to systematically evaluate the proximal, mid, and distal trachea as well as the right and left main-stem bronchi and distal airways for obstruction. This will facilitate and guide the planned interventions, including stent trial and tracheoplasty.

The patterns of pulmonary function testing and flow-volume loops are routinely used by pulmonologists for the evaluation of TBM and other lung diseases. Abnormal findings on PFTs and flow-volume loops in one study were low maximum forced expiratory flow (81.6 %), biphasic expiratory curve (19.7 %), flow oscillations (2.6 %), and notching (9.2 %) [12]. However, in this study, 17 % had no distinctive abnormalities, suggesting that PFT's and flow-volume loops are normal in a substantial number of patients with moderate to severe TBM and should not be used solely to decide whether TBM is present or clinically important [12].

Airway Stents and TBM

When faced with the diagnosis of TBM, the clinician should assess the degree of symptoms and choose therapy accordingly. Asymptomatic patients do not require treatment or further diagnostic workup. However, symptomatic patients should undergo treatment of other comorbid conditions for 4–8 weeks. These conditions frequently include GERD, sleep apnea, vocal cord dysfunction, asthma, and chronic obstructive pulmonary disease (COPD).

If symptoms persist despite an optimal trial of medical treatments, patients with diffuse disease or localized TBM should undergo a stent trial (Figs. 5.2 and 5.3). The stent is used as a temporary measure to evaluate the symptomatic changes before considering a possible surgical repair. It should be very clear to the patient that regardless of the clinical benefit, the stent is a temporizing measure and would not be left in place permanently. If after one to two weeks of stent trial, the patient has significant symptomatic improvement, it will be removed, and consideration for surgical tracheoplasty will be entertained. The use of stents for this purpose has been validated by the prospective observational trials. In a prospective study, silicone stents were used for moderate to severe diffuse TBM. Before, during, and after the stent trial, symptoms, health-related quality of life, lung function, and exercise capacity were evaluated [13]. The baseline measurements were compared to those obtained 10–14 days after stent placement. Following stent placement, 77 % of patients reported symptomatic improvement; however, complications were frequent and included obstruction, infection, migration, and severe cough. Due to the complications associated with silicone stents, it is imperative that the physician conveys a clear message to the patient regarding their temporary nature.

A standardized protocol for Y stent use in TBM was reported by Odell et al. [14]. In this study, patients with Y stent for TBM were given mucolytic agents (nebulized N-acetylcysteine) and expectorants (guaifenesin). The complication rates were compared to patients that were treated without a standardized protocol. Out of 141 patients, 98 were treated with the standardized protocol. The rate of serious complications including stent migration, obstruction, respiratory failure, and hemoptysis was statistically lower in the protocol treatment group (9 % vs. 40 % $p < 0.001$) [14]. Interestingly, shortness of breath is usually very responsive to silicone stent placement. However, cough is usually worse or unchanged due to inherent irritation of the silicone stents.

Recently, our group has tried the use of metallic (nitinol) stents in a small group of patients with severe cough due to tracheobronchomalacia (Fig. 5.2). This trial has been done with full awareness of the possible complications of metallic stent placement including granulation tissue and difficulty removing them [15]. However, when these metallic stents were promptly removed within 5–14 days, the presence of granulation was minimal, and removal was uneventful. This small group of patients reported the significant improvement in shortness of breath and cough [16]. After the successful trial, they underwent surgical tracheoplasty.

Tracheoplasty

The ultimate long-term treatment of TBM is tracheobronchoplasty with airway stabilization (Figs. 5.2 and 5.3). This surgical procedure has been prospectively studied and shown to cause symptomatic benefit in healthcare-related question-naires, dyspnea scores, and performance status [17]. In those patients with pro-hibitive surgical risk, we recommend the symptom management and discuss the possibility of a definitive stent placement. However, a proactive approach to the maintenance of the stent patency and frequent bronchoscopies are usually required.

Tracheoplasty, the preferred long-term treatment for severe TBM, entails the insertion of a polypropylene mesh to support the posterior tracheal and bronchial membrane. Unfortunately, it requires a right posterolateral thoracotomy to gain access to the thoracic trachea and bilateral main-stem bronchi. Multiple rows of sutures are used to anchor the mesh to the airway, and case duration is approxi-mately 6 h. The first 48–72 h are spent in the ICU, with an average hospital stay of 8 days [18, 19]. A successful procedure leads to a significant improvement in dyspnea, quality of life, functional status, and overall exercise capacity when compared to pre-intervention levels [19, 20].

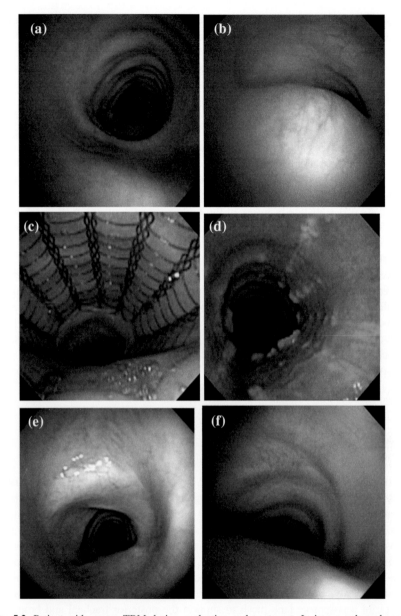

Fig. 5.2 Patient with severe TBM during evaluation and treatment. In image **a** bronchoscopic image, the proximal trachea during inhalation and in **b** during forced exhalation. Image **c** demonstrates the presence of an uncovered nitinol stent during a stent trial of one week, followed by the minimal granulation tissue seen after an uneventful removal of the stent. Image **e** and **f** demonstrate the bronchoscopic appearance of the proximal trachea during forced exhalation at 3 months and 12 months after surgical tracheoplasty

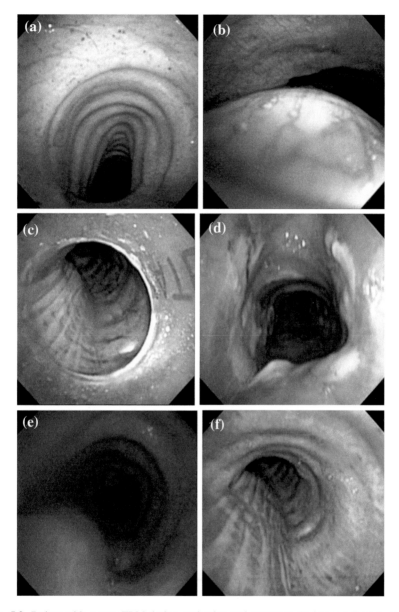

Fig. 5.3 Patient with severe TBM during evaluation and treatment. In image **a** bronchoscopic image, the proximal and mid-trachea during inhalation and in **b** during forced exhalation. Image **c** demonstrates the presence of a silicone stent during a stent trial of one week, followed by the small amount of granulation tissue seen after the removal of the stent. Images **e** and **f** demonstrate the bronchoscopic appearance of the mid-trachea during forced exhalation at 3 months and 12 months after surgical tracheoplasty

Unfortunately, complications were seen in 38 % of the cases in this series, including postoperative respiratory infections in 22 %, prolonged mechanical ventilation or reintubation, tracheostomy, atrial fibrillation, and hemothorax [19]. The mortality rate was 3 %, in spite of the multiple comorbidities and low pulmonary reserve in this patient population. At this time, this procedure is only regularly performed at high-volume centers with experienced thoracic surgeons.

Other surgical alternatives include anterior external splinting [21], circumferential external splinting [22], and suture plication of the posterior membrane [23]. However, the experience with these techniques is limited to small series involving pediatric and adult patients.

In addition, it should be mentioned that any surgical technique of tracheoplasty that involves the posterior insertion of a mesh is difficult to apply to the cervical trachea. Techniques of external splinting of the cervical malacia have also been successful in small groups of patients [24].

Finally, recurrence rates requiring repeat surgery are low, but there is a risk of progression of malacia in the untreated cervical segment of the trachea. In these cases, resection and reconstruction may be necessary [25].

Medical Management

Given the long and difficult surgery to stabilize the airway in TBM patients, there is a sizeable group with prohibitive comorbidities. In this subgroup of patients, symptom management and definitive stent use are also considered.

Although some authors have proposed the use of non-invasive mechanical ventilation (NIMV) for TBM as a pneumatic splint, this approach is fraught with difficulties. The role of NIMV is most important in the management of acute on chronic respiratory failure. Whenever these exacerbations occur, the urgent use of NIMV makes it possible to maintain airway patency and facilitates drainage of secretions.

The use of intermittent nasal pressure support during the day and of continuous pressure support (CPAP) at night are temporary bridges to more permanent treatments such as airway stents and tracheoplasty [26]. NIMV in the form of CPAP is likely to prevent prolonged mechanical ventilation and the need for tracheostomy [27]. However, there is limited evidence to their clinical benefit [26, 28].

Extensive work in TBM by Majid and cols has resulted in a proposed flowchart to guide the diagnosis and treatment of this complex condition (Fig. 5.4) [5].

Some experts have also suggested aggressive weight loss treatment [29].

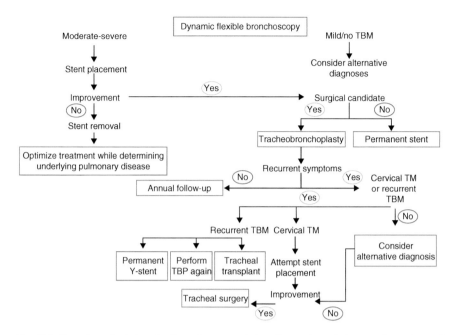

Fig. 5.4 Flowchart depicting the key elements of the diagnostic and therapeutic workup of tracheobronchomalacia. Reprinted from Barros Casas et al. [44]. With permission from Elsevier

Natural History of TBM

In children, congenital TBM is the most common congenital abnormality of the trachea [30]. Although it can be seen in healthy infants, it is more common in premature babies [31] as a result of immature tracheobronchial cartilage. Interestingly, primary tracheobronchomalacia is usually self-limited with most infants outgrowing the condition by age 2 [31–33]. In a small percentage, there is a progression to diffuse TBM [34]. In patients with vascular rings, connective tissue disorder, and congenital conditions, TBM is usually progressive and may shorten life span [35, 36].

In adults, the natural history of TBM is not completely understood. However, it is usually progressive and likely to become diffuse over time. A longitudinal study of TBM with an average follow-up of 5 years showed progression in most patients, and none showed improvement [37].

Interestingly, unmasking of a disease that was previously unrecognized has been well described. Some patients remain asymptomatic until an episode of infection, bronchitis, or pneumonia occurs. Unmasking of TBM during anesthesia and in setting of progressive hypercapneic respiratory failure has also been described [38, 39]. The underlying TBM in these cases was discovered after the failed attempts to extubate or wean off of positive-pressure mechanical ventilation. In these cases, a partial return of the structural integrity of the trachea and bronchi may be seen after the acute episode has resolved. However, recurrence is common. These patients should be evaluated in the absence of positive-pressure "airway splinting." Eventually, most of these patients have disease progression and require a thorough evaluation and treatment of comorbidities followed by a stent trial.

Future Directions

In the last few years, descriptions of the use of endobronchial laser to cause contraction scarring of the posterior wall in patients with excessive dynamic airway collapse and TBM have surfaced [40]. Other areas of interest include the use of 3D printing and modeling of airway stents in TBM patients. This technique has had excellent results in other patients with complex airway disease, but their application to TBM remains a formidable challenge [41, 42].

Novel stents with innovative materials and potentially biodegradable are being investigated [43]. Their gradual integration into the airway wall, locally increasing the rigidity of the airway while acting as a scaffold, is theoretically plausible.

References

1. Carden KA, Boiselle PM, Waltz DA, Ernst A. Tracheomalacia and tracheobronchomalacia in children and adults: an in-depth review. Chest. 2005;127:984–1005.
2. McLoud TC, Boiselle PM. Thoracic radiology. 2nd ed. Philadelphia: Mosby/Elsevier; 2010.
3. Ikeda S, Hanawa T, Konishi T, et al. Diagnosis, incidence, clinicopathology and surgical treatment of acquired tracheobronchomalacia. Nihon Kyobu Shikkan Gakkai zasshi. 1992;30:1028–35.
4. McDermott S, Barry SC, Judge EP, et al. Tracheomalacia in adults with cystic fibrosis: determination of prevalence and severity with dynamic cine CT. Radiology. 2009;252:577–86.
5. Barros Casas D, Fernandez-Bussy S, Folch E, Flandes Aldeyturriaga J, Majid A. Non-malignant central airway obstruction. Arch Bronconeumol. 2014;50:345–54.
6. Ochs RA, Petkovska I, Kim HJ, Abtin F, Brown M, Goldin J. Prevalence of tracheal collapse in an emphysema cohort as measured with end-expiration CT. Acad Radiol. 2009;16:46–53.
7. Boiselle PM, O'Donnell CR, Bankier AA, et al. Tracheal collapsibility in healthy volunteers during forced expiration: assessment with multidetector CT. Radiology. 2009;252:255–62.
8. Jokinen K, Palva T, Sutinen S, Nuutinen J. Acquired tracheobronchomalacia. Ann ClinRes. 1977;9:52–7.
9. Murgu SD, Colt HG. Description of a multidimensional classification system for patients with expiratory central airway collapse. Respirology. 2007;12:543–50.
10. Majid A, Gaurav K, Sanchez JM, et al. Evaluation of tracheobronchomalacia by dynamic flexible bronchoscopy. A pilot study. AnnAm Thorac Soc. 2014;11:951–5.
11. Lee KS, Sun MR, Ernst A, Feller-Kopman D, Majid A, Boiselle PM. Comparison of Dynamic Expiratory CT With Bronchoscopy for Diagnosing Airway Malacia: A Pilot Evaluation. Chest. 2007;131:758–64.
12. Majid A, Sosa AF, Ernst A, et al. Pulmonary function and flow-volume loop patterns in patients with tracheobronchomalacia. Respir care. 2013;58:1521–6.

13. Ernst A, Majid A, Feller-Kopman D, et al. Airway stabilization with silicone stents for treating adult tracheobronchomalacia: a prospective observational study. Chest. 2007;132:609–16.
14. Odell DD, Majid A, Gangadharan SP, Ernst A. Adoption of a standardized protocol decreases serious complications of airway stenting in patients with tracheobronchomalacia. Chest. 2010;138:784A.
15. Lund ME, Force S. Airway stenting for patients with benign airway disease and the Food and Drug Administration advisory: a call for restraint. Chest. 2007;132:1107–8.
16. Ochoa S, Cheng GZ, Folch E, Majid A. Use of Self-expanding Metallic Airway Stents in Tracheobronchomalacia. J Bronchol Intervent Pulmonol. 2015;22:e9–11.
17. Majid A, Guerrero J, Gangadharan S, et al. Tracheobronchoplasty for severe tracheobronchomalacia: a prospective outcome analysis. Chest. 2008;134:801–7.
18. Lagisetty KH, Gangadharan SP. Tracheobronchoplasty for the treatment of tracheobronchomalacia. J Thorac Cardiovasc Surg. 2012;144:S58–9.
19. Gangadharan SP, Bakhos CT, Majid A, et al. Technical aspects and outcomes of tracheobronchoplasty for severe tracheobronchomalacia. Ann Thorac Surg. 2011;91:1574–80 discussion 80-1.
20. Ernst A, Odell DD, Michaud G, Majid A, Herth FF, Gangadharan SP. Central airway stabilization for tracheobronchomalacia improves quality of life in patients with COPD. Chest. 2011;140:1162–8.
21. Cho JH, Kim H, Kim J. External tracheal stabilization technique for acquired tracheomalacia using a tailored silicone tube. Ann Thorac Surg. 2012;94:1356–8.
22. Ley S, Loukanov T, Ley-Zaporozhan J, et al. Long-term outcome after external tracheal stabilization due to congenital tracheal instability. Ann Thorac Surg. 2010;89:918–25.
23. Masaoka A, Yamakawa Y, Niwa H, et al. Pediatric and adult tracheobronchomalacia. Eur JCardio-thorac Surg. 1996;10:87–92.
24. Gobel G, Karaiskaki N, Gerlinger I, Mann WJ. Tracheal ceramic rings for tracheomalacia: a review after 17 years. Laryngoscope. 2007;117:1741–4.
25. Tracheobronchoplasty Gangadharan S. In: Dienemann HC, Hoffmann H, Detterbeck FC, editors. Chest Surgery. Berlin: Springer; 2015. p. 75–84.
26. Ferguson GT, Benoist J. Nasal continuous positive airway pressure in the treatment of tracheobronchomalacia. Am Rev Respir Dis. 1993;147:457–61.
27. Hegde HV, Bhat RL, Shanbag RD, Bharat M, Rao PR. Unmasking of tracheomalacia following short-term mechanical ventilation in a patient of adult respiratory distress syndrome. Indian J Anaesth. 2012;56:171–4.
28. Adliff M, Ngato D, Keshavjee S, Brenaman S, Granton JT. Treatment of diffuse tracheomalacia secondary to relapsing polychondritis with continuous positive airway pressure. Chest. 1997;112:1701–4.
29. Choo EM, Seaman JC, Musani AI. Tracheomalacia/Tracheobronchomalacia and hyperdynamic airway collapse. Immunol Allergy Clin North Am. 2013;33:23–34.
30. Holinger LD. Etiology of stridor in the neonate, infant and child. Ann Otol Rhinol Laryngol. 1980;89:397–400.
31. Jacobs IN, Wetmore RF, Tom LW, Handler SD, Potsic WP. Tracheobronchomalacia in children. Arch Otolaryngol-Head Neck Surg. 1994;120:154–8.
32. Baxter JD, Dunbar JS. Tracheomalacia. Ann Otol Rhinol Laryngol. 1963;72:1013–23.
33. Cogbill TH, Moore FA, Accurso FJ, Lilly JR. Primary tracheomalacia. Ann Thorac Surg. 1983;35:538–41.
34. Malhotra A, Armstrong D, Ditchfield M. Evolution of acquired tracheobronchomalacia in an infant studied by multidetector computed tomography. Pediatr Pulmonol. 2013;48:728–30.
35. Cox WL Jr, Shaw RR. Congenital Chondromalacia of the Trachea. J Thorac Cardiovasc Surgery. 1965;49:1033–9.
36. Chen H, Chang CH, Perrin E, Perrin J. A lethal, Larsen-like multiple joint dislocation syndrome. Am J Med Gen. 1982;13:149–61.
37. Nuutinen J. Acquired tracheobronchomalacia. A clinical study with bronchological correlations. Ann Clinical Res. 1977;9:350–5.

38. Katoh H, Saitoh S, Takiguchi M, Yamasaki Y, Yamamoto M. A case of tracheomalacia during isoflurane anesthesia. Anesth Analg. 1995;80:1051–3.
39. Collard P, Freitag L, Reynaert MS, Rodenstein DO, Francis C. Respiratory failure due to tracheobronchomalacia. Thorax. 1996;51:224–6.
40. Dutau H, Maldonado F, Breen DP, Colchen A. Endoscopic successful management of tracheobronchomalacia with laser: apropos of a Mounier-Kuhn syndrome. Eur J Cardio-thorac Surg. 2011;39:e186–8.
41. Morrison RJ, Hollister SJ, Niedner MF, et al. Mitigation of tracheobronchomalacia with 3D-printed personalized medical devices in pediatric patients. Sci Transl Med. 2015;7:285ra64.
42. George ZC, Erik F, Sebastian O, et al. Creating personalized airway stents via 3D printing. Am Thorac Soc. 2015;191:A3717.
43. Zopf DA, Hollister SJ, Nelson ME, Ohye RG, Green GE. Bioresorbable airway splint created with a three-dimensional printer. New Engl J Med. 2013;368:2043–5.
44. Barros Casas D, Fernandez-Bussy S, Folch E, Flandes Aldeyturriaga J, Majid A. Non-malignant central airway obstruction. Arch Bronconeumol. 2014;50(8):345–54.

Chapter 6
Tracheobronchial Amyloidosis

Gustavo Cumbo-Nacheli, Abigail D. Doyle and Thomas R. Gildea

Introduction

Tracheobronchial amyloidosis (TBA) is a disease characterized by extracellular deposition of eosinophilic, proteinaceous, and insoluble β-pleated sheets of fibers within the airways. These insoluble proteins disrupt the airway function. When the pulmonary system is involved in systemic amyloidosis, it may display different features: diffuse interstitial or alveolar septal disease, nodular disease, intra- and extrathoracic adenopathy, pleural disease, and diaphragmatic deposition. In contrast, localized pulmonary involvement manifests as nodular opacities, diffuses opacities, or tracheobronchial disease, the latter being the most common of the three [1].

In this chapter, we review the clinical features of TBA and discuss the role of radiographic imaging, bronchoscopy, and radiation therapy in the management of TBA.

Clinical Features

TBA represents only 0.5 % of all symptomatic tracheobronchial lesions [1]. Symptoms suggesting a form of obstruction, with cough, dyspnea, wheezing, hemoptysis, and hoarseness, are the most common complaints. More than half of the

G. Cumbo-Nacheli
Pulmonary and Critical Care Division, Spectrum Health Medical Group,
Grand Rapids, MI, USA

A.D. Doyle (✉)
Department of Internal Medicine, Metro Health Hospital, 5900 Byron Center Avenue,
Wyoming, MI, USA
e-mail: abigail.doyle@metrogr.org

T.R. Gildea
Pulmonary, Allergy, Critical Care and Transplant, Cleveland Clinic, Cleveland, OH, USA

© Springer International Publishing Switzerland 2016   147
A.C. Mehta et al. (eds.), *Diseases of the Central Airways*,
Respiratory Medicine, DOI 10.1007/978-3-319-29830-6_6

cases may present as obstructive pneumonia, bronchiectasis, or atelectasis [2]. Clinical features are difficult to recognize, often leading to delay in diagnosis and treatment. Routine chest radiography may be unremarkable in up to 70 % of affected patients [1, 3]. TBA tends to be misdiagnosed as asthma, COPD, and pneumonia [3]. CT of the chest often shows soft-tissue thickening and irregular narrowing of the tracheobronchial lumen, which should be further investigated by bronchoscopy [4]. Bronchoscopy with biopsy remains the gold standard for diagnosis. Although TBA nearly always presents in the absence of systemic amyloidosis, the systemic form should be ruled out with serum and urine electrophoresis, electrocardiogram, echocardiogram, and fat pad biopsy. TBA has been reported in association with Sjogren syndrome [5, 6], sarcoidosis [7], and rheumatoid arthritis [8].

Radiographic Appearance

CT findings of TBA can be defined by several characteristics that separate it from other central airways diseases. Typically, there are multiple nodular eccentric lesions in the tracheal lumen. These can occur circumferentially and may contain calcification (Fig. 6.1a–f). The posterior tracheal wall is involved in the disease process. This feature separates it from tracheopathia osteochondroplastica and relapsing polychondritis which spare the posterior wall [9]. There appear to be 2 primary appearances of TBA diffuse airway infiltration and either focal or multi-focal nodular infiltration [10]. Some have proposed a "wavy path sign" of nodular appearance along an airway in coronal views [11]. PET-CT with intense uptake of 18-fluorodeoxyglucose by the amyloid material is used to assess activity and can be used as an adjunct to bronchoscopy in follow-up [12].

Bronchoscopy

Bronchoscopy is the primary management tool for TBA from both a diagnostic and a therapeutic standpoint. Endobronchial examination shows either diffuse mucosal infiltrate or nodules (Fig. 6.2). The mucosal lesions have a tendency to have a yellowish hue and bleed easily and ooze considerably longer than typical lesions. Therefore, planning for hemorrhage management should be in place [13, 14]. Other newer imaging techniques have been used. Narrow band imaging (NBI) has been reported to show a complex vasculature and abrupt-ending large caliber vessels [13]. Probe-based confocal light endomicroscopy has also been reported to show "dappled" images of protein deposition [15].

Therapeutic bronchoscopy options include neodymium:yttrium aluminum-garnet (Nd:YAG) laser photo-resection, argon-plasma coagulation, and rigid debulking. When luminal patency is compromised balloon dilation, in some cases airway stenting has been used.

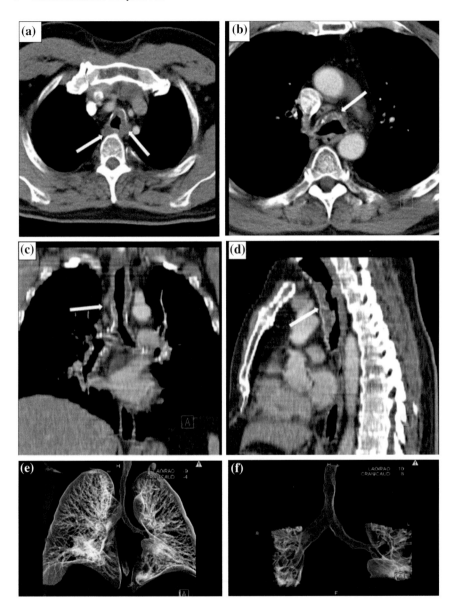

Fig. 6.1 a Axial CT image of the trachea demonstrating eccentric nodular masses along the posterolateral wall (*closed white arrow*). **b** Axial image from the same patient at the level of the carina and main-stem bronchi demonstrating diffuse circumferential wall thickening with foci of calcifications and luminal narrowing (*closed white arrow*). **c, d** Sagittal and coronal contrast-enhanced CT showing diffuse circumferential thickening of the tracheobronchial airway. **e, f** 3D external rendering showing airway narrowing, irregular tracheobronchial mucosa. Note right middle lobe subsegmental collapse. Distal airways are patent

Fig. 6.2 Bronchoscopic
findings in a case of
tracheobronchial amyloidosis

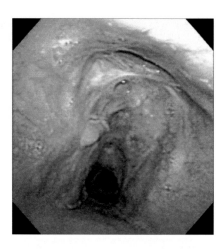

Fiorelli et al. [16] described a clinical case of a 67-year-old woman diagnosed
with TBA, who underwent rigid bronchoscopy with the removal of the mass by
mechanical resection and Nd:YAG laser coagulation, followed by placement of a
self-expanding, covered Y-stent. Her respiratory symptoms improved immediately,
and at five-month follow-up, the CT and bronchoscopic examination showed
normal patency of the tracheobronchial tree without recurrence of amyloid deposition. Resection alone may not prevent recurrences, as they often recur within
12 months after resection. A retrospective study performed by Alloubi et al. [17]
investigated the long-term outcome of six patients with primary TBA. All patients
underwent rigid bronchoscopy and received laser therapy by Nd:YAG prior to
mechanical debulking, with the hypothesis the laser therapy would decrease
intrabronchial bleeding. A satisfactory tracheal size and resolution of symptoms
were obtained after 3–5 sessions of rigid bronchoscopy in 4 of 6 patients, and the
other two patients received a silicone stent due to extreme stenosis or re-stenosis of
the trachea by tumor-like tissue without improvement after repeated bronchoscopy.
All patients had immediate symptomatic improvement, and there were no intra-
operative or perioperative deaths. Brill et al. [18] described a case of TBA successfully treated with argon-plasma laser treatment, which achieved recanalization
of the bronchus, resulting in sustained clinical improvement.

Medical Therapy

There are few reports of effective therapy for TBA. Systemic pharmacotherapy with
colchicine, melphalan, dimethyl sulfoxide (DMSO), and glucocorticoids has been
reported with modest success [2, 17]. Toxic side effects from systemic chemotherapy
render this therapeutic approach less preferable [1]. Mucolytics, antibiotics,

nebulizer treatments, and occasional courses of oral or inhaled corticosteroids may be used as adjunctive therapy in addition to bronchoscopic debulking [1].

Radiation Therapy

Low-dose external beam radiation therapy (EBRT) has been demonstrated to be effective as an adjunct to bronchoscopic management. In contrast to mechanical debulking and laser therapy, which yields immediate symptomatic improvement, EBRT has a more gradual onset of action. Advantages of EBRT include less bleeding than with bronchoscopic intervention, and higher accessibility to lesions that may not be amenable to bronchoscopic intervention. The mechanism of radiation for control of pulmonary amyloidosis is not completely understood. Some hypotheses provide improvement in localized amyloidosis due to the anti-inflammatory effects seen in early radiation, along with inhibition of localized plasma cells, as chronic inflammation is one of the important factors which stimulates amyloid formation [19]. Others hypothesize the mechanism of action could include a radiation effect on the vasculature, or the induction of immune responses against the deposits by causing local inflammation [10]. Side effects have been reportedly low, with esophagitis the main adverse event [19].

Combination therapies appear to be the most successful form of treatment for TBA patients. In a case report by Kurrus et al. [20], a multimodal approach to treatment with TBA was discussed. The patient underwent EBRT, with a dose of 20 Gy, to the distal tracheal and right main-stem bronchus. Repeat bronchoscopy showed the treated tissue to be less thickened and friable; however, there were new areas of occlusion by amyloid tumor in the right upper lobe, which was resected using a Nd:YAG laser and forceps. The bronchus intermedius was dilated and a silicone stent was placed. The right lower lobe eventually became obstructed; in contrast, the areas that had received the EBRT 7 months earlier continued to appear less thickened, red, and friable. Due to these results, they elected to treat the distal disease progression with the same dose of EBRT as used previously. Patient free of symptoms, with bronchoscopic examination essentially unchanged.

Ren and Ren 12 used EBRT with 24 Gy in 12 fractions, 5 fractions a week over 18 days on two patients diagnosed with TBA [19]. On day two, case one noticed significant improvement in dyspnea, and CT chest showed obvious abatement of the irregular thickness of the bronchial wall, and improvement of PFTs was from moderate obstruction to normal. Follow-up bronchoscopies showed abatement of the lesions, smoother mucosa, and less obstruction, and she remained symptom-free at follow-up of 54 months. Case two also noted symptomatic improvement by day two, with improvement in PFTs two months later, and stable improvement at 46 months follow-up.

A retrospective review of 10 patients with biopsy-proven airway amyloidosis (3 laryngeal and 7 TBA) who underwent EBRT at a median dose of 20 Gy showed local control in 8/10 patients at a median 6.7 years of follow-up. This was defined by CT and endoscopic evaluation showing no changes in airway wall thickening, decreased mucosal edema, and stable endobronchial pathologic findings, along with improvement in FEV1 [21]. Monroe et al. [22] described a case of extensive TBA involving the right main-stem bronchus and extending inferiorly into the right lower lobe, making surgical debulking and laser therapy difficult. The patient underwent treatment with EBRT at 24 Gy, resulting in significant improvement in respiratory status, imaging, and PFTs within 2 months. At one year, repetitive bronchoscopy showed airways to be patent. Among a cohort of 7 TBA patients with TBA treated by EBRT, all subjects displayed symptom improvement after receiving EBRT. This treatment modality was well tolerated, with the most common side effect being acute esophagitis [23].

Conclusion: Being aware of TBA in the differential diagnosis of many pulmonary symptoms and being familiar with unusual disease imaging is helpful and a key to pattern recognition for expert clinicians. There is no gold standard treatment for TBA, and management is targeted at maintaining airway patency. Treatment modalities include mechanical debulking, balloon dilation and stenting, APC, laser therapy, EBRT, and cryotherapy. The advantages of rigid bronchoscopy over flexible bronchoscopy include airway safety, ability to perform mechanical debulking, and the ease of blood and airway secretion removal [17] but add the risk of airway trauma and inciting bleeding. Being aware of the possible diagnosis and having the ability to obtain diagnostic tissue and perhaps perform simple endobronchial therapeutic procedures to improve airway lumen in a single procedure favored as an initial step but further medical evaluation, management, and consultation with radiation oncology complete comprehensive management.

References

1. Berk JL, O'Regan A, Skinner M. Pulmonary and tracheobronchial amyloidosis. Semin Respir Crit Care Med. 2002;23:155–65.
2. Berraondo J, Novella L, Sanz F, Lluch R, de Casimiro E, Lloret T. Management of tracheobronchial amyloidosis with therapeutic bronchoscopic techniques. Arch Bronconeumol. 2013;49:207–9.
3. Ding L, Li W, Wang K, Chen Y, Xu H, Wang H, Shen H. Primary tracheobronchial amyloidosis in China: analysis of 64 cases and a review of literature. J Huazhong Univ Sci Technol Med Sci. 2010;30:599–603.
4. Poovaneswaran S, Razak AR, Lockman H, Bone M, Pollard K, Mazdai G. Tracheobronchial amyloidosis: utilization of radiotherapy as a treatment modality. Medscape J Med. 2008;10:42.
5. Rodrigues K, Neves FS, Stoeterau KB, Werner Castro GR, Nobre LF, Zimmermann AF, Pereira IA. Pulmonary amyloidosis in Sjogren's syndrome: a rare diagnosis for nodular lung lesions. Int J Rheum Dis. 2009;12:358–60.
6. Inaty H, Folch E, Stephen C, Majid A. Tracheobronchial amyloidosis in a patient with sjogren syndrome. J Bronchology Interv Pulmonol. 2013;20:261–5.
7. Oka H, Ishii H, Iwasaki T, Amemiya Y, Otani S, Yoshioka D, Kishi K, Shirai R, Tokimatsu I, Kadota J. Tracheobronchial amyloidosis in a patient with sarcoidosis. Intern Med. 2009;48:1715–6.

8. Turkstra F, Rinkel RN, Biermann H, van der Valk P, Voskuyl AE. Tracheobronchomalacia due to amyloidosis in a patient with rheumatoid arthritis. Clin Rheumatol. 2008;27:807–8.
9. Obusez EC, Jamjoom L, Kirsch J, Gildea T, Mohammed TL. Computed tomography correlation of airway disease with bronchoscopy: part I–nonneoplastic large airway diseases. Curr Probl Diagn Radiol. 2014;43:268–77.
10. Acar T, Bayraktaroglu S, Ceylan N, Savas R. Computed tomography findings of tracheobronchial system diseases: a pictorial essay. Jpn J Radiol. 2015;33:51–8.
11. M'Rad S, Le Thi Huong D, Wechsler B, Monsigny M, Buthiau D, Colchen A, Godeau P. Localized tracheobronchial amyloidosis. A new case studied with x-ray computed tomographic and nuclear magnetic resonance. Review of the literature. Rev Pneumol Clin. 1988;44:260–65.
12. Soussan M, Ouvrier MJ, Pop G, Galas JL, Neuman A, Weinmann P. Tracheobronchial FDG uptake in primary amyloidosis detected by PET/CT. Clin Nucl Med. 2011;36:723–4.
13. Shaheen NA, Salman SD, Nassar VH. Fatal bronchopulmonary hemorrhage due to unrecognized amyloidosis. Arch Otolaryngol. 1975;101:259–61.
14. Zhang LQ, Zhao YC, Wang XW, Yang J, Lu ZW, Cheng YS. Primary localized tracheobronchial amyloidosis presenting with massive hemoptysis: a case report and literature review. Clin Respir J. 2015.
15. Newton RC, Kemp SV, Yang GZ, Darzi A, Sheppard MN, Shah PL. Tracheobronchial amyloidosis and confocal endomicroscopy. Respiration. 2011;82:209–11.
16. Fiorelli A, Accardo M, Galluccio G, Santini M. Tracheobronchial amyloidosis treated by endobronchial laser resection and self expanding Y stent. Arch Bronconeumol. 2013;49:303–5.
17. Alloubi I, Thumerel M, Begueret H, Baste JM, Velly JF, Jougon J. Outcomes after bronchoscopic procedures for primary tracheobronchial amyloidosis: retrospective study of 6 cases. Pulm Med. 2012;2012:352719.
18. Brill AK, Woelke K, Schadlich R, Weinz C, Laier-Groeneveld G. Tracheobronchial amyloidosis–bronchoscopic diagnosis and therapy of an uncommon disease: a case report. J Physiol Pharmacol. 2007;58(Suppl 5):51–5.
19. Ren S, Ren G. External beam radiation therapy is safe and effective in treating primary pulmonary amyloidosis. Respir Med. 2012;106:1063–9.
20. Kurrus JA, Hayes JK, Hoidal JR, Menendez MM, Elstad MR. Radiation therapy for tracheobronchial amyloidosis. Chest. 1998;114:1489–92.
21. Truong MT, Kachnic LA, Grillone GA, Bohrs HK, Lee R, Sakai O, Berk JL. Long-term results of conformal radiotherapy for progressive airway amyloidosis. Int J Radiat Oncol Biol Phys. 2012;83:734–9.
22. Monroe AT, Walia R, Zlotecki RA, Jantz MA. Tracheobronchial amyloidosis: a case report of successful treatment with external beam radiation therapy. Chest. 2004;125:784–9.
23. Neben-Wittich MA, Foote RL, Kalra S. External beam radiation therapy for tracheobronchial amyloidosis. Chest. 2007;132:262–7.

Chapter 7
Tracheobronchopathia Osteochondroplastica

Prasoon Jain and Atul C. Mehta

Introduction

Tracheobronchopathia osteochondroplastica (TO) is an uncommon disorder characterized by the development of multiple cartilaginous and bony nodules in the submucosal layer of central airways [1–3]. The nodules project into the lumen from the anterior and the lateral walls of trachea and bronchi (Fig. 7.1) causing a variety of respiratory symptoms. Typically, the posterior membranous wall of central airways is not involved with the disease process. The underlying cause of this disorder remains unknown. The clinical presentation depends on the size and distribution of the nodules. In mild cases, patients may remain asymptomatic. On the other extreme, large and confluent cartilaginous or bony nodules can cause severe airway obstruction, atelectasis, and life-threatening difficulties during intubation. In this chapter, we discuss the clinical features, diagnosis, and treatment of this rare but interesting clinical entity.

P. Jain (✉)
Louis A Johnson VA Medical Center, Clarksburg, WV 26301, USA
e-mail: prasoonjain.md@gmail.com

A.C. Mehta
Department of Pulmonary Medicine, Respiratory Institute, Cleveland Clinic,
Cleveland, OH 44195, USA
e-mail: Mehtaa1@ccf.org

A.C. Mehta
Lerner College of Medicine, Buoncore Family Endowed Chair in Lung
Transplantation, Respiratory Institute, Cleveland Clinic, Cleveland, OH, USA

© Springer International Publishing Switzerland 2016   155
A.C. Mehta et al. (eds.), *Diseases of the Central Airways*,
Respiratory Medicine, DOI 10.1007/978-3-319-29830-6_7

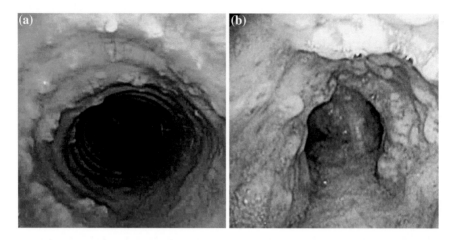

Fig. 7.1 Bronchoscopic findings in mild (**a**) and severe (**b**) tracheobronchopathia osteochondroplastica. Note extensive nodules arising from anterior and lateral wall of trachea with sparing of posterior membrane. Reprinted from [3]. With permission from Springer Science+Business Media

Historical Background

The original description of TO comes from Samuel Wilks in 1857 who reported several ossified deposits in larynx, trachea, and bronchi upon autopsy in a 38-year-old patient who died of tuberculosis [4]. In 1863, Virchow [5] proposed that cartilaginous and bony nodules in TO arise from ecchondrosis and exostosis of normal tracheobronchial cartilage. Von Schoretter is said to have seen the TO lesions for the first time in a living patient using a laryngeal mirror in 1896 [6]. The credit of first description of bronchoscopic findings of TO goes to Killian in 1897 [7]. In 1910, Aschoff-Frieburg [8] coined the term tracheopathia osteochondroplastica and proposed that these nodules arise from metaplasia of tracheal and bronchial elastic connective tissue.

Incidence

The exact incidence of TO is unknown, but by most accounts, it is exceedingly uncommon. A detailed review of the literature by Dalgaard in 1947 found 90 cases [9], and another literature review by Martin in 1974 revealed only 245 reported cases of TO [10]. Except for a series of thirty cases by Harma and Suurkari in 1977 [11] and another series of 41 cases by GERM"O"P group in 2001 [12], the majority of reports have involved a single or a handful of cases. Still, there is a possibility that TO is more common than reported because many cases go unnoticed due to the absence of any significant symptoms. Before advent of bronchoscopy, the majority of cases were detected on autopsy. In these cases, TO was most often an incidental finding, unrelated to the underlying cause of death. In one such series, findings consistent with TO were found in 2 out of 800 (0.25 %) autopsies [13]. Widespread use of chest computed tomography (CT) and flexible bronchoscopy has increasingly allowed antemortem detection of TO in live patients. The incidence of TO is reported to vary from 0.02 to 0.77 % of bronchoscopies performed for unrelated indications [14–21].

Pathology

Table 7.1 summarizes the pathologic findings of TO. Several autopsy studies provide a detailed description of pathological findings in TO [13, 22]. Most commonly, the disease process involves the lower two-third of trachea. Involvement of the main-stem and lobar bronchi is also common. Very seldom, segmental bronchi may also be involved. Isolated involvement of main-stem bronchi without involvement of trachea has been described in some cases. The involvement of larynx in TO is uncommon but has been reported by several authors [22, 23]. On gross examination, the tracheal wall is thickened and the nodules are visible over the mucosal surface of anterior and lateral wall sparing the posterior membranous wall. Many of the nodules have stony hard consistency. Microscopic examination of the trachea shows bony and cartilaginous nodules within the submucosa and lamina propria of trachea and bronchi (Fig. 7.2). The nodules vary in size and shape. In some cases, there are only a few small nodules [24], while in other cases, the nodules are too numerous to count, becoming confluent in certain areas. Partial ossification of cartilaginous nodules is a common finding [22]. Interestingly, many but not all nodules show an anatomical continuity with the perichondrium of the cartilaginous ring. Some bony nodules contain marrow space with fatty tissue and a

Table 7.1 Pathological findings in tracheobronchopathia osteochondroplastica	*Gross examination*
	• Thickening of tracheal wall
	• Multiple nodules arising from anterior and lateral wall of trachea and bronchi
	• Many nodules have stony hard consistency
	• Absence of mucosal ulceration
	• Sparing of posterior wall of trachea
	Microscopic examination
	• Cartilaginous nodules in submucosa
	• Bony nodules in submucosa
	• Fatty and hematopoietic marrow within ossified nodules
	• Calcification
	• Squamous metaplasia

Fig. 7.2 Histological findings in tracheobronchopathia osteochondroplastica, illustrating submucosal calcification, ossification, and cartilage formation. Reprinted from [3]. With permission from Springer Science +Business Media

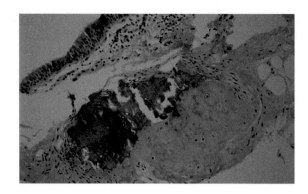

small amount of hematopoietic cells. The overlying epithelium frequently demonstrates squamous metaplasia. The inflammatory reaction is conspicuously minimal or absent.

Small biopsies obtained during flexible bronchoscopy may reveal many of the typical pathological findings described above, but it is not possible to retrieve a diagnostic specimen in every instance. It is also unrealistic to expect a classical pathological description of TO even when adequate bronchoscopic biopsies are obtained. This is well illustrated in a series of 41 patients, in which histopathology of bronchoscopic biopsies was diagnostic in 28 of 40 (70 %) of patients [12]. Bony nodules in submucosa was the most common finding, seen in 23 (58 %) of patients. Other findings included cartilaginous nodules in 15 (38 %), calcification in 8 (20 %), and squamous metaplasia in 19 (48 %) patients.

Etiology and Pathogenesis

The events that lead to development of TO are currently unknown. For more than a century, the debate has centered around two different views to explain how cartilaginous and bony nodules develop within the submucosa of central airways in TO. According to one of these theories advanced by Virchow [5], the new formations in this disorder represent ecchondrosis or exostosis arising from tracheal cartilage. A direct anatomical continuity between these lesions and the perichondrium of tracheal cartilage on serial sections, especially in early stages of the disease process, lends some support to this view [13, 24]. However, not every nodule is connected to the tracheal cartilage. The presence of isolated bony and cartilaginous islands can be explained by thinning, stretching, and eventual separation as the nodules elongates after their origin from the perichondrium of tracheal cartilage [25]. Aschoff [8] in 1910 proposed an alternative theory, according to which the cartilaginous and bony nodules arise from metaplasia of elastic connective tissue normally present in the submucosal layer of trachea. According to Dalgaard [9], the undifferentiated connective tissue cells found in close relation to submucosal elastic fibers are the parent cells from which TO lesions originate. Additional support for Aschoff's proposal also comes from the frequent presence of elastic fibers in close relationship to the nodules on detailed pathological examination [22]. However, sparing of posterior tracheal membrane, which is rich in elastic fibers, cannot be explained on the basis of this theory.

Even more mysterious are the cellular mechanisms that eventually lead to the formation of cartilaginous and bony nodules in TO. It is not difficult to imagine that chondrogenesis and osteogenesis in such an unusual site would involve a complex interplay between several cells, growth factors, and regulatory pathways. In this context, there is some indication that bone morphogenic protein (BMP) and transforming growth factor beta-1 (TGF-β-1) are involved in pathogenesis of TO. Bone morphogenic proteins belong to TGF-β superfamily and are known to play a critical role in embryogenesis and tissue homeostasis. An important property of BMP is its ability to promote differentiation of mesenchymal stem cells into osteoprogenitor cells [26]. There is also evidence for role of BMP in the development of cartilaginous tissue [27]. Apart from promoting formation of cartilage and bone, BMP also plays important role in mineralization and formation of hematopoietic marrow. In this regard, BMP is shown to have an active role not only where the normal bones are found in the body but also at ectopic sites outside the skeleton [28].

Many biological actions of TGF-β and BMP converge as they share similar cellular receptors and intracellular transduction pathways [29]. TGF-β stimulates the production of extracellular matrix proteins by chondrocytes [30] and is shown to induce formation of bone [31]. In this regard, TGF-β seems to complement BMP through different phases of bone formation [32]. Since the key pathological features of TO include formation of cartilage and bone at ectopic site in the tracheal submucosal layer, it is not unreasonable to speculate that BMP and TGF-β may have some role in pathogenesis of this disorder.

This possibility was addressed in one study in which immunohistochemical methods were used to identify the presence of bone morphogenic protein-2 (BMP-2) and TGF-β-1 in 2 autopsy cases of TO [33]. Significant amount of BMP-2 activity was located in the mesenchymal cells around the osteocartilaginous nodules. BMP-2 immunoreactivity was also located in the chondroblasts, the new cartilage, and the immature matrix of the cartilage. Although a significant BMP-2 activity was noted in the newly formed nodules, no significant BMP-2 was found in the adjacent normal tracheal cartilage. TGF-β-1 was detected in the chondrocytes and osteocytes of the submucosal nodules. TGF-β-1 activity was also found in bronchial epithelial cells. Based on these findings, the authors speculated that BMP-2 and TGF-β-1 have synergistic role in promoting formation of osteocartilaginous nodules in TO.

What initiates the development of TO lesions has not been identified. Except for a single report of TO in a mother and daughter [34], there are no other reports of familial occurrence or genetic predisposition. No other factor has been conclusively linked to the development of TO, although many possibilities have been raised, as discussed below.

Concurrent finding of amyloidosis in certain cases has led some investigators to suggest that TO may be a late stage of primary tracheobronchial amyloidosis [35–39]. Some support to this view comes from a series of 32 patients with tracheobronchial amyloidosis in which 7 (22 %) cases also had bronchoscopic and biopsy evidence of TO lesions [40]. Similarly, in a series of 41 patients with TO, 16 biopsy specimens specifically were examined for amyloidosis with Congo red stain and 2 (13 %) biopsies disclosed the presence of amyloidosis [12]. While coexistence of such rare entities in some patients justifiably provide a reason to associate TO and amyloidosis, there are several points against this proposal. First, the presence of amyloidosis has been reported only a small fraction of all reported cases of TO. We find no cases of tracheobronchial amyloidosis among additional 97 patients from 7 case series of TO [11, 16–20, 41]. Similarly, except for one report [40], no patients with tracheo-bronchial amyloidosis has been reported to have a simultaneous diagnosis of TO in a number of case series [42–45]. Further, posterior membrane of trachea is frequently involved with tracheobronchial amyloidosis where as it is characteristically spared in TO. Taken together, there is no persuasive evidence to establish an etiologic link between TO and tracheobronchial amyloidosis.

In contrast, the association between ozena and TO appears more than coinci-dental. Ozena is a chronic nasal disease characterized by the progressive atrophic rhinitis, atrophy of underlying bone and turbinates, thick mucopurulent nasal secretions that form crusts that emit foul odor [46]. The characteristic pathological changes in ozena include chronic inflammation, squamous metaplasia, ciliary destruction, bone destruction, and formation of crusts. *Klebsiella ozaenae* is fre-quently isolated from nasal secretions, but it is still unsettled whether or not it is the underlying cause of the problem.

Frequent clinical association and similarity in the histological appearance of nasal and the tracheal mucosa has led many investigators to speculate that ozena increases the future risk of developing TO [47–49]. Several recent case series appear to support this view. In a series of 18 patients from Scandinavia, ozena or recurrent maxillary sinusitis was reported in 6 (33 %) of patients with TO [20]. Although no data were provided, TO was stated to be more severe when two conditions were present simultaneously. Symptoms of atrophic rhinitis, sinusitis, or pharyngitis were reported in 29 % of patients in another series of 41 patients with TO [12]. *K. ozaenae* was isolated from bronchial secretions in 8 (20 %) of these patients. In another report, atrophic rhinitis was detected in 2 (20 %) patients in a series of 10 patients with TO from Iran [18]. The most convincing association between these two entities comes from a series of 30 patients from Finland in which 23 patients had atrophic rhinitis and 4 (13 %) patients had *K. ozaenae* on culture of tracheal secretions [11]. Interestingly, 6 of these patients revealed purulent and crusty secretions over the tracheal mucosa reminiscent of atrophic rhinitis and ozena. The authors used the term tracheozaena to describe these findings. These findings do raise a possibility that *K. ozaenae* is somehow involved in pathogenesis of TO. In an experimental study, exposure to *K. ozaenae* led to the development of an amorphous material causing irregular clumping of nasal mucosal cilia. The damaging effect of the bacteria on ciliary function in the nose was proposed as a possible cause for the development of atrophic rhinitis and ozena [50]. It can be argued that similar events take place in tracheal mucosa of TO patients with *K. ozaenae* infection.

Although these reports make a convincing case, any association between ozena and TO cannot be taken as an evidence of cause and effect. It can be argued that a primary defect in mucosal defenses due to squamous metaplasia and loss of cilia could itself favor colonization and proliferation of *K. ozaenae* and other bacteria in the trachea. Thus, tracheal and bronchial infections with *K. ozaenae* may represent a complication and not the cause of TO. Regardless, these observations do provide a strong rationale for the physicians to diligently look for TO when atrophic rhinitis is detected and perform a thorough nasal and upper airway examination when TO is diagnosed.

No other consistent causative factor has been identified. Tracheal cultures have isolated *Mycobacterium avium*-intercellulare [51, 52], *M. gordanae*, and *M. tuberculosis* [12] in several reported cases, but there is no reason to believe that these infections are in any way related to pathogenesis of TO. Same can be said about a report of tracheal botyromycosis in a patient with underlying TO [53]. There is a single report of selective IgA deficiency with frequent sino-pulmonary infections in a patient with TO [54], but systematic investigations have revealed no abnormality in immunoglobulin or complement levels and cell mediated immunity [11]. No underlying endocrine problem has been found in patients with TO. Calcium and phosphate levels are usually within normal range. Occurrence of dermatomyositis, multiple myeloma, and other systemic disorders in some reports is coincidental [12]. A case of TO in a patient with underlying silicosis has been reported, but there is no reason to postulate a link between these two entities [55]. Report of ectopic calcification of falx cerebri in a 31-year-old patient is interesting but does not appear related to TO [56]. Finally, persuasive case for cause and effect relationship cannot be made on the basis of infrequent and isolated reports of non-Hodgkin lymphoma [57] and lung cancer [17, 58] in patients with TO.

Clinical Features

The clinical features of TO are highly variable. In early and mild disease, patients are asymptomatic and the diagnosis is established on the basis of incidental radiologic or bronchoscopic findings. On the other extreme are cases in which extensive involvement of air passages seriously compromised the airway lumen and caused rapidly progressive respiratory failure needing urgent interventions [59, 60]. The majority of diagnosed cases fall somewhere in-between these two extremes. The age distribution is highly variable. The diagnosis is usually made in fifth through seventh decade of life. However, many patients have been diagnosed in the second through fourth decade of life [11, 12, 18, 41]. In fact, in pediatric literature, the disease has been described in patients as young as 5 and 9 years of age [61, 62]. Quite possibly, the disease progresses slowly and remains asymptomatic for several

Table 7.2 Clinical
presentation of
tracheobronchopathia
osteochondroplastica

• Cough
• Sputum production
• Hemoptysis
• Dyspnea
• Wheezing
• Hoarseness
• Ozena or recurrent sinusitis
• Recurrent lower respiratory tract infections
• Atelectasis
• Acute respiratory distress and stridor
• Unexpected difficulty during intubation
• Incidental finding on bronchoscopy or CT study

years before the clinical symptoms surface in later years of life. Even so, it can be seen that in many reported cases, non-specific respiratory symptoms were ignored for several years before the correct diagnosis was made. There is no difference in distribution of cases according to gender or ethnicity. Smoking does not seem to increase the risk of TO. No environmental exposure or genetic predisposition is consistently identified in patients with TO.

Table 7.2 lists the presenting features and symptoms of TO. There are no pathognomonic signs and symptoms. Many patients are entirely asymptomatic, and it is not unusual to have diagnosis made incidentally on thoracic imaging or flexible bronchoscopy [11, 12].

Chronic cough is the most common presenting symptom experienced by 50–70 % of patients [12, 18, 41]. Some patients report chronic cough for several years or decades before correct diagnosis is made [19, 63]. While cough is usually associated with other pulmonary symptoms such as hemoptysis, dyspnea, and chest discomfort, in some instances chronic cough is the sole manifestation of the disease [12]. Cough is usually dry but up to one-third of patients report significant sputum production. Purulent sputum production is due to superimposed bacterial infection and is easily mistaken for acute bronchitis, chronic obstructive pulmonary disease (COPD) exacerbation, or bronchiectasis.

Dyspnea is reported by 20–90 % of patients with TO. The severity of dyspnea depends on degree of airway involvement [12, 18–20, 41]. Although dyspnea is usually mild in majority of cases, 11 of 41 (27 %) of patients in one series had rapidly progressive breathlessness [12]. Sometimes, emergent endotracheal intubation or tracheostomy is needed in TO patients presenting with stridor and acute respiratory failure.

Hemoptysis is the third most common symptom, reported by 20–60 % of patients [12, 18, 20, 41]. Intermittent mild hemoptysis in these patients is usually secondary to ulceration of mucosa overlying a prominent bony or cartilaginous nodule. Hemoptysis is usually self-limiting and is of limited clinical relevance. However, this is one symptom for which there is low threshold for performing bronchoscopy, thus providing opportunity to detect an otherwise unsuspected diagnosis. Massive hemoptysis is unusual and should suggest an alternative diagnosis.

The nasal and sinus symptoms are reported by at least one-third of patients [12, 20]. Symptoms of atrophic rhinitis or ozena are common, as discussed in the previous sections. Many patients experience recurrent episodes of acute sinusitis. Hoarseness and dysphonia are reported by up to 20 % of patients [12, 19]. Persistent hoarseness is uncommon but is seen when larynx and subglottis are involved with the disease process [23, 41, 64]. Laryngeal cancer should be excluded in such cases with careful direct laryngeal examination. Difficulty in swallowing has also been reported in some patients with TO.

There are several reports of recurrent lower respiratory tract infections, fever and pneumonia as presenting symptoms of TO [41, 65–67]. In one study, bronchial cultures were positive in 61 % of patients with TO [12]. The most common organisms isolated are *K. ozaenae*, *Pseudomonas aeruginosa,* and *Staphylococcus aureus*. Quite possibly, a defect in local mucosal defense due to squamous metaplasia and impaired mucociliary clearance is the root cause of bacterial colonization, which in turn increases the risk of recurrent pneumonia in these patients.

Extensive endobronchial obstruction has also caused lobar atelectasis and recurrent pneumonia in some patients with TO. For example, Meyer and associates described a patient suffering from right middle lobe atelectasis for 6 years which was later proven to be due to severe and diffuse involvement of the middle lobe bronchus with TO [68]. Similarly, Hodges and Israel have reported two patients with TO who presented with right middle lobe collapse. In each case, the opening of right middle lobe bronchus was more than 90 % occluded with TO lesions [69]. In both of these reports, although right middle lobe bronchus was most severely affected, typical TO nodules were also seen throughout the trachea and bronchi. Lobar atelectasis as the sole manifestation of TO is unusual but is reported. In one case, the patient developed right upper lobe atelectasis due to complete occlusion of the corresponding bronchus with a hard mass lesion later proven to be TO on pathological examination on surgical specimen [70]. In second case, an isolated TO lesion caused complete occlusion of sub-segmental (right 3b bronchus) resulting in post-obstructive pneumonia [71]. The most unusual feature in these cases was complete absence of TO lesions elsewhere in the tracheobronchial tree.

Several reports have also drawn attention to unexpected difficulties during planned endobronchial intubation for general anesthesia in TO [72, 73]. Grating sensation has been felt during attempts at passage of endotracheal tube into the trachea [74]. In some cases, the failure to pass endotracheal tube through the trachea has forced the providers to cancel the planned surgery [75, 76]. In one reported case, single-lung ventilation failed because nodular outgrowths projecting into airway lumen prohibited sufficient occlusion of right main-stem bronchus by the balloon blocker [77]. Laryngeal mask airway has been successfully used in one patient with failed prior intubation who required general anesthesia for an intra-abdominal surgery [78].

Patients with failed prior intubation in above reports showed narrowing of trachea on a subsequent bronchoscopy. Interestingly, none of these patients had any prior clinical symptoms on preoperative evaluation. Evidently, there are patients who never develop clinically significant symptoms despite severe involvement of central airways with TO.

Non-specific signs such as wheezing, rhonchi, and crackles can be appreciated in 30–60 % of TO patients, but these findings are not helpful in suspecting correct underlying diagnosis. Stridor and tachypnea are sometimes observed in patients with severe tracheal narrowing and impending respiratory failure [59].

Laboratory Investigations

Routine laboratory tests including calcium and phosphate levels are normal in TO [11, 67]. Serum immunoglobulin and complement levels are also normal. No serological tests or systemic endocrine abnormalities have been identified. Based on current data, extensive laboratory testing is not indicated in suspected or confirmed patients with TO.

Cultures of respiratory secretions are indicated in patients who present with lower respiratory tract infection. Identification of offending organism may help clinicians to choose most appropriate antibiotic therapy. Microbiologic evaluation in asymptomatic patients is unlikely to have any meaningful value.

Imaging

Chest radiograph has a limited value in diagnosis of TO. In isolated cases, chest radiographs have been reported to exhibit diffuse and irregular narrowing of airways, and scalloping or thickening of tracheal wall, best appreciated on lateral films [79–81]. Tracheal calcification is rarely seen on plain films. In one series, chest radiograph from 38 TO patients showed narrowing of trachea in 8 (21 %), calcification in 4 (11 %), atelectasis in 4 (11 %), and pneumonia in 10 (26 %) of patients [12].

In actual clinical practice, chest radiographs are rarely helpful since the findings on chest radiograph are usually subtle and are easily overlooked. It is also not uncommon to have normal chest radiograph despite a significant involvement of central airways with the disease process [19, 41]. Non-specific findings on chest radiography are common in TO but are insufficient to persuade clinician to consider TO as a diagnostic possibility [16, 20].

Chest CT scan is more helpful than chest radiograph and is the imaging modality of choice. The most common CT finding is the presence of multiple calcified and non-calcified nodules arising from inner anterior and lateral walls of trachea and projecting into the lumen without involving the posterior wall [82–85] (Fig. 7.3). The nodules vary from 3 to 8 mm in diameter. Thickening of tracheal wall is

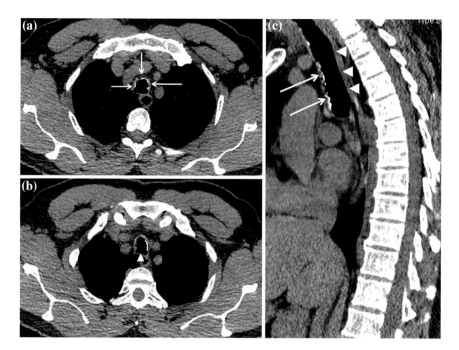

Fig. 7.3 Chest CT showing irregular calcified nodules involving anterior and lateral walls of trachea (*arrows*) with sparing of posterior tracheal wall (*arrowheads*). Reprinted from [107]. With permission from Springer Science+Business Media

another commonly reported finding. In one series, CT was performed in 31 TO patients [12]. 74 % of patients had submucosal nodules, 61 % had submucosal calcification, and 10 % had tracheal stenosis. Even though CT is the most accurate imaging modality to determine the extent and distribution of the lesions, diagnosis can be overlooked in early stages and especially in patients with minimal involvement [18].

In some reports, repeated CTs have been performed presumably to assess future course of disease, but value of this practice is uncertain [86]. Follow-up CTs in one case series showed progression of lesions in 2 of 20 (10 %) of patients [12]. We do not recommend serial CTs in these patients as it would unnecessarily expose these patients to diagnostic radiation and, in the absence of new symptoms, would not provide any useful clinical information.

Findings on magnetic resonance imaging (MRI) have also been reported in one patient. These included diffuse irregular mural thickening of the trachea with the absence of contrast enhancement, sparing of the posterior wall, and low-signal dots on T1- and T2-weighted spin echo, suggestive of calcification within the tracheo-bronchial walls [87]. However, MRI does not provide any unique perspective about the disease process and is less sensitive than CT in detecting submucosal calcification. Therefore, there is no reason to perform MRI in patients with suspected TO.

Pulmonary Function Tests

Pulmonary function tests can be normal in early stages but may disclose obstructive ventilator defect when airway lumen is significantly compromised. In a series of 41 patients, pulmonary function tests were performed in 28 patients [12]. Airflow obstruction was detected in 11 (39 %), and restrictive defect was found in 5 (18 %) patients. Peak flows were reduced in 9 of 14 (64 %) patients. Spirometry was normal in 43 % of patients. In another series, 7 of 8 patients had obstructive ventilator defect and one remaining patient had a combined obstructive and restrictive defect [19]. Obstructive defect has also been reported by others [17, 20, 41]. Longitudinal assessments of pulmonary functions in one study showed no deterioration of spirometric parameters over a mean follow-up period of 4.2 years [88]. Reversibility after bronchodilator administration is sometimes reported [17, 19], but airway hyper-responsiveness on formal methacholine challenge test is not found [88]. Flow volume loop showed expiratory plateau in 3 of 16 (19 %) and inspiratory plateau in 2 of 16 (13 %) patients in one series [12]. Others have reported similar findings in a small number of patients [41]. Flow volume loop has been suggested to be a useful parameter to follow in TO [89], but data on its ability to detect progression of disease are rather limited.

Bronchoscopy

Bronchoscopy is the gold standard for diagnosis of TO. The most characteristic finding is the presence of multiple bony or cartilaginous nodules arising from the anterior and lateral wall of the airways and sparing the posterior tracheal membrane [1–3] (Fig. 7.1). The nodules measure 1–10 mm in diameter. Larger and confluent nodules can be seen to project into the airway lumen causing a variable degree of airway obstruction. The distribution of nodules is said to be "scattered" when few nodules are present with areas of normal mucosa between them, "diffuse" when numerous nodules are covering entire airway surface without intervening normal mucosa and "confluent" when the nodules are seen to coalesce and fuse together [12]. Sometimes, the bronchoscopic findings of this disorder have been compared to cobble stone appearance, rock garden, and stalactite cave. The overlying mucosal membrane may appear normal, but thinning of mucosa [41], ulceration, and hemorrhagic changes [12] can be appreciated in some patients. The presence of excessive amounts of serous, mucoid, or purulent secretions in the central airways is not unusual. Although the disease process is said to be most profuse in the distal two-third of the trachea [19], nodules are usually widely distributed and can involve nearly every part of central airways [12]. Several cases with involvement of larynx, subglottis, and proximal trachea can be found in the published literature [12, 23–41, 90]. The rigidity of airway wall limits the dynamic movement of airways with respiration seen in normal subjects. In heavily involved areas, it may be difficult to advance the bronchoscope through the narrow air passages. It is ill-advised to force the bronchoscope through such areas. In one instance, bronchoscope was reported to get stuck requiring considerable force to retrieve the scope out of the air passages [31]. Difficulty may also be encountered during passage of rigid bronchoscope. A grating sound sometimes heard as rigid instrument is advanced through the airways containing large bony projections. Similar grinding of flexible scope against the hard nodules has also been described in some reports [12].

Bony hard consistency makes it difficult to obtain diagnostic biopsies using standard bronchoscopic techniques. The biopsy forceps tends to slip and slide away from the lesion, and small mucosal fragments are all that can be retrieved in many cases. Repeat bronchoscopy may be needed after failure to obtain diagnostic specimen on the first attempt. For instance, in one series, endobronchial biopsies were obtained in 28 of 40 (70 %) of patients [12]. Diagnostic specimen was obtained on first bronchoscopy in 22 of 40 (55 %) patients. Remaining 18 of 40 (45 %) patients required additional bronchoscopy to obtain diagnostic tissue. Many patients required repeated bronchoscopies before the histological diagnosis could be secured. Larger biopsy forceps via rigid bronchoscope may have better success in obtaining diagnostic biopsy specimens.

In one case, mucosa was reported to have a smooth and continuous green appearance on autofluoresecence bronchoscopy, as expected in healthy tracheobronchial lining [91]. In another interesting case report, probe-based confocal laser endomicroscopy (pCLE) over the airway nodules showed a mottled and brightly autofluorescing submucosa and not the regular and cross-hatched healthy basement membrane as seen in normal subjects [92]. Future studies are indicated to address the predictive value of autofluorescence bronchoscopy and optical biopsy techniques in diagnosis of TO.

Atypical presentation of TO in some cases may not allow immediate diagnosis to be made on the basis of visual inspection, thus posing a considerable diagnostic challenge. For example, in one reported case, bronchoscopy in a 20-year-old patient showed a 3.2-cm endoluminal mass attached to the anterior wall of trachea causing near-total occlusion of the lumen [93]. No other submucosal nodules were identified either proximal or distal to the tracheal mass. Histological examination of the lesion obtained after primary surgical resection of the lesion revealed findings consistent with TO. In another atypical case, a patient presenting with chronic and mild hemoptysis showed three discrete localized and vascular appearing growths involving right middle, left upper, and left lower lobe openings, later proven to be TO on histological examination. There were no usual TO findings elsewhere on bronchoscopic examination in this case either [94]. We have already alluded to reports of TO presenting with isolated mass lesions blocking lobar or segmental bronchi causing lobar or segmental atelectasis [70, 71]. In the absence of typical bronchoscopic findings in such atypical cases, biopsy evidence is needed to establish the diagnosis. Fortunately, such cases are exceptions rather than the rule. Overwhelming majority of patients has classical bronchoscopic appearance which is sufficient for instant diagnosis in the bronchoscopy room.

Curiously, in one case, considerable difficulty was experienced in performing transbronchial needle aspiration in a TO patients with unrelated mediastinal lymph node enlargement [95]. The difficulty in the insertion of needle through the airway wall was presumably due to the presence of calcified nodules in the submucosal layer of the tracheal wall.

Diagnosis

There are no pathognomonic signs or symptoms of TO. It is therefore not surprising that diagnosis in pre-bronchoscopy era was exclusively made on autopsy. As clinical presentation is non-specific in a vast majority of patients, the most critical prerequisite for diagnosing TO is high index of suspicion that can only come from awareness of the disease entity. Bronchoscopy is most likely to provide diagnosis in early stages since radiologic findings as well as abnormalities on pulmonary function testing may be subtle or absent. In advanced stages, chest CT can provide useful clues to the underlying diagnosis, but diagnostic confirmation still requires direct inspection of tracheobronchial tree with bronchoscopy.

There is a debate whether histological evidence is essential for diagnosis of TO. To some extent, this debate is fueled by technically difficulties in obtaining representative biopsies during flexible bronchoscopy. According to one view, characteristic bronchoscopic appearance is sufficient and histological evidence is not necessary for diagnosing TO [2]. However, there are others who disagree and suggest that histological confirmation is essential in order to exclude other conditions such as tracheobronchial amyloidosis that can be mistaken for TO, especially by inexperienced operators [3, 15]. We share the latter view and perform bronchoscopic biopsies as much as possible to secure a firm histological diagnosis if characteristic endobronchial features are not present.

Delay in diagnosis of TO is very common. Failure to include TO in differential diagnosis and lack of familiarity with the disease entity are the main causes of delays in diagnosis. According to some accounts, TO is among the most common conditions that are identified on bronchoscopy performed for chronic and refractory cough. For example, in one study, bronchoscopy was performed in 25 patients with chronic and persistent cough [96]. The underlying cause of cough could be identified with bronchoscopy in 7 (28 %) of patients. TO was diagnosed in 2 of these patients. Similar findings were reported in another study in which 82 bronchoscopies were performed for the evaluation of chronic and unexplained cough [97]. Diagnosis was established on bronchoscopy in 9 (11 %) of 82 patients. TO was the leading diagnosis, found in 7 (8.5 %) of the bronchoscopies. In majority of these cases, the involvement of airways with the disease process was relatively mild, not sufficient to cause significant airway obstruction or abnormal CT findings.

   Asthma is the most common incorrect diagnoses made in patients with TO [41]. Many such patients have received anti-asthma therapy for several years before correct diagnosis is identified [98, 99]. In order to avoid this pitfall, it is a sound practice to question the validity of asthma diagnosis when the clinical features are atypical, response to therapy is inadequate, and methacholine challenge test is negative. It is useful to remember asthma mimics such as TO under such circumstances. Flexible bronchoscopy is appropriate for further evaluation of many of these patients.

   Calcification of tracheal and bronchial cartilage, which is seen most often in older women, is sometimes mistaken for TO. Calcium deposit is seen in anterior and lateral wall without involvement of the posterior wall due to the absence of cartilage in this location. However, the inner lining of trachea is thin and smooth in age-related calcification of tracheal cartilage in contrast to thickened and nodular appearance in TO. On direct inspection, tracheal and bronchial mucosa is normal in patients with age-related calcification of cartilage, whereas it shows typical nodular changes as described above. In most cases, the distinction between age-related calcification of tracheal cartilage and TO can be made on the basis of radiological findings, and bronchoscopy is not needed for this purpose.

   Primary tracheobronchial amyloidosis should be excluded in every patient suspected to have TO. CT findings of tracheobronchial amyloidosis include concentric, smooth, or nodular thickening of submucosa with or without calcification [42]. Bronchoscopy may also reveal diffuse and nodular changes in tracheal and bronchial mucosal lining. One distinguishing feature is frequent involvement of posterior tracheal wall in amyloidosis, which is characteristically uninvolved in TO. Positive staining of endobronchial biopsy specimens with Congo red stain in tracheobronchial amyloidosis is also helpful in differential diagnosis.

   Patients with relapsing polychondritis can develop thickening of anterior and lateral wall of trachea due to inflammation and calcification of the tracheal cartilage with sparing of the posterior tracheal wall [100]. However, the inner wall of trachea appears smooth on CT, and the mucus membrane does not show nodular changes on bronchoscopic examination in relapsing polychondritis, which is very different from nodular appearance seen in TO. Further, it is common to detect tracheobronchomalacia on CT and bronchoscopy in relapsing polychondritis [101], whereas the airway wall shows a characteristic rigidity in TO. The presence of extra-pulmonary manifestations such as joint pain, uveitis, and inflammation of cartilage at other sites in relapsing polychondritis is also helpful in differential diagnosis.

   Endobronchial tuberculosis, sarcoidosis, and tracheobronchial papillomatosis sometimes also feature in the differential diagnosis, but these conditions are easily differentiated from TO on the basis of bronchoscopic appearance, cultures, and histological examination of the biopsy material. Bony hard submucosal nodules are not found on bronchoscopy in these conditions.

Treatment

There is no medical therapy that can remove the existing lesions, prevent formation of new nodules, or prevent future progression of the disease. Fortunately, most patients have minimal or no symptoms and do not require any therapy. Humidification, mucolytics agents, inhaled bronchodilators, and antibiotic therapy are indicated for management of recurrent pulmonary infections [2, 3]. The results of sputum cultures may help with the selection of most appropriate antibiotics. Oral or inhaled corticosteroids have no established role and must be avoided as much as possible. It is not uncommon for several TO patients to have received inhaled and oral corticosteroids for several years for presumed treatment-resistant asthma. All efforts must be made to discontinue corticosteroids in such patients.

Interventional bronchoscopic procedures are needed in a minority of patients who develop severe symptoms due to advanced central airway obstruction. The most common approach is to perform laser photoresection and mechanical debulking of the airways using rigid bronchoscope and large biopsy forceps [18, 41, 59, 102]. Adequate removal of nodules may not be feasible with flexible bronchoscope. Application of laser usually does not vaporize the calcified nodules but makes it easier to extract the lesions with the biopsy forceps. Temporary placement of silicone stent has been needed in some cases [59]. Metallic stents should not be used. In one reported case, bronchoscopic cryotherapy was used to control low-grade chronic hemoptysis [41]. With proper patient selection, successful application of the interventional bronchoscopy procedures has yielded excellent long-term results in severe and symptomatic TO [103]. Unfortunately, in the absence of specific guidelines, the selection of patient for interventional therapy is mostly driven by personal experience and local practices. This is illustrated well by comparing the treatment modalities in two different series of TO patients. In one series of 41 patients, the majority of patients received only symptomatic treatment [12]. Only one patient received laser treatment and one patient required tracheostomy for management of respiratory symptoms. In contrast, in a series from Iran, all 10 patients received laser photoresection, 5 patients underwent core-out procedure with rigid bronchoscope and one patient had airway stent placement [18].

Utmost restraint must be exercised in selecting appropriate patients for interventional bronchoscopy. The fundamental purpose of these procedures is to restore the airway lumen and to relieve symptoms. In the absence of symptoms, interventional bronchoscopic procedures cannot be expected to provide any meaningful benefit to the patients. Interventional bronchoscopy procedures are complicated and expensive and are not without complications. Such procedures must be offered only after a thorough risk–benefit analysis.

Bronchoscopic therapies may not be feasible in some patients who have severe disease and need relief from troubling symptoms [31]. Surgical treatment may be needed in some of these patients. In one report, 4 such patients with severe disease not suitable for interventional bronchoscopic procedures underwent linear tracheoplasty operation [104]. No major complications were encountered. Excellent long-term results were achieved in all patients undergoing the surgery. Respiratory obstruction was relieved, and patients were able to resume normal daily activities. Modified slide tracheoplasty has provided successful long-term outcome in another patient with severe involvement of proximal half of trachea with the disease process [105]. Surgical excision and end-to-end anastomosis of a section of trachea have also been performed in one case with limited but high-grade involvement of central airways [60]. Thus, surgery is a viable option for those who have severe symptoms that cannot be relieved with less invasive options. However, such operations are complicated and must only be performed by an experienced surgeon in an advanced medical facility.

Anesthesia should be carefully planned in patients with known or suspected TO. It is ill-advised to force the ETT if resistance is met as it can cause trauma, bleeding, and inflammatory edema resulting in further airway compromise.

Prognosis

The majority of TO patients follows a benign clinical course. Usually, patients continue to experience mild and non-specific respiratory symptoms after the diagnosis. Clinical course is often punctuated by superimposed lower respiratory tract infection and bacterial pneumonia. Several reported patients have shown no clinical deterioration for as long as 20 years after the diagnosis [63]. Very occasionally, patients have been reported to develop rapidly progressive symptoms and acute respiratory distress [106].

In one series, a repeat bronchoscopy after initial diagnosis was performed in 18 patients [12]. The disease burden remained stable in 10 (55 %) patients. Progression was noted in 8 (45 %) patients, but it was clinically significant only in 3 (17 %) of patients. No regression of lesions was observed.

It must again be stressed that no form of therapy is known to alter the natural history of TO. Therefore, the fundamental purpose of bronchoscopic procedures and surgery is relief of distressing respiratory symptoms. There is no reason to pursue such therapies in asymptomatic or minimally symptomatic patients.

Summary

TO is an uncommon and benign disease characterized by the development of multiple cartilaginous and bony nodules in the anterior and lateral walls of central airways without involving the posterior wall. The underlying cause of TO is still unknown. Most commonly, the disease is diagnosed in 5th to 7th decade of life. The clinical presentation is non-specific with chronic cough, sputum production, intermittent hemoptysis, and breathlessness. In many instances, the diagnosis is discovered as an incidental finding on CT or bronchoscopy performed for unrelated indications. A few patients do develop severe airway compromised and present with severe respiratory distress, hypoxemia, and stridor. Chest CT is the most useful imaging technique, but early disease can easily be missed on CT. Bronchoscopy is the gold standard for diagnosis. The presence of hard nodules arising from anterior and lateral wall of central airways provides strong indication of diagnosis instantly in the bronchoscopy suite. Whether biopsy is essential for diagnosis is a debatable matter. No treatment is needed in asymptomatic or minimally symptomatic patients. Excellent long-term results have been achieved with laser photoresection and mechanical debulking in symptomatic patients with advanced central airway obstruction. Surgery may be needed in some patients who are not suitable for interventional bronchoscopic procedures. However, the majority of patients follows a benign clinical course and requires no specific therapy.

References

1. Prakash U. What is tracheobronchopathia osteochondroplastica? J Bronchol. 2001;8:75–7.
2. Prakash U. Tracheobronchopathia osteochondroplastica. Semin Respir Crit Care Med. 2002;23:167–75.
3. Abu-Hijleh M, Lee D, Braman SS. Tracheobronchopathia osteochondroplastica: a rare large airway disorder. Lung. 2008;186:353–9.
4. Wilks S. Ossific deposits on the larynx, trachea and bronchi. Trans Pathol Soc Lond. 1857;8:88.
5. Virchow R. Die krankhaften Geschwulste. Berlin: Hirschwald; 1863. p. 442–3.
6. Muckleston HS. On so called multiple osteoma of tracheal mucus membrane. Laryngoscope. 1909;19:881–93.
7. Killian G. Ein unter Schwebelaryngoskopie entferter grosser subglottischer Tumor. Laryngol Gesellsch. 1914;17:7.
8. Aschoff-Frieburg L. Ueber tracheopathia osteoplastica. Verh Dtsch Pathol. 1910;14:125–7.
9. Dalgaard JB. Tracheopathia chondro-osteoplastica. A case elucidating the problems concerning development and ossification of elastic cartilage. Acta Pathol Microbiol Scand. 1947;24:118–34.
10. Martin CJ. Tracheobronchopathia osteochondroplastica. Arch Otolaryngol. 1974;100:290–3.
11. Harma RA, Suukari S. Tracheopathia chondro-osteoplastica. A clinical study of thirty cases. Acta Otolaryngol. 1997;84:118–23.
12. Leske V, Lazor R, Coetmeur D, Crestani B, Chatte G, Cordier J-F. Tracheobronchopathia osteochondroplastica. A study of 41 patients. Medicine. 2001;80:378–90.
13. Pounder DJ, Pieterse AS. Tracheopathia osteoplastica: report of four cases. Pathology. 1982;14:429–33.
14. van Nierop MA, Wagennar SS, van den Bosch JM, Westermann CJ. Tracheobronchopathia osteochondroplastica. Report of four cases. Eur J Respir Dis. 1983;64:129–33.
15. Parez-Rodriguez E, Nunez N, Alvarado C, et al. Diagnosis of tracheopathia osteochondroplastica. Chest. 1990;97:763.
16. Briones-Gomez A, Cases-Viedma E, Cordero-Rodriguez PJ, Pietro-Rodriguez M, Sanchis-Aldas JL. Tracheopathia osteoplastica. Series of six cases. J Bronchol. 2000;7:301–5.
17. Bioque JC, Feu N, Rubio JM, et al. Tracheobronchopathia osteochonderoplastica. Clinical study and follow-up in nine cases. J Bronchol. 2001;8:78–83.

18. Jabbardarjani HR, Radpey B, Kharabian S, Masjedi MR. Tracheobronchopathia osteochondroplastica: presentation of ten cases and review of literature. Lung. 2008;186:293–7.
19. Lundgren R, Stjernberg NL. Tracheobronchopathia osteochondroplastica. A clinical bronchoscopic and spirometric study. Chest. 1981;80:706–9.
20. Vilkman S, Keistinen T. Tracheobronchopathia osteochondroplastica. Report of a young man with severe disease and retrospective review of 18 cases. Respiration. 1995;62:151–4.
21. Jindal S, Nath A, Neyaz Z, Jaiswal S. Tracheobronchopathia osteochondroplastica. A rare or an overlooked entity. Radiol Case. 2013;7:16–25.
22. Way SPB. Tracheopathia osteoplastica. J Clin Pathol. 1967;20:814–20.
23. Paaske PB, Tang E. Tracheopathia osteoplastica in the larynx. J Laryngol Otol. 1985;99:305–10.
24. Pounder DJ, Pieterse AS. Tracheopathia osteoplastica. A study of minimal lesion. J Pathol. 1982;138:235–9.
25. Young R, Sandstrom R, Mark G. Tracheopathia osteochondroplastica: clinical, radiologic and pathologic correlation. J Thoracic Cardiovasc Surg. 1980;79:537–41.
26. Miyazono K, Kamiya Y, Morikawa M. Bone morphogenic protein receptors and signal transduction. J Biochem. 2010;147:35–51.
27. Tsumaki N, Yoshikawa H. The role of bone morphogenetic proteins in endochondral bone formation. Cytokines Growth Factor Rev. 2005;16:279–85.
28. Shi S, de Gorter JJ, Hoogaars WMH, 't Hoen PAC, Ten Dijeke P. Overactive bone morphogenic protein signaling in heterotopic ossification and Duchene muscular dystrophy. Cells Mol Life Sci. 2013;70:407–23.
29. Miyazoneo K, Kusanagi K, Inoue H. Divergence and convergence of TGF-β/BMP signaling. J Cell Physiol. 2001;187:265–7.
30. Robey PG, Young MF, Flander KC, et al. Osteoblasts synthesize and respond to transforming growth factor type beta (TGF-β) in vitro. J Cell Biol. 1987;105:457–63.
31. Bonewald LF, Dallas SL. Role of active and latent transforming growth factor-beta in bone formation. J Cell Biochem. 1994;55:350–7.
32. Chen G, Deng C, Li YP. TGF-β and BMP signaling in osteoblast differentiation and bone formation. Int J Biol Sci. 2012;8:272–88.
33. Tajima K, Yamakawa M, Katagiri T, Sasaki H. Immunohistochemical detection of bone morphogenetic protein-2 and transforming growth factor beta-1 in tracheopathia osteochondroplastica. Virchow Arch. 1997;431:359–63.
34. Prakash UB, McCullough AE, Edell ES, Nienhuis DM. Tracheopathia osteoplastica: familial occurrence. Mayo Clin Proc. 1989;64:1091–6.
35. Sakula A. Tracheobronchopathia osteoplastica. Its relationship to primary tracheobronchial amyloidosis. Thorax. 1968;23:105–10.
36. Jones AW, Chatterji AN. Primary tracheobronchial amyloidosis with tracheobronchopathia osteoplastica. Br J Dis Chest. 1977;71:268–72.
37. Alroy GG, Lichtig C, Kaftori JK. Tracheopathia osteoplastica: end stage of primary lung amyloidosis. Chest. 1972;61:465–8.
38. Kirbas G, Dagli CE, Tanrikulu AC, et al. Unusual combination of tracheobronchopathia osteochondroplastica and AA amyloidosis. Yonsei Med J. 2009;50:721–4.
39. Phillips MJ. Tracheopathia osteoplastica. Proc Roy Soc Med. 1976;69:18–9.
40. Piazza C, Cavaliere S, Foccoli P, Toninelli C, Bolzoni A, Peretti G. Endoscopic management of laryngo-tracheobronchial amyloidosis: a series of 32 patients. Eur Arch Otorhinolaryngol. 2003;260:349–54.
41. Nienhuis DM, Prakash UBS, Edell ES. Tracheobronchopathia osteochondroplastica. Ann Otol Rhinol Laryngol. 1990;99:689–94.
42. O'Regan A, Fenlon HM, Beamis JF, Steele MP, Skinner M, Berk JL. Tracheobronchial amyloidosis. The Boston University experience from 1984 to 1999. Medicine. 2000;79:69–79.
43. Diaz-Jimenez JP, Rodriguez A, Ballarin JIM, Castro MJ, Argemi TM, Manresa F. Diffuse tracheobronchial amyloidosis. J Bronchol. 1999;6:13–7.

174   P. Jain and A.C. Mehta

44. Capizzi SA, Betancourt E, Prakash UBS. Tracheobronchial amyloidosis. Mayo Clin Proc. 2000;75:1148–52.
45. Hui AN, Koss MN, Hochholzer L, et al. Amyloidosis presenting in the lower respiratory tract: clinicopathologic, radiologic, immunohistochemical, and histochemical studies on 48 cases. Arch Pathol Lab Med. 1986;110:212–8.
46. Shehata MA. Atrophic rhinitis. Am J Orolaryngol. 1996;17:81–6.
47. Vaheri E, Vaheri E. Tracheopathia osteoplastica. Acta Otolaryngol. 1967;64:251–5.
48. Jepsen O, Sorensen H. Tracheopathia osteoplastica and ozaena. Acta Otolaryngol. 1960;51:79–83.
49. Clee MD, Anderson JM, Johnston RN. Clinical aspects of tracheobronchopathia osteochondroplastica. Br J Dis Chest. 1983;77:308–14.
50. Ferguson J, McCaffrey TV, Kern EB, Martin WJ. Effect of Klebsiella ozaenae on ciliary activity in vitro: implication in the pathogenesis of atrophic rhinitis. Otolaryngol Head Neck Surg. 1990;102:207–11.
51. Al-Ajam MR, Al-Khasawneh KR, Galli WP. Tracheobronchopathia osteochondroplastica. J Bronchol Intervent Pulmonol. 2010;17:149–51.
52. Baugnee PE, Delaunois LM. Mycobacterium avium-intercellulare associated with tracheobronchopathia osteochondroplastica. Eur Respir J. 1995;8:180–2.
53. Shih J-Y, Hsueh P-R, Chang Y-L, et al. Tracheal botryomycosis in a patient with tracheopathia osteochondroplastica. Thorax. 1998;53:73–6.
54. Dincer HE, Dunitz JM. Tracheobronchopathia osteochondroplastica and selective IgA deficiency. J Bronchol Intervent Pulmonol. 2012;19:54–6.
55. Pinheiro GA, Antao VCS, Muller NL. Tracheobronchopathia osteochondroplastica in a patient with silicosis. CT, bronchoscopy and pathology findings. J Comput Assist Tomogr. 2004;28:801–3.
56. Rizzo S. Tracheobronchopathia osteochondroplastica associated with calcification of falx cerebri and rhinobronchial syndrome with nasal polyposis. J Bronchol. 1998;5:128–31.
57. Karlikaya C, Yuksel M, Kilicli S, Candan L. Tracheobronchopathia osteochondroplastica. Respirology. 2000;5:377–80.
58. Erelel M, Yakar F, Bingol ZK, Yakar A. Tracheopathia osteochondroplastica. Two unusual cases. J Bronchol Intervent Pulmonol. 2010;17:241–3.
59. Datau H, Musani AI. Treatment of severe tracheobronchopathia osteochondroplastica. J Bronchol. 2004;11:182–5.
60. Khan AM, Shim C, Simmons N, et al. Tracheobronchopathia osteochondroplastica. A rare cause of tracheal stenosis—TPO stenosis. J Thorac Cardiovasc Surg. 2006;132:714–6.
61. Sant'Anna CC, Pires-de-Mello P, Morgado Mde F, March Mde F. Tracheobronchopathia osteochondroplastica in a 5 year old girl. Indian Pediatr. 2012;49:985–6.
62. Simsek PO, Ozcelik U, Demirkazik F, et al. Tracheobronchopathia osteochondroplastica in a 9-year old girl. Pediatr Pulmonol. 2006;41:95–7.
63. Huang C-C, Kuo C-C. Chronic cough: tracheobronchopathia osteochondroplastica. CMAJ. 2010;182:E859.
64. Pinto JA, da Silva LC, Perfeito DJP, Soares JDS. Osteochondroplastic tracheobronchopathy —report of 2 cases and bibliographic review. Braz J Otolaryngol. 2010;76:789–93.
65. Brend N, Harrison AC, Hartnett BJS, Lawson J, Marlin GE. Tracheobronchopathia osteochondroplastica. Aust NZ J Med. 1979;9:188–92.
66. Los H, Schramel FMNH, van der Harten JJ, Golding RP, Postmus PE. An unusual cause of recurrent fever. Eur Respir J. 1997;10:504–7.
67. Castella J, Puzo C, Cornudella R, Curell R, Tarres J. Tracheobronchopathia osteochondroplastica. Respiration. 1981;42:129–34.
68. Meyer CN, Dossing M, Broholm H. Tracheobronchopathia osteochondroplastica. Respir Med. 1997;91:499–502.
69. Hodges MK, Israel E. Tracheobronchopathia osteochondroplastica presenting as right middle lobe collapse. Diagnosis by bronchoscopy and computerized tomography. Chest. 1988;94:842–4.

70. Doshi H, Thankachen R, Philip MA, Kurien S, Shukla V, Korula RJ. Tracheobronchopathia osteochondroplastica presenting as an isolated nodule in the right upper lobe bronchus with upper lobr collapse. J Thorac Cardiovasc Surg. 2005;130:901–2.
71. Shigematsu Y, Sugio K, Yasuda M, et al. Tracheobronchopathia osteochondroplastica occurring in a subsegmental bronchus and causing obstructive pneumonia. Ann Thorac Surg. 2005;80:1936–8.
72. Smith DC, Pillai R, Gillbe CE. Tracheopathia osteochondroplastica. A cause of unexpected difficulty in tracheal intubation. Anesthesia. 1987;42:536–8.
73. Coetmeur D, Bovyn G, Leroux P, Niel-Duriez M. Tracheobronchopathia osteochondroplastica presenting at the time of a difficult intubation. Respir Med. 1997;91:496–8.
74. Gurunathan U. Tracheobronchopathia osteochondroplastica: a rare cause of difficult intubation. Br J Anesthesia. 2010;104:787–8.
75. Tadjeddein A, Khorgami Z, Akhlaghi H. Tracheobronchopathia osteochondroplastica: a cause of difficult intubation. Ann Thorac Surg. 2006;81:1480–2.
76. Warner MA, Chestnut DH, Thompson G, Bottcher M, Tobert D, Nofftz M. Tracheobronchopathia osteochondroplastica and difficult intubation: case report and perioperative recommendations for anesthesiologists. J Clin Anesthesia. 2013;25:659–61.
77. Martens PR, Van den Brande FG. Failure of one-lung ventilation because of tracheopathia osteoplastica during a heartport procedure with EZ blocker. J Cardiothorac Vasc Anesth. 2010;26:e35.
78. Ishii H, Fugihara H, Ataka T, et al. Successful use of laryngeal mask airway for a patient with tracheal stenosis with tracheobronchopathia osteochondroplastica. Anesth Analg. 2002;95:781–2.
79. Howland WJ Jr, Good CA. Radiographic features of tracheopathia osteochondroplastica. Radiology. 1958;71:847–50.
80. Secrest PG, Kendig TA, Beland AJ. Tracheobronchopathia osteochondroplastica. JAMA. 1964;36:815–8.
81. Ozmen I, Kongar NA, Oruc K, Kiziltas S, Yilmaz A, Calisir HC. Tracheobronchopathia osteochondroplastica. An unusual presentation. J Bronchol Interent Pulmonol. 2010;17:80–3.
82. Zack JR, Rozenshtein A. Tracheobronchopathia osteochondroplastica: report of three cases. J Comput Assist Tomogr. 2002;26:33–6.
83. Mariotta S, Pallone S, Pedicelli G, Bisetti A. Spiral CT and endoscopic findings in a case of tracheobrochopathia osteochondroplastica. J Comput Assist Tomogr. 1997;21:418–20.
84. White BD, Kong A, Khoo E, Southcott AM. Computerized tomography diagnosis of tracheobronchopathia osteochondroplastica. Autralas Radiol. 2005;49:319–21.
85. Restrepo S, Pandit M, Villami MA, Rojas IC, Perez JM, Gascue A. Tracheobronchopathia osteochondroplastica: helical CT findings in 4 cases. J Thorac Imaging. 2004;19:112–6.
86. Al-Busaidi N, Dhuloya D, Habibullah Z. Tracheobronchopathia osteochondroplastica. Case report and literature review. SQU Med J 2012;12:109–12.
87. Hantous-Zannad S, Sebai L, Zidi A, et al. Tracheobronchopathia osteochondroplastica presenting as a respiratory insufficiency: diagnosis by bronchoscopy and MRI. Eur J Radiol 2003;113–6.
88. Tukiainen H, Torkko M, Terho EO. Lung function in patients with tracheobronchopathia osteochondroplastica. Eur Respir J. 1988;1:632–5.
89. Bergeron D, Cormier Y, Desmeules M. Tracheobronchopathia osteochondroplastica. Am Rev Respir Dis. 1976;114:803–6.
90. Smid L, Lavrencak B, Zargi M. Laryngo-tracheo-bronchopathia chondro-osteoplastica. J Laryngol Otol. 1992;106:845–8.
91. Cumbo-Nacheli G, Gildea TR. Autofluorescence pattern in tracheobronchopathia osteochondroplastica. J Bronchol Intervent Pulmonol. 2010;17:368–9.
92. Newton R, Kemp S, Zoumot Z, Yang G-Z, Darzi A, Shah PL. An unusual case of hemoptysis. Thorax. 2010;65:309.

93. Raess PW, Cowan SW, Haas AR, et al. Tracheopathia osteochondroplastica presenting as a single dominant tracheal mass. Ann Diag Pathol. 2011;15:431–5.
94. Riker DR, Campagna AC, Beamis JF. Tracheobronchopathia presenting as hemoptysis associated with vascular endobronchial tumors. J Bronchol. 2007;14:212–4.
95. Rial MB, Fernandez-Villar A, Fernandez VL, et al. Tracheobronchopathia osteochondroplastica: cause of difficult transbronchial needle aspiration. J Bronchol. 2008;15:287–9.
96. Sen RL, Walsh TE. Fiberoptic bronchoscopy for refractory cough. Chest. 1991;99:33–5.
97. Decalmer S, Woodcock A, Greaves M, Howe M, Smith J. Airway abnormalities at flexible bronchoscopy in patients with chronic cough. Eur Respir J. 2007;30:1138–42.
98. Hayes D. Tracheopathia osteoplastica misdiagnosed as asthma. J Asthma. 2007;253–5.
99. Park SS, Shin DH, Lee DH, Jeon SC, Lee JH, Lee JD. Tracheopathia osteoplastica simulating asthmatic symptoms. Diagnosis by bronchoscopy and computerized tomography. Respiration. 1995;62:43–5.
100. Lee KS, Ernst A, Trentham D, Lunn W, Feller-Kopman DJ, Boiselle P. Prevalence of functional airway abnormalities in relapsing polychondritis. Radiology. 2006;240:565–73.
101. Ernst A, Rafeq S, Boiselle P, et al. Relapsing polychondritis and airway involvement. Chest. 2009;135:1024–30.
102. Gleich LL, Rebeiz EE, Pancratov MM, Shapshay SM. The holmium YAG laser assisted otolaryngologic procedures. Arch Otolayrngol Head Neck Surg. 1995;121:1162–6.
103. Tibesar RJ, Edell ES. Tracheopathia osteoplastica: effective long term management. Otolaryngol Head Neck Surg. 2003;129:303–4.
104. Grillo HC, Wright CD. Airway obstruction owing to tracheopathia osteoplastica: treatment by linear tracheoplasty. Ann Thorac Surg. 2005;79:1676–81.
105. Kutlu CA, Yeginsu A, Ozalp T, Baran R. Modified slide tracheoplasty for the management of tracheobronchopathia osteochondroplastica. Eur J Cardiothorac Surg. 2002;21:140–2.
106. Molloy AR, McMohan JN. Rapid progression of tracheal stenosis associated with tracheopathia osteo-chondroplastica. Intensive Care Med. 1988;15:60–2.
107. Acar T. Computed tomography finding of tracheobronchial system disease: a pictorial essay. Jpn J Radiol. 2015;33(2):51–8.

Chapter 8
Endobronchial Tuberculosis

Pyng Lee

Introduction

Involvement of the trachea and major bronchi by tuberculosis was first described by Morton in 1698 [1]. Endobronchial tuberculosis (EBTB), defined as tuberculous infection of the tracheobronchial tree, is not uncommon. Endobronchial involvement was reported in 42 % of 1000 autopsies of patients with tuberculosis [2] and 10–38.8 % of living patients undergoing rigid bronchoscopy [3–5].

EBTB continues to be a major public health problem because its diagnosis is often delayed, and airway stenosis and its attendant complications such as post-obstructive pneumonia, atelectasis, hemoptysis, wheezing, and dyspnea can develop during the course of treatment [6–8]. Owing to HIV infection, poverty, aging population, migration, multidrug resistance, failure in health systems, and rise in diabetes, a resurgence of tuberculosis is observed globally, which accounts for 8.8 million new cases and 1.8 million TB-related deaths each year [9, 10]. It is also likely that HIV may be associated with a higher incidence of EBTB [11, 12]. In this chapter, the pathogenesis, clinical presentation, diagnosis, and current treatment of EBTB are discussed.

Pathogenesis

The pathogenesis of EBTB is not fully understood and is thought to arise from direct implantation of the tubercle bacilli onto the tracheobronchial tree from adjacent pulmonary parenchymal lesion. This theory is supported by finding tuberculosis

P. Lee (✉)
Division of Respiratory and Critical Care Medicine, National University Hospital,
National University of Singapore, 1E Kent Ridge Road,
Singapore 119228, Singapore
e-mail: pyng_lee@nuhs.edu.sg; pynglee@hotmail.com

© Springer International Publishing Switzerland 2016
A.C. Mehta et al. (eds.), *Diseases of the Central Airways*,
Respiratory Medicine, DOI 10.1007/978-3-319-29830-6_8

affecting the bronchus opposite to the airway that drains the tuberculous cavity. Another proposed mechanism is direct airway infiltration by adjacent tuberculous mediastinal lymph node, which is more commonly seen in children. Lymphatic and hematogenous spread to endobronchial tree is rare [13–15]. The clinical course of EBTB can be variable and complex, and is dependent on the interaction between mycobacteria, host immunity, and anti-tuberculous drugs [16, 17].

Clinical Features

EBTB appears to occur more frequently in women in their second and third decades of life even though they have a lower incidence of pulmonary TB [6, 13, 16, 17]. One explanation is the implantation of mycobacteria from infected sputum occurs more frequently in females as they do not expectorate sputum well due to socio-cultural circumstances. Clinical features depend on the type and stage of EBTB. Some patients are asymptomatic, while most complain of productive cough, fever, hemoptysis, hoarseness, chest pain, and generalized weakness [6]. Wheezing can be detected by auscultation in a third of patients erroneously managed as asthma with steroids and decreased air entry in a quarter [8, 18–20]. Diagnosis of EBTB is difficult to establish because similar symptoms can occur as part of pulmonary TB or other respiratory diseases.

Radiology

Chest X-ray can be normal as these lesions are not detectable unless airway obstruction has occurred causing distal atelectasis. Interestingly, the lower or middle lung lobes are affected slightly more often than upper lobes which would favor the direct implantation theory of EBTB by gravity (Fig. 8.1) [6, 8, 16, 18]. Pleural effusions and military tuberculosis may be observed [14, 21]. Computed tomography (CT) is more useful in demonstrating bronchial wall irregularities and lymphadenopathy associated with bronchial lesion, and 3D CT reconstruction for degree and the extent of tracheobronchial stenosis especially if surgery or bronchoscopic intervention is planned (Fig. 8.2a–c) [22, 23].

Laboratory Tests

Sputum smear for acid-fast bacilli (AFB) is positive in 17 % and increases to 79 % when combined with bronchoscopic specimens [6, 18]. This finding is unexpected as EBTB is presumed to yield higher sputum AFB smear positivity. One possible explanation is that sputum expectoration may be difficult due to mucus entrapment

Fig. 8.1 CXR showing left
lower lobe collapse

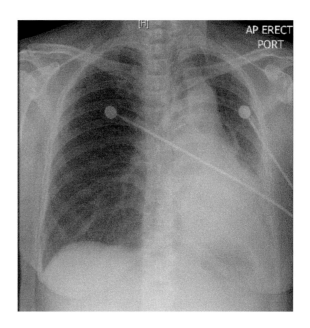

by proximal granulation tissue. Alternatively, mucosal ulceration, which is not seen
in every patient with EBTB, may be necessary for positive AFB smear. Polymerase
chain reaction (PCR) for mycobacteria tuberculosis is increasingly applied to
improve the diagnosis of EBTB [24, 25].

Bronchoscopy and Histopathology

EBTB affects the trachea, main bronchi, and upper bronchi (Fig. 8.3). The presence
of caseating granuloma or acid-fast bacilli is diagnostic for EBTB. Biopsy specimens are diagnostic for EBTB. In some instances, endobronchial biopsies show
non-caseating granuloma, but the presence of Langhan's giant cells in these cases is
helpful in establishing the underlying diagnosis and in excluding sarcoidosis,
fungal, or other granulomatous diseases (Fig. 8.4). Chung and coworkers classified
EBTB into 7 categories (% prevalence): non-specific bronchitis (8 %), actively
caseating (43 %), granular (11 %), edematous hyperemic (14 %), ulcerative (3 %),
tumorous (10.5 %), and fibrostenotic (10.5 %). Serial bronchoscopy was performed
from the diagnosis of EBTB to the completion of anti-tuberculous treatment, and
actively caseating, edematous-hyperemic, tumorous, and fibrostenotic lesions
(Fig. 8.3) demonstrated higher risk of progression to tracheobronchial stenosis
usually within 3 months [6, 26].

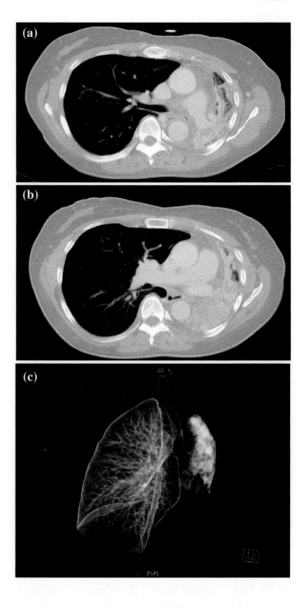

Fig. 8.2 a CT scan of left main bronchial stricture, distal lingular, and lower lobe collapse. **b** CT scan of left lower lobe collapse. **c** 3D CT reconstruction showing LMB stricture with left lung collapse

The classification of EBTB can be explained pathologically by disease progression. The initial lesion is characterized by erythema and lymphocytic infiltration which corresponds to non-specific bronchitis. As the disease advances, submucosal tubercles develop giving it a granular appearance (granular), while marked mucosal edema describes the edematous-hyperemic type. It can undergo caseous necrosis

(a)   (c)

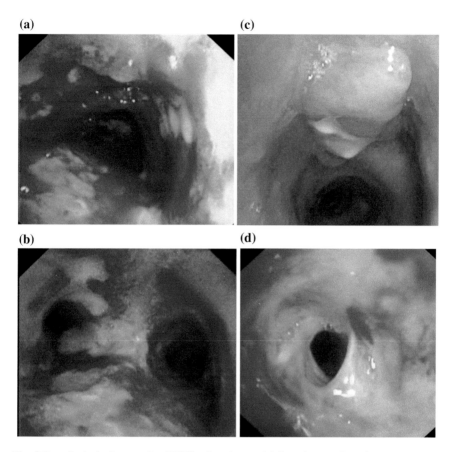

(b)   (d)

Fig. 8.3 a, b Actively caseating EBTB of trachea and left main-stem bronchus. **c** Tumorous EBTB of right upper lobe. **d** Fibrostenotic EBTB of left main bronchus

(actively caseating) or becomes ulcerative if the inflammation continues. The actively caseating or ulcerative lesion can either evolve into hyperplastic–inflammatory polyp (tumorous type) or heal by fibrostenosis [15, 27, 28]. Moreover, the associated intrathoracic tuberculous lymph node can erode and protrude into the airway akin to tumorous EBTB [11, 14, 28]. Rikimaru and coworkers have further divided the ulcerative type into active (stage A), healing (stage H), and scarring (stage S). Only stage A lesions were observed before anti-tuberculous treatment. During 1 and 2 months of therapy, 76 % of ulcerative lesions were in stage A or H, and thereafter, 63 % were in stage S of which one-third of patients developed inflammatory polyps [29].

Fig. 8.4 **a** Mycobacteria stain bright red with Ziehl–Neelsen stain bronchial aspirate. **b** Histology of tumorous EBTB. Medium power view: bronchial wall cartilage and several granulomas with some associated necrosis

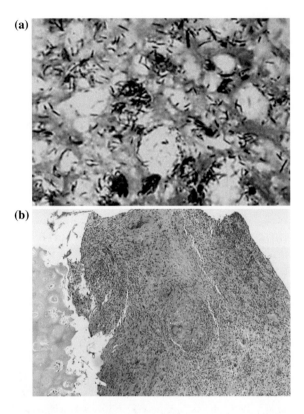

(a)

(b)

Treatment

Active and fibrous subtypes must be differentiated. Fibrous disease is considered as inactive TB, but it can lead to bronchial stenosis which can be a challenging sequel to EBTB during or after treatment.

Active EBTB

The most important goal of treatment is in the eradication of tubercle bacilli without selecting drug-resistant mycobacteria. The second most important goal is in the prevention of tracheobronchial stenosis. Chemotherapy eradicates tubercle bacilli except for multidrug-resistant TB, while the sequel of tracheobronchial stricture is atelectasis with dyspnea or obstructive pneumonia. Tracheobronchial strictures can develop despite prompt anti-tuberculous therapy [6, 8, 16, 26], and previously topical silver nitrate application has been attempted for ulcerative EBTB [30, 31] and electrosurgery via rigid bronchoscopy for tumorous or polypoidal lesions [32]. A recent systematic review and meta-analysis conclude that steroids could be effective in reducing mortality for all forms of tuberculosis including PTB [33]. However, the role of corticosteroids in preventing fibrostenosis consequent to EBTB remains controversial. Two prospective, randomized, placebo-controlled studies of children with endobronchial obstruction from enlarged tuberculous hilar lymph nodes demonstrated the significant improvement in the group treated with steroids [34, 35]. However, only one such randomized study is available in adults which did not show any difference in the rate of bronchial strictures between the steroid-treated and placebo groups. It was a small study, and timing of initiation of systemic steroids could contribute to the negative results. There are case reports that show favorable response to both systemic and endoscopic injection of steroids [36].

Shim recommends steroids for the edematous-hyperemic, actively caseating, and tumorous types as these tend to progress to tracheobronchial stenoses. Prednisolone at 1 mg/kg is prescribed for 4–6 weeks followed by slow taper for the same duration [37]. In 1963, Nemir et al. [38] observed that short course of prednisone of less than 4 months was effective adjunct to the anti-tuberculous therapy for EBTB. Song et al. [39] also observed good response if steroids were initiated within 3 months of symptoms and concluded that steroids were beneficial in early-phase EBTB, but had no impact on bronchial stenosis. Rikumaru et al. [40] observed that heal time for ulcerative EBTB was shorter, and bronchial stenosis less severe if patients were treated with twice daily aerosol therapy of streptomycin 100 mg, dexamethasone 0.5 mg, and naphazoline 0.1 mg in addition to anti-tuberculous therapy. Um et al. [41] found that age >45 years, fibrostenotic subtype, and >90 days between symptom onset and the initiation of anti-tuberculosis chemotherapy were independent predictors of persistent airway stenosis, and oral corticosteroids (prednisolone equivalent ≥30 mg/d) did not reduce the frequency of airway stenosis. It is apparent that steroids do not affect the regression of fibrostenotic lesions, but ameliorate inflammation and edema in the early phase of EBTB.

Fibrous EBTB

An important sequel of EBTB is bronchial stenosis which causes atelectasis and secondary obstructive pneumonia. Patients present with dyspnea and wheezing. As steroids are unable to reverse stenosis, airway patency must be restored by surgery or bronchoscopic intervention. Surgical resection of an atelectatic lung with stenotic main-stem bronchus (pneumonectomy) has been normal practice (Fig. 8.5a, b), but lung-sparing surgery such as sleeve resection, carina resection, and end-to-end anastomosis is increasingly performed [42–44]. Bronchoscopic techniques that

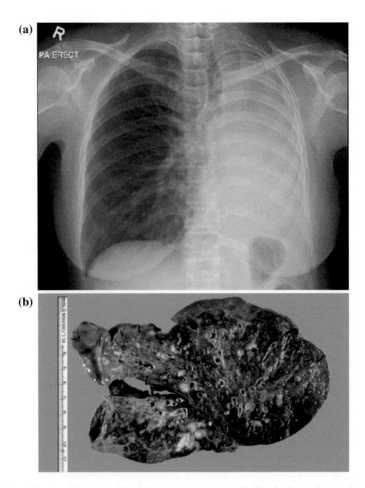

Fig. 8.5 a Chest radiograph after left pneumonectomy. **b** Surgical specimen shows lung atelectasis with areas of caseous necrosis

include laser, electrosurgery, argon plasma coagulation, cryotherapy, and balloon bronchoplasty have been applied singly or in combination to restore airway patency (Fig. 8.6a–h) [45–54]. Silicon stents are deployed following airway recanalization and dilatation as adjunct to the management of complex strictures (Fig. 8.7a, b) [55–57]. Metallic stents should be avoided since they are difficult to remove due to airway epithelization [57, 58]. Complications after dilatation and stenting include airway perforation, stent migration, and stent-related obstructing granuloma, which can cause subcutaneous emphysema, pneumothorax, pneumomediastinum, mediastinitis, dyspnea, and hemoptysis [58]. A patient who received silicon stent for post-TB complex stricture developed obstructing granuloma that was successfully

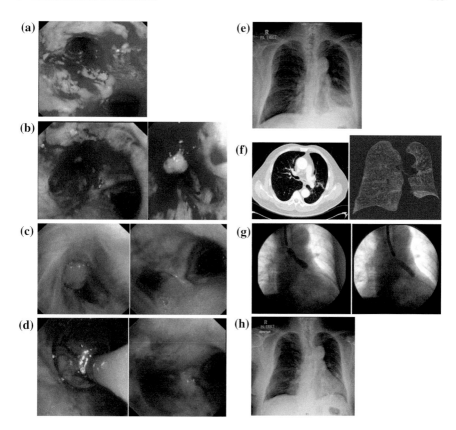

Fig. 8.6 a Actively caseating EBTB left main bronchus. **b** Bronchoscopy after 3 months of anti-tubercular treatment showed progression to tumorous EBTB of left main bronchus. **c** After completion of anti-tubercular treatment, bronchoscopy showed tumorous EBTB with stricture of left main bronchus. **d** Balloon bronchoplasty of left main bronchus was performed. **e** Pre-dilation chest radiograph showed left lower lobe collapse–consolidation. **f** Chest computed tomography with 3D reconstruction showed left main bronchial stricture. **g** Fluoroscopy during balloon bronchoplasty of left main bronchial stricture. **h** Chest radiograph post-balloon bronchoplasty shows re-expansion of left lower lobe

treated with laser and topical mitomycin C application [59]. It is challenging to determine who will respond to interventional procedures and who will need surgery. Lee and coworkers reported that with interventional treatment, only 30 % of patients experienced successful re-expansion defined as recovery of lung volume >80 % of estimated original volume; these patients were younger median age 22 years versus 34 years. The presence of parenchymal calcification as well as bronchiectasis within the atelectasis showed higher tendency for failure, while mucus plugging, extent of airway narrowing, volume loss on CT, and endobronchial TB activity at the time of intervention did not affect lung re-expansion [60].

Fig. 8.7 **a** Fibrostenotic left
main stricture, **b** radial cuts
applied with electrosurgical
knife, dilated with balloon
bronchoplasty and silicon
stent placement

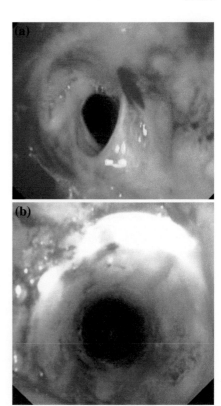

Conclusions

Diagnosis of EBTB is often delayed as it is difficult to detect on chest radiograph.
Symptoms of hemoptysis, wheezing, and dyspnea as well as chest X-ray finding of
atelectasis should alert the physician of EBTB. EBTB is divided into 7 categories
based on bronchoscopic appearances, and actively caseating, edematous-
hyperemic, tumorous, and fibrostenotic lesions demonstrate higher risk of progression to tracheobronchial stenosis. Airway strictures occur in up to two-thirds of
EBTB, and steroids when instituted early can prevent progression to tracheobronchial stenosis. Aerosol therapy comprising of streptomycin and corticosteroid
is also an effective adjunct to anti-tuberculous treatment. 3D reconstruction CT is
not only useful in the planning of bronchoscopic intervention or surgery and it can
also be a means to follow-up EBTB during therapy instead of bronchoscopy.
Patients with airway strictures consequent to EBTB will require surgery or bronchoscopic procedures which may include laser, electrocautery, argon plasma
coagulation or cryotherapy, balloon bronchoplasty, or stent.

References

1. Hudson EH. Respiratory tuberculosis–clinical diagnosis. In: Heaf ERG, editors. Symposium on tuberculosis. London: Cassell & Co.;1957. p. 321–464.
2. Auerbach O. Tuberculosis of the trachea and major bronchi. Am Rev Tuberc. 1949;60:604–20.
3. Judd AR. Tuberculous tracheobronchitis. J Thorac Surg. 1947;16:512–23.
4. MacRae DM, Hiltz JE, Quinlan JJ. Bronchoscopy in a sanatorium. Am Rev Tuberc. 1950;61:355–68.
5. Jokinen K, Palva T, Nuutinen J. Bronchial findings in pulmonary tuberculosis. Clin Otolaryngol. 1997;2:139–48.
6. Lee JH, Park SS, Lee DH, et al. Endobronchial tuberculosis: clinical and bronchoscopic features in 121 cases. Chest. 1992;102:990–4.
7. Albert RK, Petty TL. Endobronchial tuberculosis progressing to bronchial stenosis. Chest. 1976;70:537–9.
8. Hoheisel G, Chan BK, Chan CH, et al. Endobronchial tuberculosis: diagnostic features and therapeutic outcome. Respir Med. 1994;88:593–7.
9. Dye C, Watt CJ, Bleed DM, et al. Evolution of tuberculosis control and prospects for reducing tuberculosis incidence, prevalence and deaths globally. J Am Med Assoc. 2005;293:2767–75.
10. World Health Organization. 47th World Health Assembly: Provisional Agenda Item 19. Tuberculosis Programme—Progress Report by the Director-General. Document WHA47/1994/A47/12. Geneva, Switzerland: World Health Organization;1994.
11. Judson MA, Sahn SA. Endobronchial lesion in HIV infected individuals. Chest. 1994;105:1314–23.
12. Calpe JL, Chiner E, Larramendi CH. Endobronchial tuberculosis in HIV infected patients. AIDS. 1995;9:59–64.
13. Smart J. Endobronchial tuberculosis. Br J Tuberc Dis Chest. 1951;45:61–8.
14. Matthews JI, Matarese SL, Carpenter JL. Endobronchial tuberculosis simulating lung cancer. Chest. 1984;86:642–4.
15. Smith LS, Schillaci RF, Sarlin RF. Endobronchial tuberculosis: serial fiberoptic bronchoscopy and natural history. Chest. 1987;91:644–7.
16. Kim YH, Kim HT, Lee KS, et al. Serial fiberoptic bronchoscopic observations of endobronchial tuberculosis before and early after antituberculous chemotherapy. Chest. 1993;103:673–7.
17. Chan HS, Pang JA. Effect of corticosteroids on deterioration of endobronchial tuberculosis during chemotherapy. Chest. 1989;96:1195–6.
18. Ip MS, So SY, Lam WK, Mok CK. Endobronchial tuberculosis revisited. Chest. 1986;89:727–30.
19. Kurasawa T, Kuze F, Kawai M, et al. Diagnosis and management of endobronchial tuberculosis. Intern Med. 1992;31:593–8.
20. Williams DJ, York EL, Norbert EJ, et al. Endobronchial tuberculosis presenting as asthma. Chest. 1988;93:836–8.
21. Rikumaru T, Kinosita M, Yano H, et al. Diagnostic features and therapeutic outcome of erosive and ulcerous endobronchial tuberculosis. Int J Tuberc Lung Dis. 1998;2:558–62.
22. Lacrosse M, Trigaux JP, van Beers BE, et al. 3D spiral CT of the tracheobronchial tree. J Coput Assist Tomogr. 1995;19:341–7.
23. Lee KS, Yoon JH, Kim TK, et al. Evaluation of tracheobronchial disease with helical CT with multiplanar and three-dimensional reconstruction: correlation with bronchoscopy. Radiographics. 1997;17:555–67.
24. Lee SH, Kim SW, Lee S. Rapid detection of mycobacterium tuberculosis using a novel ultra-fast chip-type real-time PCR system. Chest. 2014. doi:10.1378/chest.14-0626. (Epub ahead of print).
25. Kim CH, Woo H, Hyun IG, et al. A comparison between the efficiency of the Xpert MTB/RIF assay and nested PCR in identifying mycobacterium tuberculosis during routine clinical practice. J Thorac Dis. 2014;6:625–31.

26. Chung HS, Lee JH. Bronchoscopic assessment of the evolution of endobronchial tuberculosis. Chest. 2000;117:385–92.
27. Salkin D, Cadden AV, Edson RC. The natural history of tuberculous tracheobronchitis. Am Rev Tuberc. 1943;47:351–9.
28. Medlar EM. The behavior of pulmonary tuberculosis lesions: a pathological study. Am Rev Tuberc. 1955;71:1–244.
29. Rikimaru T, Tanaka Y, Ichikawa Y, et al. Endoscopic classification of tracheobronchial tuberculosis with healing processes. Chest. 1994;105:318–9.
30. Sharp JC, Gorham CB. Routine bronchoscopy in tuberculosis. Am Rev Tuberc. 1940;41:708–18.
31. Judd AR. Tuberculous tracheobronchitis. J Thorac Surg. 1947;16:512–23.
32. Packard JS, Davison FW. Treatment of tuberculous tracheobronchitis. Am Rev Tuberc. 1938;38:758–68.
33. Critchley JA, Young F, Orton L, et al. Corticosteroids for prevention of mortality in people with tuberculosis: a systematic review and meta-analysis. Lancet Infect Dis. 2013;13:223–37.
34. Nemir RL, Cardiba FV, Toledo R. Prednisone as an adjunct in the chemotherapy of lymph node-bronchial tuberculosis in childhood: a double-blind study. Am Rev Respir Dis. 1967;95:402–10.
35. Topper M, Malfrost A, Derde MP, et al. Corticosteroids in primary tuberculosis with bronchial obstruction. Arch Dis Child. 1990;65:1222–6.
36. Park IW, Choi BW, Hue S. Prospective study of corticosteroid as an adjunct in the treatment of endobronchial tuberculosis in adults. Respirology. 1997;2:275–81.
37. Shim YS. Endobronchial tuberculosis. Respirology. 1996;1:95–106.
38. Nemir RL, Cardona J, Lacoius A, et al. Prednisone therapy as an adjunct in the treatment of lymph node, bronchial tuberculosis in childhood. A double blind study. Am Rev Respir Dis. 1963;88:189–98.
39. Song JH, Han SK, Heo IM. Clinical study on endobronchial tuberculosis. Tuberc Respir Dis. 1985;32:276–82.
40. Rikimaru T, Kinosita M, Yano H, et al. Diagnostic features and therapeutic outcome of erosive and ulcerous endobronchial tuberculosis. Int J Tuberc Lung Dis. 1998;2:558–62.
41. Um SW, Yoon YS, Lee SM, et al. Predictors of persistent airway stenosis in patients with endobronchial tuberculosis. Int J Tuberc Lung Dis. 2008;12:57–62.
42. Nakamoto K, Tse CY, Hong B, et al. Carina resection for stenotic tuberculous tracheitis. Thorax. 1988;43:492–3.
43. Bisson A, Bonnette P, El Kadi NB, et al. Tracheal sleeve resection for iatrogenic stenoses (subglottic laryngeal and tracheal). J Thorac Cardiovasc Surg. 1992;104:882–7.
44. Lei Y, Tian-Hui Z, Ming H, et al. Analysis of the surgical treatment of endobronchial tuberculosis (EBTB). Surg Today. 2014. (Epub ahead of print).
45. Liu AC, Mehta AC, Golish JA. Upper airway obstruction due to tuberculosis: treatment by photocoagulation. Postgrad Med. 1985;78:275–8.
46. Dumon JF, Reboud E, Garbe L, et al. Treatment of tracheobronchial lesions by laser photoreaction. Chest. 1982;81:278–84.
47. Tong MC, van Hasselt CA. Tuberculous tracheobronchial strictures: clinicopathological features and management with the bronchoscopic carbon dioxide laser. Eur Arch Otorhinolaryngol. 1993;250:110–4.
48. Hooper RG, Jackson FN. Endobronchial electrocautery. Chest. 1985;87:712–4.
49. Morice RC, Ece T, Ece F, et al. Endobronchial argon plasma coagulation for treatment of hemoptysis and neoplastic airway obstruction. Chest. 2001;119:781–7.
50. Jin F, Mu D, Xie Y, et al. Application of bronchoscopic argon plasma coagulation in the treatment of tumorous endobronchial tuberculosis: historical controlled trial. J Thorac Cardiovasc Surg. 2013;145:1650–3.
51. Mathur PN, Wolf KM, Busk MF, et al. Fiberoptic bronchoscopic cryotherapy in the management of tracheobronchial obstruction. Chest. 1996;110:718–23.
52. Nakamura K, Terada N, Ohi M, et al. Tuberculous bronchial stenosis: treatment with balloon bronchoplasty. AJR Am J Roentgenol. 1991;157:1187–8.

53. Sheski FD, Mathur PN. Long-term results of fiberoptic bronchoscopic balloon dilation in the management of benign tracheobronchial stenosis. Chest. 1998;114:796–800.
54. Mehta AC, Lee FY, Cordasco EM, et al. Concentric tracheal and subglottic stenosis. Management using the Nd-YAG laser for mucosal sparing followed by gentle dilatation. Chest. 1993;104:673–7.
55. Dumon JF. A dedicated tracheobronchial stent. Chest. 1990;97:328–32.
56. Petrous M, Kaplan D, Goldstraw P. Bronchoscopic diathermy resection and stent insertion: a cost effective treatment for tracheobronchial obstruction. Thorax. 1993;48:1156–9.
57. Iwamoto Y, Miyazawa T, Kurimoto N, et al. Interventional bronchoscopy in the management of airway stenosis due to tracheobronchial tuberculosis. Chest. 2004;126:1344–52.
58. Lee P, Kupeli E, Mehta AC. Airway stents. Clin Chest Med. 2010;31:141–50.
59. Penafiel A, Lee P, Hsu A, Eng P. Topical Mitomycin-C for obstructing endobronchial granuloma. Ann Thorac Surg. 2006;82:22–3.
60. Lee JY, Chin AY, Kim TS, et al. CT scan features as predictors of patient outcome after bronchial intervention in endobronchial TB. Chest. 2010;138:380–5.

Chapter 9
Endobronchial Fungal Infections

Atul C. Mehta, Tanmay S. Panchabhai and Demet Karnak

Introduction

Endobronchial fungal infections (EBFIs), though infrequent, are being recognized with increasing frequency with widespread use of flexible bronchoscopy. Predisposing causes of EBFIs are listed in Table 9.1. These infections are most likely a consequence of initial colonization in patients receiving immunosuppressive therapy [1] or those who are on continuous mechanical ventilation [2]. Lung or other solid organ transplantation and diabetes mellitus are other major risk factors for EBFI. The purpose of this chapter is to highlight the presentation of EBFI and its associated complications and mortality and to outline suggested management therapies.

Salient clinical features of EBFIs are summarized in Table 9.2. *Aspergillus* species, *Coccidioides immitis*, Zygomycetes, *Candida* species, *Cryptococcus neoformans*, and *Histoplasma capsulatum* are the most common agents that cause EBFI [3]. Although full demographic information is incomplete in patients with EBFIs, coccidioidomycosis was reported more frequently in younger patients, with a mean age of 30 years. Most EBFIs seemed to occur in males and male/female

A.C. Mehta
Lerner College of Medicine, Buoncore Family Endowed Chair in Lung Transplantation, Respiratory Institute, Cleveland Clinic, Cleveland, OH, USA
e-mail: Mehtaa1@ccf.org

A.C. Mehta
Department of Pulmonary Medicine, Respiratory Institute, Cleveland Clinic, Cleveland, OH, USA

T.S. Panchabhai
Advanced Lung Disease and Lung Transplant Programs, Norton Thoracic Institute, St. Joseph's Hospital and Medical Center, Phoenix, AZ, USA

D. Karnak
Department of Chest Disease, Ankara University School of Medicine, Mamak Street, 06100 Ankara, Turkey

© Springer International Publishing Switzerland 2016
A.C. Mehta et al. (eds.), *Diseases of the Central Airways*, Respiratory Medicine, DOI 10.1007/978-3-319-29830-6_9

Table 9.1 Predisposing factors for fungal infections

Acute leukemia or lymphoma during myeloablative chemotherapy
Bone marrow or peripheral blood stem cell transplantation
Solid organ transplantation on immunosuppressive therapy
Prolonged corticosteroid therapy
Acquired immunodeficiency syndrome
Prolonged neutropenia from various causes
Congenital immune deficiency syndromes
Postsplenectomy state
Genetic predisposition
Living in a building with ongoing construction
Diabetic ketoacidosis
Travel to endemic region

Table 9.2 Fungal infections and clinical features

Infection type	Clinical features
Aspergillosis	• Fever • Cough and dyspnea • Hemoptysis—blood vessel invasion • Expectorated fungal casts—like the shape of the bronchial tree • Hypoxia • Signs of airway dehiscence-lung transplant patients • Parenchymal invasion—with tracheobronchial and pseudomembranous forms • Pseudomembranous form—usually fatal despite treatment
Coccidioidomycosis	• Dyspnea and stridor from parenchymal disease and extrinsic compression from enlarged lymph nodes
Zygomycosis	• Rapid and sometimes indolent course, asymptomatic • Severe fatal diffuse pulmonary infection—who inhaled a large inoculum • Contiguous structure involvement such as the mediastinum and heart • Hemoptysis and death—angioinvasive form • Affects large bronchi • Dyspnea and hemoptysis from bronchoarterial fistulas
Candidiasis	• In immunocompromised cases—with other fungi such as *Aspergillus* and *Mucor*
Cryptococcosis	• Dyspnea and hemoptysis • Fever, cough, and headache • Acute respiratory distress syndrome • Seen also in immunocompetent host

Histoplasmosis	• Asymptomatic
	• Self-limiting influenza-like illness
	• Symptoms based on:
	    – the extent of exposure,
	    – underlying lung disease,
	    – general immune status and specific immunity
	• Mediastinal lymph nodes—most common site of involvement
	• Expectoration of broncholiths: a rare manifestation

(M/F) ratios for each type of EBFI listed above was as follows: aspergillosis (1.7/1), coccidioidomycosis (3.8/1), zygomycosis (2.5/1), candidiasis (2/1), and crypto-coccosis (3.5/1). Interestingly, histoplasmosis has been reported more frequently in female patients, with an M/F ratio of 0.4/1 [3]. Endemic fungal infections seem to be more common in men than in women, perhaps because estrogen may have an inhibitory effect on the growth cycle of fungi [4].

Endobronchial Aspergillosis

Aspergillus species commonly colonize airways in immunosuppressed patients and have been recovered from as many as 57 % patients with cystic fibrosis [5]. *Aspergillus* species remain the primary fungal cause of infection in patients' postlung transplantation with infection rates ranging up to 22 % [6, 7]. Most *aspergillus* infections fit into the category of invasive pulmonary aspergillosis and up to 20 % of patients have simultaneous tracheobronchial involvement [8, 9]. *A. fumigatus*, *A. flavus*, *A. nidulans*, and *A. niger* are the types of aspergillosis infections most commonly reported in the literature.

Aspergillus **spp.** in the tracheobronchial and pulmonary systems may present with a wide variety of manifestations [10]. Alveolar macrophages normally are capable of killing the *aspergillus* conidia. If these cells are low in number or are defective, the *Aspergillus* conidia will begin to germinate and form hyphae. During hyphal growth, the fungus produces various metabolites, such as complement inhibitors, proteases, and mycotoxins that help to negate host defenses [10]. Predisposing factors which support hyphal growth include immunosuppressive drugs, radiation therapy, antilymphocytic therapy, hematopoietic malignancy, granulocytopenia, uremia, diabetes mellitus, aplastic anemia, and miliary tubercu-losis (Table 9.1) [11]. The mechanisms by which lung transplant recipients have a unique predilection for aspergillosis are as follows: direct exposure of the trans-planted organ to the environment, impairment in local host defenses (i.e., mucociliary clearance and cough reflex), disruption of lymphatic drainage, ischemic airway injury, altered alveolar phagocytic function, and overall greater requirement of immunosuppression all of which can cause airway colonization and disease process by *Aspergillus* [12, 13]. Patients who undergo pulmonary resection surgery could also develop bronchial stump aspergillosis. Bronchial stump infections by *Aspergillus* can be reduced by using unbraided nylon monofilament instead of silk sutures [14].

The various forms of tracheobronchial aspergillosis include invasive tracheo-bronchitis, ulcerative tracheobronchitis, and pseudomembranous tracheobronchitis. Histopathological examination is key to distinguish these entities from one another.

Fever is not a common symptom as the patients are usually immunocompro-mised. Most patients present with worsening dyspnea or hemoptysis, the latter occurs due to direct invasion of the blood vessel wall (Table 9.2).

Table 9.3 Radiologic features in the endobronchial fungal infections

Infection type	Radiologic features
Aspergillosis	• Air crescent sign—aspergilloma • Halo sign—invasive aspergillosis • Tracheal or bronchial wall thickening • Proximal bronchiectasis • Airway plaques and patchy centrilobular nodules branching linear–nodular areas having a "tree-in-bud" appearance • Segmental lung collapse—obstructive fungal casts
Coccidioidomycosis	• Pulmonary infiltrates including pneumonia • Nodules with cavities • Miliary pattern • Hilar or mediastinal lymphadenopathy
Zygomycosis	• Focal consolidation • Mass effect • Signs of infarction • Cavitary lesion • Air crescent sign
Candidiasis	• No specific findings • Normal chest X-ray
Cryptococcosis	• Well-defined, small, non-calcified nodules • Lobar infiltrates • Hilar or mediastinal adenopathy • Pleural effusions • Fungus ball appearance • Abscess with air-fluid level
Histoplasmosis	• Solitary nodule to fibrocystic disease • Fibrosing mediastinitis • Interstitial markings • Lymph node enlargement—calcification • Splenic calcifications—prior histoplasmosis

Although varied radiographic findings are seen in different forms of pulmonary **aspergillosis**, in the appropriate clinical setting, the presence of the "air crescent sign" of aspergilloma or the "halo sign" of invasive aspergillosis on computed tomography of the chest may support clinical suspicion of EB aspergillosis (Table 9.3) [10, 15]. Tracheal or bronchial wall thickening, proximal bronchiectasis, airway plaques, and patchy centrilobular nodules or branching linear nodular areas having a "tree-in-bud" appearance may be other direct or indirect signs of tracheobronchial aspergillosis on a high-resolution CT. Obstructive bronchial aspergillosis can cause lobar or segmental lung collapse due to obstructive fungal casts [16, 17].

Among lung transplant recipients, tracheobronchial aspergillosis may be diagnosed on routine surveillance bronchoscopies. The pseudomembranous form is the most severe condition and is usually fatal despite treatment with antifungal agents. Tracheobronchial aspergillosis is an obstructive form of bronchial aspergillosis [17]. Patients with obstructive bronchial aspergillosis can expectorate fungal casts in the shape of the bronchial tree. Aspergillosis is often found in EB mucosa in association with other presentations of *Aspergillus* infection and hence its nature (primary or secondary) is difficult to establish [10, 18]. In a review of pulmonary aspergillosis, tracheobronchial aspergillosis was described in 16 % of patients. Of these, invasive tracheobronchitis, ulcerative tracheobronchitis, and pseudomembranous tracheobronchitis were reported in 7, 10, and 7 % of patients, respectively. Obstructive bronchial aspergillosis was seen in 5 % of patients. Parenchymal invasion was seen with tracheobronchial and pseudomembranous forms in 7 and 6 % of patients, respectively [3]. Combined forms of tracheobronchial and allergic bronchopulmonary aspergillosis together and obstructive bronchial aspergillosis and organizing pneumonia were found very rarely. Aspergilloma with EB involvement was the least common combination (4 %) [14, 19].

Data regarding the utility of the galactomannan antigen assay, the beta-D-glucan assay, or the polymerase chain reaction (PCR) for the diagnosis of invasive aspergillosis in the lung transplant recipients are limited [20]. Using an index cutoff value of ≥1, the assay had a sensitivity of 60 % and a specificity of 98 % [6]. A retrospective study compared performance of an *Aspergillus* real-time PCR assay with the galactomannan assay in 150 BAL specimens from lung transplant recipients who underwent bronchoscopy for surveillance or diagnostic evaluation [21]. The sensitivity and specificity of an *Aspergillus fumigatus*-specific PCR were 85 and 96 %, respectively, and the sensitivity and specificity of the galactomannan assay (using a cutoff value ≥0.5) were 93 and 89 %, respectively. Beta-D-glucan is a cell wall component of all fungi. Serum assays for beta-D-glucan to screen for invasive fungal infections including *Aspergillus* spp., Candida spp., Pneumocystis, and other fungi are available. However, they have not been adequately studied in lung transplant recipients.

Coccidioidomycosis

Coccidioidomycosis is an endemic fungal infection with approximately 100,000 cases being newly diagnosed every year and 0.5 % progressing to disseminated coccidioidomycosis [21]. This infection occurs after inhalation of arthroconidia and can be seen in any age group. The true incidence of endobronchial involvement is, however, unknown. Coccidioidomycosis is reported in 1–8 % of all cases of solid organ transplantation in endemic areas [22]. Infection by *C. immitis* is also common in other groups of immunosuppressed patients [23]. Spores of *C. immitis* (3–5 μm) can travel as far as the terminal airways or even the alveoli. Once an arthroconidium is inhaled, it transforms to a spherical structure of 70 μm or larger with internal septations. Within each of the subcompartments of spherical structures, individual cells, called endospores, evolve. After several days, mature spherules rupture, releasing endospores, which are capable of producing more spherules. Cell-mediated or humoral immunity of normal individuals can block the last step of dissemination using macrophages and complement activation [24]. However, immunocompromised hosts, especially infants, pregnant females, diabetic patients, non-Caucasians, and patients with human immunodeficiency virus (HIV), are considered to be at increased risk of developing the disease [22]. Patients at particular risk for coccidioidomycosis include African Americans and patients with low CD4 cell counts (<200–250 cells/μL), or those with a history of oropharyngeal or esophageal candidiasis. Patients on protease inhibitor therapy may have a reduced risk [1].

In **coccidiomycosis**, dyspnea and stridor are the most common symptoms due to either the parenchymal disease or extrinsic compression of the airway by the enlarged lymph nodes [3]. **Coccidioidomycosis** produces a wide variety of pulmonary infiltrates including pneumonia and nodules with cavities or miliary pattern [24]. In a review, 16 % of patients had disease confined to trachea and/or mainstem bronchus without evidence of parenchymal disease, but 37 % of them had infiltrates. One patient later developed cavitary lesion and 31 % of them had hilar or mediastinal lymphadenopathy [3].

Zygomycosis

Zygomycosis (Mucormycosis) is an opportunistic infection from fungi of the class Zygomycetes. Of all the species causing infections in humans (*Mucor, Rhizopus, Absidia*, and *Chlamydoconidia*), *Mucor* is the most common culprit. It is a ubiquitous organism, abundantly present in soil and decaying matter. It enters the body by inhalation of aerosolized spores [19, 25]. In over 90 case reports of pulmonary mucormycosis, 34 % had endobronchial (EB) involvement and *Mucor* was isolated in over 64 % cases [3]. **Zygomycetes** have an enzyme, ketone reductase that allows them to thrive in high-glucose environments and hence patients with uncontrolled diabetes are at higher risk. Iron overload and deferoxamine therapy also increase the risk of mucormycosis [26]. The deferoxamine–iron chelate, called feroxamine, is absiderophore for the Zygomycetes; increased iron uptake by the fungus stimulates fungal growth and may lead to clinical infection. The increased serum iron in diabetic patients from impaired transferrin binding may also contribute to their increased risk of infection. The most common underlying condition in EB mucormycosis was diabetes mellitus (65 %) in one study [26]. Hematologic malignancies, prolonged neutropenia, treatment with corticosteroids or deferoxamine, bronchogenic cancer, renal transplantation and acquired immunodeficiency syndrome were other reported risk factors [19, 25]. The pace of **mucormycosis** is usually rapid, yet there are a few descriptions of an indolent course. Most healthy individuals with low-inoculum exposure remain asymptomatic for a considerable period of time. However, patients who inhale a large inoculum often develop a severe and potentially fatal diffuse pulmonary infection [27]. Lungs are the most common site of *Mucor* infection, which may then spread to contiguous structures such as the mediastinum and heart. As it is an angioinvasive organism, infarction is its hallmark and hemoptysis is a common clinical symptom as well as cause of death. If EB involvement occurs, it mainly affects large bronchi and is also associated with high mortality [27, 28]. Patients with EB disease mainly present with dyspnea and hemoptysis; the latter can sometimes be massive due to angioinvasion leading to bronchoarterial fistulas (19 %) [3].

In patients with EB mucormycosis, radiographic findings are usually non-specific and can vary from focal consolidation to mass effect [27–29]. Specific radiologic signs of infarction, or cavitary lesions including air crescent sign, have seldom been reported [3].

Endobronchial Candidiasis

Candida species are normal commensals of the human skin and gastrointestinal tract. Esophageal and laryngeal candidiasis are well described in the literature, but EB candidiasis is less commonly recognized. One study, however, found that 57 % of EB involvements were among lung transplant recipients. Most EB infections are caused by *Candida albicans* and produce unilateral bronchial involvement. Tracheal involvement with *C. albicans* has been reported in 2 cases, and there is a single published case report of *C. parapsilosis* with fungus ball formation [3]. Conditions that predispose to the development of **Candidiasis** are age, endocrine disorders, malignancy, alteration of immunologic status, antibiotic therapy, neutropenia, and aplastic anemia. In immunocompromised hosts, *Candida* infection can occur in association with other fungi such as *Aspergillus* and *Mucor* [30]. Clinical manifestations of EB infection with candida range from those related to local mucosal infections to widespread dissemination with multisystem organ failure [31].

For EB **candidiasis**, there are no specific radiographic findings mentioned in the literature [32]. Almost every case reported in the literature had a normal chest radiograph.

Cryptococcosis

Cryptococcosis is caused by the yeast-like fungus *C. neoformans*. Thought it can be found worldwide, it has a higher prevalence in the USA and in Australia [16]. The reported incidence of new cases of cryptococcosis is 1.9 in males and 0.26 in females per 100,000 in endemic regions such as California, and 0.02–0.03 in other parts of the USA [33]. Humans become infected by inhaling basidiospores which have small polysaccharide capsules that facilitates its deposition in the alveoli and terminal bronchioles [34]. The incidence of direct airway involvement is unknown. In total, 8.3 % of patients with acquired immunodeficiency syndrome and disseminated disease were reported to have EB involvement [35]. Predisposing factors for *C. neoformans*, include HIV infection, malignancy, cirrhosis, renal failure, chronic lung diseases, diabetes mellitus, sarcoidosis, stem cell and solid organ transplantation, sickle cell disease, and steroid therapy [34]. However, in patients with EB disease, only 23 % were had underlying diseases of myocarditis, diabetes mellitus, and acquired immunodeficiency syndrome but without evidence of disseminated disease. Conversely, 17 % of immunocompetent cases had dissemination to the central nervous system besides the EB involvement suggesting high virulence of the organism. In EB **cryptococcosis**, dyspnea and hemoptysis were the most common symptoms. If systemic infection exists, fever, cough, and headache can also be seen in addition to these manifestations. Some patients may develop acute respiratory distress syndrome. In most cases of EB involvement, the disease is identified incidentally on abnormal chest radiographs, biopsy of lung masses, or cultures of lung specimens obtained for other reasons [34].

Residence in endemic areas, the organism load, and depressed immune status positively correlate with the severity of disease [36, 37]. In one review, 81 % were from endemic areas, and all were immunocompetent [3].

The radiographic findings of pulmonary **cryptococcosis** vary from well-defined, small, non-calcified nodules, with or without cavitation to lobar infiltrates and hilar or mediastinal adenopathy. Pleural effusions have also been occasionally reported [33]. In EB cryptococcosis, "fungus ball" has been reported in 46 % of the cases. Abscess with an air-fluid level was also seen in 15 % of the patients with EB involvement.

Histoplasmosis

Histoplasmosis is the most common endemic respiratory mycosis in the central USA and in Latin America. In the USA, it is most often encountered in the Midwestern states in the Ohio, Missouri, and Mississippi River valleys. Individuals are infected by inhaling the aerosolized microconidia form of the fungus. Infection is mostly self-limited; only 1 % of affected individuals develop chronic disease [36, 37]. Airway involvement from histoplasmosis can be direct or indirect, though direct invasion of the airways is relatively uncommon. In most cases, airways are indirectly involved by either enlarged or calcified lymph nodes or fibrosing mediastinitis [3]. Residence in endemic areas for **histoplasmosis**, organism load, and depressed immune status positively correlate with severity of disease [3, 37, 38] (Table 9.1).

Most people infected by **histoplasmosis** remain asymptomatic, yet around 10–40 % can develop self-limiting influenza-like illness. The duration of symptoms depends upon the extent of exposure, underlying lung disease, general immune status, and specific immunity to *H. capsulatum*. Mediastinal lymph nodes are the most common site of involvement, while EB involvement is rare [39]. In a review, patients presented mainly with hemoptysis (72 %) mainly related to fibrosing mediastinitis. Expectoration of broncholiths is also a rare manifestation of EB histoplasmosis [3].

Histoplasma polysaccharide antigen (HPA) test is an initial test for the diagnosis of disseminated histoplasmosis that takes 2–4 weeks for completion. Detection of circulating HPA in urine, serum, and other body fluids has an increasingly important role in the rapid diagnosis of disseminated histoplasmosis. Sensitivity is greater in urine than in serum, and the sensitivity of the urine assay for the diagnosis of disseminated histoplasmosis is approximately 90 %. In patients who have other fungal infections, including coccidioidomycosis, blastomycosis, paracoccidioidomycosis, and penicilliosis, false positive reactions for HPA in urine may occur. The HPA test is often negative in isolated pulmonary disease. In such patients, direct examination and culture of sputum, BAL, or transbronchial biopsy can be performed. Bone marrow, lymph node, liver, or a skin or mucous membrane lesion provides other diagnostic sources [40].

Radiographic findings of pulmonary **histoplasmosis** are non-specific and varied. They can vary from a solitary nodule to fibrocystic disease. There are no radiologic markers of EB involvement except for those related to fibrosing mediastinitis. Interstitial markings and lymph node enlargement are the most prominent features [35, 36]. A non-specific infiltrative pattern (72 %), lymph node enlargement (63 %), and calcification (36 %) all have been detected. The presence of splenic calcifications may also suggest prior histoplasmosis.

Pseudallescheria boydii Infection

Pseudallescheria boydii (*Scedosporium apiospermum*) is a saprophytic mold that is ubiquitous and found in multiple environmental sources. It has been classically associated with mycetoma [41]. More recently, it has been reported to cause infections in solid organ transplant recipients and also colonize the airways of lung transplant recipients. An inherent resistance to amphotericin B is a characteristic of this group of fungi and early identification along with therapy with newer azoles is key in the management [41, 42]. In bone marrow transplant recipients, *Pseudallescheria boydii* has been reported to be associated with increased mortality, early infection, and fungemia. Treatment with voriconazole in this patient population has shown a trend toward improved mortality (Fig. 9.1) [41, 42].

Fig. 9.1 *Pseudallescheria boydii* infection involving the right bronchial anastomosis in a lung transplant recipient for cystic fibrosis

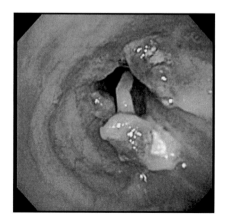

Bronchoscopy

According to the published literature, lesions of EBFI predominantly involve the lobar and segmental bronchi unilaterally (70 %), while bilateral (15 %) and tracheal involvement (9 %) are uncommon. The characteristics of the lesions include yellowish white necrotic plaques, ulcerative lesions, irregular–sessile nodules, granulomatous lesions, EB masses (hemorrhagic or non-hemorrhagic), hyperemic mucosa and bronchial stenosis, and anastomotic infection, especially in transplant patients (Fig. 9.1; Table 9.2) [3, 18, 20].

More specifically, obstructive bronchial aspergillosis can be described when thick mucous plugs loaded with *Aspergillus* are found in the airways, with little mucosal inflammation or invasion (Fig. 9.2). In invasive tracheobronchitis, necrotic white mucosa can be seen [18]. In the ulcerative form, there is focal fungal invasion ulcer of the tracheobronchial mucosa and/or cartilage [18, 43, 44]. The

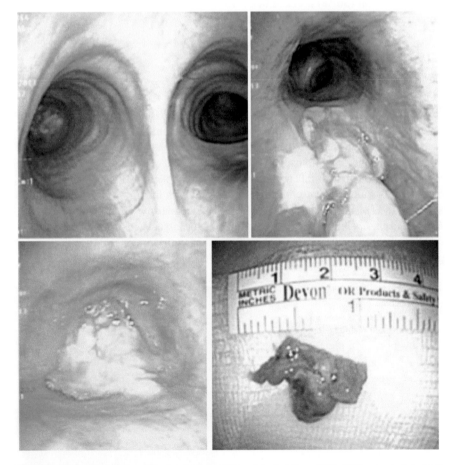

Fig. 9.2 Obstructive *Aspergillus* tracheobronchitis. Adapted from [17]. With permission from American College of Chest Physicians

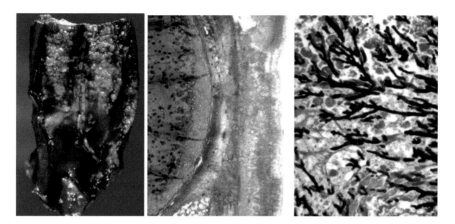

Fig. 9.3 Pseudomembranous tracheobronchial aspergillosis: an autopsy specimen of a lung transplant recipient. Histological examination confirming the presence of the fungus

pseudomembranous form is characterized by extensive inflammation and invasion of the bronchial mucosa with a pseudomembrane composed of necrotic debris and hyphae [12, 45, 46] (Fig. 9.3). In patients with *A. niger*, black pigmentation can also be seen. In addition, white masses of calcium oxalate crystals are also present. The fungus produces oxalic acid with an affinity to bind tissue calcium forming these crystals (Fig. 9.4).

Proliferation of **coccidioidomycosis** accounts for the inflammatory appearance of the bronchi in endobronchial coccidioidomycosis. Bronchitis and bronchiolitis have been reported in association with parenchymal lesions and are occasionally accompanied by inflammatory debris filling the lumen, or mucosal ulceration [14].

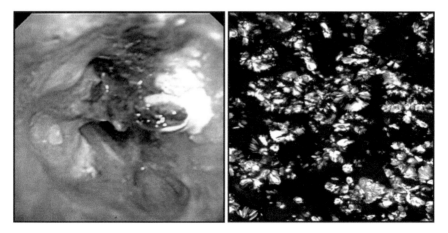

Fig. 9.4 Dark black pigments of *Aspergillus niger* and white calcium oxalate crystals involving the right upper lobe bronchus of a lung transplant recipient

Fig. 9.5 Candidial plaques in
a 68-year-old male postlung
transplantation

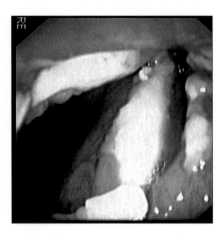

Other reported EB abnormalities are sessile–irregular and submucosal nodules
(45 %). In patients with mediastinal or hilar lymphadenopathy, extrinsic compression of the airways has also been reported [3].

In endobronchial zygomycosis, the disease presented as a mass lesion in 32 % of
patients or a grayish white fibrinous plug obstructing the bronchus in 26 %. It also
caused sloughing of mucosa, granular lesions, ulcers, stenotic lesions, or pseudomembrane formation in about 39 % patients [47].

In *Candidiasis*, multiple white plaques are a characteristic feature of mucosal
invasion on EB examination [31]. Pseudomembrane formation and hemorrhagic
bronchitis are other common presentations (Fig. 9.5).

The most common presentation of EB **cryptococcosis** is a white or hemorrhagic
mass. Intense mucosal inflammation, gelatinous mass, nodules, plaques, pseudomembranes, and/or ulcerative lesions have also been reported.

Endobronchial **histoplasmosis** can present as mild–severe stenosis of the trachea, carinae, or main bronchi from the enlarged or calcified lymph nodes. EB
disease can be due to compression caused by a calcified lymph node between the
bronchus and a vessel or esophagus. Chronic compression between calcified lymph
nodes, the airways, and the esophagus can cause disruption of the bronchial and
esophageal wall leading to the development of a bronchoesophageal fistula.
Fibrosing mediastinitis can cause hyperemia, or mucosal edema with diffuse
spider-like microvasculature in the airways due to distal obstruction of the bronchial
blood vessels (Fig. 9.6). Direct EB involvement may mimic tumor [3]. The most
prominent finding of EB histoplasmosis in a review was hyperemic mucosa in
27 %. Masses, mucosal hemorrhage, and broncholiths were other EB findings [3].
(Table 9.4)

Fig. 9.6 Bronchoscopic view
of fibrosing mediastinitis
(**a**, **b**). Note the presence of
erythema, mucosal edema,
and prominent blood vessels

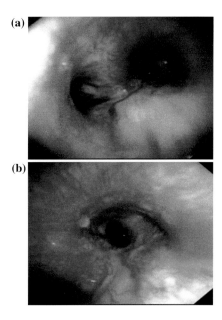

(a)

(b)

Table 9.4 Bronchoscopic findings in various endobronchial fungal infections

Infection type	Bronchoscopic findings
Aspergillosis	• Bronchial stenosis • Yellowish white necrotic plaques • White masses/nodules of calcium oxalate crystals • Obstructive—mucous plugs • Invasive tracheobronchitis—necrotic white mucosa • Ulcerative form—ulcer of the tracheobronchial mucosa and/or cartilage • Pseudomembranous-extensive inflammation and invasion with a pseudomembrane composed of necrotic debris and hyphae • Edematous irregular mucosa • *A. niger*—black pigmentation, white calcium oxalate crystals
Coccidioidomycosis	• Nodules (sessile, irregular, submucosal) • Hyperemia • Cobble stone appearance • White raised lesion • Mucosal ulceration • Extrinsic compression—mediastinal or hilar lymphadenopathy
Zygomycosis	• Mass lesion • Grayish white fibrinous plug • Sloughing of mucosa • Granular lesions • Ulcer • Stenosis • Pseudomembrane formation
Candidiasis	• White plaques over the vocal cords, airways • Pseudomembrane formation • Hemorrhagic mucosa
Cryptococcosis	• White or hemorrhagic mass • Intense mucosal inflammation

(continued)

Table 9.4 (continued)

Infection type	Bronchoscopic findings
	• Gelatinous mass, nodules, plaques, pseudomembranes, and/or ulcerative lesions
Histoplasmosis	• Mild–severe stenosis of the trachea, carina or main bronchi—due to enlarged or calcified lymph nodes (compression—the bronchus and a vessel or esophagus) • Chronic compression—disruption of the bronchial and esophageal wall leading to the development of a bronchoesophageal fistula • Fibrosing mediastinitis—hyperemia, or mucosal edema with diffuse spider-like microvasculature in the airways due to distal obstruction of the bronchial blood vessels • Hyperemic mucosa • Masses, mucosal hemorrhage, and broncholiths

Pathology

Fungi are eukaryotic one-celled organisms that rarely cause diseases. These are more complex than bacteria. Tubular aggregates of fungi are called "hyphae." If it shows constriction, it is called "pseudohyphae." Discrete fungal cells called yeast or spores and spore-forming bodies are known as "conidia" or "sporangia." Demonstration of fungi in the tissue or culture growth lead to diagnosis. Some fungi can be visible on hematoxylin and eosin stains. Gomori methenamine silver (GMS), Grocott silver stain, and periodic acid–Schiff (PAS) stains are needed for screening and confirmation. A diagnosis of a particular fungus can be made based on the morphology and size [48] (Table 9.5).

Diagnosis

Bronchial washings and/or brushings provide a diagnosis in 36 % of patients. Bronchoalveolar lavage (BAL) culture is positive in 25 % of cases. The time required for fungal growth in culture is usually several weeks when incubated at

Table 9.5 Diagnostic features of fungi

Organism	Morphology (diameter)	Yeast	Hyphae	Pseudohyphae
Aspergillus	45° dichotomous branching (3–6 μm)	–	+ septate	–
Coccidiosis	Spherules with endospores (20–60 μm)	–	–	–
Mucormyces	Broad, irregular wide-angle branching (10–20 μm)	–	+ pauciseptate	–
Candida	Dimorphic yeast	+	±	+
Cryptococcus	Budding yeast with capsule (2–20 μm)	+	–	–
Histoplasma	Budding yeast (2–5 μm)	+	–	–

25–30 °C. The specimen is inoculated into media like Sabouraud's dextrose agar-containing cycloheximide and chloramphenicol. The cycloheximide is left out if a mold requires identification. Culture identifies the organism responsible for the infection and is very helpful in selecting the most suitable treatment [3].

Endobronchial biopsy of the lesion can be diagnostic in 46 % of patients. Serology could be diagnostic in as many as 20 % of cases among all patients with coccidioidomycosis, aspergillosis, and cryptococcosis [3]. Diagnosis is established at necropsy in as many as 12 % of patients.

Aspergillosis is known to be a common colonizer of the respiratory tract; thus, sputum cultures are not reliable. A tissue diagnosis is most definitive; however, when this is not available, multiple positive cultures in appropriate clinical context may suggest the diagnosis. Serological test for the detection of galactomannan antigen has been reported to have 81 % sensitivity and 89 % specificity [49]. However, far lower sensitivity (30 %) has been reported in lung transplant recipients with invasive aspergillosis [50]. PCR and nucleic acid sequence-based amplification are other advanced methods for establishing the diagnosis of aspergillosis and may support EB involvement [23]. Histopathological examination and culture of EB biopsies in 35 %, bronchial washing, and brushing material in 40 % and BAL in 28 % of patients are the main confirmatory tests for EB aspergillosis. Presumptive diagnosis of respiratory tract disease can be made in the absence of a tissue biopsy if *Aspergillus* spp. are cultured from a respiratory sample, a compatible lesion or syndrome is present, and no alternative causative process is identified. Although serum galactomannan antigen testing and PCR-based techniques may be useful, they have not been studied in patients with HIV infection.

The diagnosis of EB coccidioidomycosis is established by demonstration of spherules on a wet preparation of the EB specimen. Potassium hydroxide solution, calcofluor staining, or Papanicolaou staining are usually used for this purpose [51]. The diagnosis of coccidioidomycosis was made by surgical, laryngoscopic, or EB biopsy of an airway lesion in 3, 5, and 66 % of the patients, respectively. A bronchial brush of a lesion provided the diagnosis rarely. Skin and paravertebral mass biopsy may also lead to diagnosis. Culture of BAL is reported to be positive in 32 % cases and exclusively diagnostic in 13 %. Although serology was available in 74 % of the patients, it was helpful for presumptive diagnosis in only 3 % of the patients [3]. Thus, it is not recommended as a diagnostic test due to impaired serologic responses among immunocompromised hosts [24]. The mainstays of diagnosis of coccidioidomycosis are histopathological identification and cultures [52]. In cases of pulmonary coccidioidomycosis, results of culture of respiratory specimens (sputum, BAL fluid, or transbronchial biopsy) are frequently positive. The diagnosis can also be established by demonstration of the typical spherule on histopathological examination of involved tissue.

In endobronchial **mucormycosis**, biopsy reveals characteristic broad, non-septate hyphae with right-angle branching on calcofluor white or methenamine silver stains. However, the absence of hyphae does not rule out the diagnosis in a proper clinical setting. Sputum or BAL specimens may also show the characteristic hyphae. In published cases of EB mucormycosis, bronchial washing and brushings were diagnostic in 52 % of the cases and EB biopsy was diagnostic in 45 % patients. However, in 26 % patients the diagnosis was established at necropsy [3].

To establish the diagnosis of primary pulmonary **candidiasis**, the following criteria have been proposed: (1) *Candida* cultured from bronchoscopic material; (2) negative mycobacterial culture; (3) no other etiology for pulmonary disease, and (4) *Candida* demonstrated on the biopsy specimen [3, 28]. However, there are no established criteria to confirm airway candidiasis. Primary pulmonary candidiasis may be associated with EB involvement. However, ruling out of other organisms causing airway involvement is essential.

Cryptococcus species are rare pathogens colonizing the airways. Encapsulated yeast forms in sputum, BAL, and tissue establish the diagnosis of cryptococcosis. The serum antigen titer is also indicative of infection and suggests extrapulmonary spread [53]. Cryptococcal antigen testing has been reported to be of more utility in the immunocompromised host since its presence does not require immune response by the host. Examination of the cerebrospinal fluid is a standard part of the evaluation in immunocompromised hosts with pulmonary cryptococcosis [34]. In EB cryptococcosis, serology in 77 % of the patients, EB biopsy in 69 %, other bronchoscopic material in 46 %, and BAL culture in 15 % were helpful in making the diagnosis. Blood fungal cultures are also specific and should be performed. The diagnosis of pulmonary cryptococcosis can be made by culture of sputum, BAL fluid, pleural fluid, and transbronchial biopsy specimen. The measurement of cryptococcal antigen in the BAL can be a rapid, simple way to make the diagnosis [54].

In the appropriate clinical setting, detection of the **histoplasmosis** on a bronchoscopy specimen culture or glycoprotein antigen detection in urine or serum by complement fixation helps establish the diagnosis. Low-level positive antibody titers, however, may relate to past rather than active infection. Involvement of the airways is confirmed by bronchoscopy or by verifying the lesion by biopsy via appropriate specimen recovery [3]. In 82 % of the patients, diagnosis was established by the EB biopsy.

Differential Diagnosis

For fungus ball, the air crescent sign is often considered to be characteristic of mycetomas but has also been described in bronchogenic carcinoma, retained foreign body following thoracotomy, hemorrhage into a cavity, Wegener's granulomatosis, sclerosing haemangioma, echinococcal cyst, tuberculosis, and Rasmussen aneurysm in a tuberculous cavity [55]. The air crescent sign may also be seen in angioinvasive aspergillosis, where it corresponds pathologically to a space caused by retraction of an area of retracted infarcted lung (Table 9.6) [56].

Table 9.6 Differential diagnosis for pulmonary fungal infections

Lung cancer
Bacterial, atypical or viral pneumonia
Aspiration pneumonia
Pneumocystis jirovecii pneumonia
Eosinophilic pneumonia
Hypersensitivity reaction caused by fungal antigen— e.g., allergic asthma, allergic bronchopulmonary aspergillosis, and extrinsic allergic alveolitis
Chemical pneumonitis—e.g., chemical worker's lung
Coal worker's pneumoconiosis
Löffler's disease (marked eosinophilia and benign, transient, migratory or recurrent pulmonary infiltrates with minimal constitutional upset)
Adult respiratory distress syndrome
Causes of pulmonary fibrosis
Tuberculosis
Pulmonary edema
Helminthic infections

Complications

Complications of EBFI are disease dissemination to other sites (i.e., brain, meninges, skin, liver, spleen, kidneys, adrenals, heart, and eyes). Sepsis syndrome and blood vessel invasion can also be seen which can lead to hemoptysis, pulmonary infarction, myocardial infarction, cerebral emboli, cerebral infarction, or blindness. Other complications associated with EBFI are listed in Table 9.7 [3].

Treatment

Suggested treatment for EB **aspergillosis** is similar to that for invasive aspergillosis, which includes intravenous AmB (1–1.5 mg/kg/day), liposomal AmB (5 mg/kg/day), and/or 400 mg/day of oral itraconazole. Voriconazole, a new triazole, is also being used with increasing frequency with the loading dose of 6 mg/kg every 12 h; followed by maintenance dose of 4 mg/kg every 12 h (400 mg every 12 h for 2 doses then 200 mg every 12 h for oral voriconazole). Duration of therapy is guided by clinical response. It may be extend to several weeks to a year. The ultimate response of these patients to antifungal therapy is largely related to host factors, such as correction of neutropenia and neutrophil function and reduction of immunosuppression [57, 58]. Other possible therapies include caspofungin alone (though some experts have raised concerns about its efficacy in severe disease) or in combination with voriconazole, intravenous AmB, or liposomal AmB. The role of

Table 9.7 Complications of endobronchial fungal infection

Complications
Disease dissemination to other sites (brain, meninges, skin, liver, spleen, kidneys, adrenals, heart, and eyes)
Sepsis syndrome
Blood vessel invasion leading to hemoptysis, pulmonary infarction, myocardial infarction, cerebral emboli, cerebral infarction, or blindness
Bronchopleural or tracheoesophageal fistulas
Fibrosing mediastinitis (histoplasmosis)
Broncholithiasis (histoplasmosis)
Lung cavitation
Development of mycetoma in a lung cavity
Bronchopleural or tracheoesophageal fistulas
Mediastinal fibrosis
Calcification in pulmonary tree
Immunologic reaction to fungal antigens.
Associated rheumatological complex/pericarditis with endemic fungal pneumonias
Fungal endocarditis
Progressive respiratory failure

aerosolized AmB in therapy remains controversial, although authors have reported it to be effective [58–60]. Local instillation directly to the cavity for fungus ball or pleural space can also be advocated [61]. Further studies are needed to determine optimal therapy. Liposomal and standard AmB inhaled formulations have been studied more extensively in the context of prophylaxis in lung transplantation [58]. Posttransplant antifungal prophylactic or preemptive therapies are used in many transplant centers, especially in patients with cystic fibrosis where *Aspergillus* is a common colonizer [23, 51].

In **coccidioidomycosis**, therapies utilized in reported cases have generally followed the Infectious Diseases Society of America (IDSA) guidelines. These include intravenous AmB (0.5–0.7 mg/kg/day), oral ketoconazole (400 mg/day), oral or intravenous fluconazole (400–800 mg/day), or oral itraconazole (200 mg twice a day) either singly or in combination. According to these guidelines, a total intravenous AmB dose of 1.5–3.0 g is followed by oral azole therapy lasting from 3 to 24 months depending on the response. Among immunocompromised hosts, lifelong suppressive therapy may be required. Surgical resection may also be required for localized refractory lesions or those associated with significant hemoptysis [59]. In 38 EB coccidioidomycosis cases, 26 (68 %) patients received a course of intravenous AmB 10 (26 %), 2 cases oral ketoconazole, 8 cases oral fluconazole, and 3 cases itraconazole before or after the course of AmB. Two patients received multiple azoles and another 2 received fluconazole therapy alone. Therapy duration was at least 12 months.

Mucor species are resistant to azoles and echinocandins. The recommended therapy is high-dose intravenous AmB or liposomal AmB, as well as surgical or EB resection, in appropriate clinical settings [3]. As *Mucor* is angioinvasive and a rapidly growing fungus, surgical intervention should be early and aggressive. Concomitant systemic treatment is also required [62]. In a large review, 85 % of patients who underwent surgical treatment survived their disease.

Management of EB candidiasis is similar to systemic infection. Systemic therapy for primary candidiasis consists of either intravenous AmB or liposomal AmB in severely ill patients or oral fluconazole in milder presentations [18]. Caspofungin is a more recent alternative, particularly for azole-resistant yeasts. In our literature search, 8 patients (57 %) received intravenous AmB and/or aerosolized AmB, 5 (36 %) patients received fluconazole and remaining 2 (14 %) received itraconazole (14 %).

In pulmonary *cryptococcosis*, recommended therapy is intravenous AmB (0.7 mg/kg/day) plus flucytosine (100 mg/kg/day) as induction therapy for 3–4 weeks, followed by oral fluconazole [3]. The optimal duration of maintenance therapy with fluconazole is unclear. In immunocompromised hosts, at least a 6–12-month course of therapy should be considered. It is recommended that all HIV-infected individuals continue maintenance therapy for life. Itraconazole is an acceptable prophylactic alternative [63]. There are no specific recommendations for the treatment of EB disease. Hence, a regimen similar to that for systemic infection should be acceptable. Therapy duration varied from 3 to 18 months. With appropriate therapy, 62 % of patients were alive at the time of reporting [3].

According to the IDSA guidelines for pulmonary **histoplasmosis**, if the patient is critically ill, intravenous AmB (0.7–1.0 mg/kg/day) is considered, with the total AmB treatment amount less than 35 mg/kg. After stabilization of symptoms, the patient can be switched to oral itraconazole for up to 12 months. If symptomatic major airway obstruction takes place, then 40–80 mg prednisone daily for 2 weeks should be considered [64]. While it is well known that there is generally no added benefit of antifungal treatment in broncholithiasis or fibrosing mediastinitis, such treatment should be considered in patients with elevated erythrocyte sedimentation rate or complement fixation titers for *H. capsulatum* over 1:32, as these patients may have active ongoing infection [3, 39]. Prognosis of the patient with EB histoplasmosis is relatively good. In cases reported to date, all patients with EB histoplasmosis were alive at the time of report, after appropriate therapy. Surgical approaches, including lobectomy, segmentectomy, or closure of the bronchoesophageal fistula, were required in 72 % of the cases. Only 18 % received oral antifungal therapy while steroids were used in 45 %.

Therapeutic bronchoscopy may be required in as many as 30 % of patients with EB fungal infections. Such procedures were performed to excise or vaporize the mass lesions in 5 %, to stop hemoptysis in 6 % and to place a stent or perform balloon dilatation for stenotic airways in 8 and 9 %, respectively [3].

Prevention

HIV-infected patients are routinely treated with prophylactic <u>antifungal</u> drugs to try to avoid infection with opportunistic fungal pathogens, particularly *C. neoformans*. Transplant patients may also benefit from prophylactic antifungal agents. Itraconazole has shown some benefits as prophylaxis against invasive fungal infections in transplant patients. Patients likely to have prolonged neutropenia should avoid activities that increase exposure to environmental fungal spores, such as gardening or working with potted plants and fresh flowers, cleaning, building work, and handling uncooked vegetables [65].

Treatment Outcomes

Forty-five percentage of the lung transplant recipients with EB aspergillosis may require bronchoplasty for stenosis. EB involvement with *Aspergillus* may indicate a poor prognosis [44, 66]. Nine percentage of EB aspergillosis with invasive disease and concomitant massive hemoptysis is associated with grave prognosis. For **Aspergillosis**, if the suture material from prior surgery is present in the EB tree, it should be removed with scissors or burned with laser photoablation [67].

In **Mucormycosis**, if disease is not detected early enough, mortality is very high. Of the 31 reports, 77 % were treated with intravenous AmB (1 mg/kg/day), 42 % of the patients underwent surgery, and 3 % had endoscopic removal of a plug with rigid bronchoscope. Reported mortality was 52 % [3]. In **candidiasis**, reported mortality was 21 % [3].

For **coccidioidomycosis**, airway disease may require stent, tracheostomy, and surgical management to prevent complete obstruction of the airway [3].

In **histoplasmosis**, a broncholith, if detected free in the bronchus, can be removed via bronchoscope. In patients with hemoptysis from fibrosing mediastinitis, hemostasis can be achieved by argon plasma coagulation or laser photoresection using a flexible bronchoscopy [63]. As reported in the literature, therapeutic bronchoscopy was required in 18 % using argon plasma coagulation or Nd-YAG laser for hemoptysis. This presentation also required bronchial artery embolization 27 % [3].

Prognosis

An exhaustive review of literature reveals that complete cure can be achieved in 36 % of patients with aspergillosis, 11 % with coccidioidomycosis, 35 % with zygomycosis, 78 % with candidiasis, 62 % with cryptococcosis, and 100 % with histoplasmosis [3].

Overall, reported mortality from EB aspergillosis is approximately 48 %. For coccidioidomycosis, even if AmB was used, 3 patients died, 4 were alive, and the survival status of 31 patients was unknown [3].

Although extended follow-up was not available for all patients, 48 % with aspergillosis, 8 % with coccidioidomycosis, 52 % with zygomycosis with 21 % candidiasis, and 31 % with cryptococcosis had expired despite appropriate therapy [3].

Summary and Recommendations

EBFI usually occurs by inhalation of fungal organisms. Its true incidence and prevalence remains unknown. Immunocompromised individuals are affected much more than immunocompetent ones. Serologic examination may support the clinical suspicion. In most patients with EBFI, bronchoscopic examination correlates with the radiographic findings. Bronchospasm, pneumothorax, and bleeding are seen as complications in very small percentages with flexible bronchoscopy [3, 68]. Bronchoscopic descriptions of airway lesions include mass lesions, yellowish white or reddish polypoid lesions, fragile mucosa, plaques, and ulcerative lesions. Tissue necrosis-mimicking tumors may cause yellowish white pseudomembranous-type lesions especially in patients with aspergillosis and zygomycosis. Fungal organisms can also cause granulomas. Washing, brushing, and BAL or biopsy is required to confirm the diagnosis. Interventional bronchoscopic techniques may be required for removal of the deceased tissue. Fungal infections should feature in the differential diagnosis of any kind of EB disease, especially in an immunocompromised host.

References

1. Zainuddin B. Steroid therapy in obstructive airway disease. Respirology. 1997;2:17–31.
2. Azoulay E, Cohen Y, Zahar JR, Garrouste-Orgeas M, Adrie C, Moine P, de Lassence A, Timsit JF. Practices in non-neutropenic ICU patients with Candida-positive airway specimens. Intensive Care Med. 2004;30:1384–9.
3. Karnak D, Avery RK, Gildea TR, Sahoo D, Mehta AC. Endobronchial fungal disease. An under-recognized entity. Respiration. 2007;74(1):88–104.
4. Smith JA, Kauffman CA. Pulmonary fungal infections. Respirology. 2012;17(6):913–26.
5. Kosmidis C, Denning DW. The clinical spectrum of pulmonary aspergillosis. Thorax. 2015;70 (3):270–7.
6. Mehrad B, Paciocco G, Martinez FJ, Ojo TC, Iannettoni MD, Lynch JP 3rd. Spectrum of Aspergillus infection in lung transplant recipients: case series and review of the literature. Chest. 2001;119:169–75.
7. Singhal P, Usuda K, Mehta AC. Post-lung transplantation *Aspergillus niger* infection. J Heart Lung Transpl. 2005;24:1446–7.
8. Sancho JM, Ribera JM, Rosell A, Munoz C, Feliu E. Unusual invasive bronchial aspergillosis in a patient with acute lymphoblastic leukemia. Haematologica. 1997;82:701–2.

9. Singh N, Husain S. Aspergillus infections after lung transplantation: clinical differences in type of transplant and implications for management. J Heart Lung Transpl. 2003;22:258–66.

10. Franquet T, Muller NL, Gimenez A, Guembe P, La de Torre J, Bague S. Spectrum of pulmonary aspergillosis. Histologic, clinical, and radiologic findings. Radiographics. 2001;21:825–37.

11. Mehta AC, Dar MA, Ahmad M, Weinstein AJ, Golish JA. Thoracic aspergillosis (Part III). Invasive pulmonary and disseminated aspergillosis. Cleve Clin Q. 1984;51:655–65.

12. Higgins R, McNeil K, Dennis C, Parry A, Large S, Nashef SA, Wells FC, Flower C, Wallwork J. Airway stenoses after lung transplantation: management with expanding metal stents. J Heart Lung Transpl. 1994;13:774–8.

13. Nunley DR, Gal AA, Vega JD, Perlino C, Smith P, Lawrence EC. Saprophytic fungal infections and complications involving the bronchial anastomosis following human lung transplantation. Chest. 2002;122:1185–91.

14. Noppen M, Claes I, Maillet B, Meysman M, Monsieur I, Vincken W. Three cases of bronchial stump aspergillosis: unusual clinical presentations and beneficial effect of oral itraconazole. Eur Respir J. 1995;8:477–80.

15. Ruhnke M, Eichenauer E, Searle J, Lippek F. Fulminant tracheobronchial and pulmonary aspergillosis complicating imported *Plasmodium falciparum* malaria in an apparently immunocompetent woman. Clin Infect Dis. 2000;30:938–40.

16. George AS, Scott ED. Fungal diseases of the lung. 3rd ed. Washington: Lippincott Williams & Wilkins; 2000. p. 123.

17. Panchabhai TS, Bandyopadhyay D, Alraiyes AH, Mehta AC, Almeida FA. A 60-year-old woman with cough, dyspnea and atelectasis 19 years after liver transplantation. Chest. 2015;148(4):e122–5.

18. Kim JS, Rhee Y, Kang SM, Ko WK, Kim YS, Lee JG, Park JM, Kim SK, Kim SK, Lee WY, Chang J. A case of endobronchial aspergilloma. Yonsei Med J. 2000;41:422–5.

19. Clarke A, Skelton J, Fraser RS. Fungal tracheobronchitis. Report of 9 cases and review of the literature. Medicine (Baltimore). 1991;70:1–14.

20. Kimura M, Schnadig VJ, McGinnis MR. Chlamydoconidia formation in zygomycosis due to Rhizopus species. Arch Pathol Lab Med. 1998;122:1120–2.

21. Wheat LJ, Garringer T, Brizendine E, Connolly P. Diagnosis of histoplasmosis by antigen detection based upon experience at the histoplasmosis reference laboratory. Diagn Microbiol Infect Dis. 2002;43(1):29–37.

22. Chaturvedi V, Ramani R, Gromadzki S, Rodeghier B, Chang HG, Morse DL. Coccidioidomycosis in New York State. Emerg Infect Dis. 2000;6:25–9.

23. Blair JE, Balan V, Douglas DD, Hentz JG. Incidence and prevalence of coccidioidomycosis in patients with end-stage liver disease. Liver Transpl. 2003;9:843–50.

24. Polesky A, Kirsch CM, Snyder LS, LoBue P, Kagawa FT, Dykstra BJ, Wehner JH, Catanzaro A, Ampel NM, Stevans DA. Airway coccidioidomycosis—report of cases and review. Clin Infect Dis. 1999;28:1273–80.

25. Baker RD. Pulmonary mucormycosis. Am J Pathol. 1956;32:287–307.

26. Boelaert JR, Fenves AZ, Coburn JW. Deferoxamine therapy and mucormycosis in dialysis patients: report of an international registry. Am J Kidney Dis. 1991;18:660–7.

27. Al-Majed S, Al-Kassimi F, Ashour M, Mekki MO, Sadiq S. Removal of endobronchial mucormycosis lesion through a rigid bronchoscope. Thorax. 1992;47:203–4.

28. Spear RK, Walker PD, Lampton LM. Tracheal obstruction associated with a fungus ball. A case of primary tracheal candidiasis. Chest. 1976;70:662–3.

29. Hamilos G, Samonis G, Kontoyiannis DP. Pulmonary mucormycosis. Semin Respir Crit Care Med. 2011;32(6):693–702.

30. Pappas PG. Guidelines for the treatment of candidiasis. Infectious Diseases Society of America. Clin Infect Dis. 2004;38:161.

31. Bhaskaran A, Hosseini-Moghaddam SM, Rotstein C, Husain S. Mold infections in lung transplant recipients. Semin Respir Crit Care Med. 2013;34(3):371–9.

32. Hosseini-Moghaddam SM, Husain S. Fungi and molds following lung transplantation. Semin Respir Crit Care Med. 2010;31(2):222–3330.
33. Friedman GD, Jeffrey Fessel W, Udaltsova NV, Hurley LB. Cryptococcosis. The 1981–2000 epidemic. Mycoses. 2005;48:122–5.
34. Long RF, Berens SV, Shambag GR. Case reports. An unusual manifestation of pulmonary cryptococcosis. Br J Radiol. 1972;45:757–9.
35. Christoph I. Pulmonary *Cryptococcus neoformans* and disseminated *Nocardia brasiliensis* in an immunocompromised host. Case report. N C Med J. 1990;51:219–20.
36. Dalys JS, Mark EJ. Case records of the Massachusetts General Hospital. Weekly clinicopathological exercises. Case 14-2002. A 51-year-old woman with recurrent hemoptysis. N Engl J Med. 2002;346:1475–82.
37. Chandler FW, Watts JC. Fungal infections. In: Dail DH, Hammer SP, editors. Pulmonary pathology. New York: Springer; 1988. p. 189–257.
38. Boyle KE, Parish JM, Lyng PJ, Viggiano RW, Wesselius LJ, Ocal IT, Vikram HR. Pseudomemmbranous tracheobronchitis caused by Rhizopus sp. after allogeneic stem cell transplantation. J Broncchol Intervent Pulmonol. 2014;21:166–9.
39. Hadjiliadis D, Howell DN, Davis RD, Lawrence CM, Rea JB, Tapson VF, Perfect JR, Palmer SM. Anastomotic infections in lung transplant recipients. Ann Transpl. 2000;5:13–9.
40. McKinsey DS, McKinsey JP. Pulmonary histoplasmosis. Semin Respir Crit Care Med. 2011;32(6):735–44.
41. Sahi H, Avery RK, Minai OA, Hall G, Mehta AC, Raina P, Budev M. Scedosporium apiospermum (*Pseudoallescheria boydii*) infection in lung transplant recipients. J Heart Lung Transpl. 2007;26(4):350–6.
42. Husain S, Muñoz P, Forrest G, Alexander BD, Somani J, Brennan K, Wagener MM, Singh N. Infections due to Scedosporium apiospermum and Scedosporium prolificans in transplant recipients: clinical characteristics and impact of antifungal agent therapy on outcome. Clin Infect Dis. 2005;40(1):89–99.
43. Stanzani M, Orciuolo E, Lewis R, Kontoyiannis DP, Martins SL, St John LS, Komanduri KV. *Aspergillus fumigatus* suppresses the human cellular immune response via gliotoxin-mediated apoptosis of monocytes. Blood. 2005;105:2258–65.
44. Hines DW, Haber MH, Yaremko LS. Pseudomembranous tracheobronchitis caused by aspergillosis. Am Rev Respir Dis. 1991;143:1408–11.
45. Pervez NK, Kleinerman J, Kattan M, Freed JA, Harris MB, Rosen MJ, Schwartz IS. Pseudomembranous necrotizing bronchial aspergillosis. A variant of invasive aspergillosis in a patient with hemophilia and acquired immune deficiency syndrome. Am Rev Respir Dis. 1985;131:961–3.
46. Al-Abbadi MA, Russo K, Wilkinson EJ. Pulmonary mucormycosis diagnosed by bronchoalveolar lavage: a case report and review of the literature. Pediatr Pulmonol. 1997;23:222.
47. Cagle PT, Allen TC, Kerr KM. Transbronchial and endobronchial biopsies. In: Haque A, Sienko A, Cagle PT, editors. Fungus. Philadelphia, USA: Lippincott Williams and Wilkins; 2009. p. 61–2.
48. Wheat LJ. Rapid diagnosis of invasive aspergillosis by antigen detection. Transpl Infect Dis. 2003;5:158–66.
49. Husain S, Kwak EJ, Obman A, Wagener MM, Kusne S, Stout JE, McCurry KR, Singh N. Prospective assessment of Platelia Aspergillus galactomannan antigen for the diagnosis of invasive aspergillosis in lung transplant recipients. Am J Transpl. 2004;4:796–802.
50. Rogers TR, Haynes KA, Barnes RA. Value of antigen detection in predicting invasive pulmonary aspergillosis. Lancet. 1990;336:1210.
51. Ampel NM, Nelson DK, Chavez S, Naus KA, Herman AB, Li L, Simmons KA, Pappagianis D. Preliminary evaluation of whole-blood gamma interferon release for clinical assessment of cellular immunity in patients with active coccidioidomycosis. Clin Diagn Lab Immunol. 2005;12(6):700–4.

52. Jensen WA, Rose RM, Hammer SM, Karchmer AW. Serologic diagnosis of focal pneumonia caused by *Cryptococcus neoformans*. Am Rev Respir Dis. 1985;132:189–91.
53. Baughman RP, Rhodes JC, Dohn MN, Henderson H, Frame PT. Detection of cryptococcal antigen in bronchoalveolar lavage fluid: a prospective study of diagnostic utility. Am Rev Respir Dis. 1992;145(5):1226–9.
54. Wheat LJ, Conces D, Allen SD, Blue-Hnidy D, Loyd J. Pulmonary histoplasmosis syndromes: recognition, diagnosis, and management. Semin Respir Crit Care Med. 2004;25:129–44.
55. Shameem M, Bhargava R, Ahmad Z, Fatima N, Malik A. Endobronchial aspergilloma—presenting as solitary pulmonary nodule. Respir Med. 2010;3:111–2.
56. Bochud PY, Chien JW, Marr KA, Leisenring WM, Upton A, Janer M, et al. Toll-like receptor 4 polymorphisms and aspergillosis in stem-cell transplantation. N Engl J Med. 2008;359 (17):1766–77.
57. Stevens DA, Kan VL, Judson MA, Morrison VA, Dummer S, Denning DW, Bennett JE, Walsh TJ, Patterson TF, Pankey GA. Practice guidelines for diseases caused by Aspergillus. Infectious Diseases Society of America. Clin Infect Dis. 2000;30:696–709.
58. Boettcher H, Bewig B, Hirt SW, Moller F, Cremer J. Topical amphotericin B application in severe bronchial aspergillosis after lung transplantation: report of experiences in 3 cases. J Heart Lung Transpl. 2000;19:1224–7.
59. Galgiani JN, Ampel NM, Catanzaro A, Johnson RH, Stevens DA, Williams PL. Practice guideline for the treatment of coccidioidomycosis. Infectious Diseases Society of America. Clin Infect Dis. 2000;30:658–61.
60. Oppenheim BA, Herbrecht R, Kusne S. The safety and efficacy of AmpB colloidal dispersion in the treatment of invasive mycosis. Clin Infect Dis. 1995;21:1145.
61. Stratakos G, Zakynthinos S. Adjuvant endobronchial amphotericin B for refractory invasive pulmonary aspergillosis: evidence is scarce but promise does exist. Respiration. 2007;74 (6):609–10.
62. Saag MS, Graybill RJ, Larsen RA, Pappas PG, Perfect JR, Powderly WJ, Sobel JD, Dismukes WE. IDSA practice guidelines for he management of cryptococcal disease. Infectious Diseases Society of America. Clin Infect Dis. 2000;30:710–8.
63. Wheat J, Sarosi G, McKinsey D, Hamill R, Bradsher R, Johnson P, Loyd J, Kauffman C. Practice guidelines for the management of patients with histoplasmosis. Infectious Diseases Society of America. Clin Infect Dis. 2000;30:688–95.
64. Playford EG, Webster AC, Sorrell TC, Craig JC. Systematic review and meta-analysis of antifungal agents for preventing fungal infections in liver transplant recipients. Eur J Clin Microbiol Infect Dis. 2006;25(9):549–61.
65. Sole A, Morant P, Salavert M, Peman J, Morales P. Valencia Lung Transplant Group: Aspergillus infections in lung transplant recipients: risk factors and outcome. Clin Microbiol Infect. 2005;11:359–65.
66. Helmi M, Love RB, Welter D, Cornwell RD, Meyer KC. Aspergillus infection in lung transplant recipients with cystic fibrosis: risk factors and outcomes comparison to other types of transplant recipients. Chest. 2003;123:800–8.
67. Manali ED, Saad CP, Krizmanich G, Mehta AC. Endobronchial findings of fibrosing mediastinitis. Respir Care. 2003;48:1038–42.
68. Karnak D, Köksal D, Beder S, Kayacan OA. Rare cause of empyema in a non-immunocompromised case and successful combined treatment. Postgrad Med J. 2004;80(941):184–6.

Chapter 10
Recurrent Respiratory Papillomatosis

Joseph Cicenia and Francisco Aécio Almeida

Causes and Pathophysiology of RRP

Recurrent respiratory papillomatosis (RRP) was first recognized by Sir Morell Mackenzie in the late 1800s when he identified papillomas as a distinct lesion in the larynx of children [1]. It was not until 1923, however, that Ullman demonstrated laryngeal papillomatosis was infectious by inoculating his arm with laryngeal papillomas from a 6-year-old boy and developing characteristic lesions several months later [2]. It was not until the 1980s that Mounts and other confirmed human papilloma virus (HPV) as the cause of RRP [3]. HPV is a DNA virus that is categorized into over 180 genotypes, each of which results in different clinical manifestations based on their tissue preference, virulence, and capacity to result in malignant transformation. HPV types 6 and 11 account for most cases (>95 %) of RRP [4]. Other HPV types have been rarely been implicated in the development of RRP, including HPV-16, HPV-18 (which are those types typically associated with cervical cancer), HPV-31, and HPV-33 [5].

  HPV has a propensity for infecting epithelial cells by infecting stem cells within the basal layer of the epithelial mucosa. HPV has eight genes coding for six early phase proteins (E1, E2, E4, E5, E6, and E7) and two late phase proteins (L1 and L2). The early phase proteins interact with host cell proteins resulting in cell transformation that disrupt normal cell growth and function, including altered cell cycle function and resistance to apoptosis. These alterations result in keeping the cell in a DNA replicative state and promoting unimpeded proliferations. It appears the infectivity of HPV is related to host immune factors, with those predisposed to developing disease having an impaired HPV-specific T-cell response [6] in the face of HPV-induced downregulation of inflammatory cytokines, including IL1-A, IL-18,

J. Cicenia (✉) · F.A. Almeida
Pulmonary Medicine, Respiratory Institute, Cleveland Clinic,
9500 Euclid Avenue, M2-137, Cleveland, OH 44195, USA
e-mail: cicenij@ccf.org

© Springer International Publishing Switzerland 2016   215
A.C. Mehta et al. (eds.), *Diseases of the Central Airways*,
Respiratory Medicine, DOI 10.1007/978-3-319-29830-6_10

and IL-31 [7]. Furthermore, HPV-mediated upregulation of IL-8 is thought to promote angiogenesis needed for papillomatosis propagation. Additionally, interactions of these early proteins with p53, a potent tumor suppressor gene, are thought to be responsible for the increased risk of oncogenic transformation of HPV-infected cells [8]. The binding potential of these proteins to p53, and other tumor suppressor genes, across HPV subtypes seems to relate to the malignant potential of each, some of which are high (HPV-16) and some of which are low (HPV-11 and HPV-6) [9]. Histologically, HPV appears as a pedunculated mass with fingerlike projections with a central fibrovascular core covered by stratified squamous epithelium. Early in its course, the papillomas are flat and have a velvety appearance; with time, these lesions become exophytic with a typical cauliflower-like appearance.

Epidemiology

RRP occurs in patients of all ages and has been separated into juvenile- and adult-onset variants based on the age of onset before or after the age of 18, respectively. The incidence of adult-onset RRP (AO-RRP) has been reported to be between 3 and 10 per 1,000,000 [10], and juvenile-onset RRP incidence seems to be about half that [11]. AO-RRP most commonly presents between ages of 20 and 40 years, with men being affected more than women [12, 13]. Though juvenile-onset RRP is often due to vertical transmission, AO-RRP is thought to be an acquired infection via oral sex. Data in support of sexual transmission in adults are conflicting; not all patients with AO-RRP provide a history of oral sex [14, 15]. Some hypothesize that AO-RRP represents reactivation of latent infection acquired during childhood [16]. The role of laryngeal irritants (such as tobacco smoke and gastroesophageal acid reflux) in the development of RRP is also controversial and thus not definitively linked. In the oropharynx, it is speculated that HPV enters the basal layer of the tonsillar epithelium and infects crypt cells, progressing to the infection of the vocal folds, a process which may be enhanced by local microtrauma caused by phonation [17].

Clinical Manifestations

Symptoms of RRP typically mask the disease since they are initially non-specific. Symptoms include hoarseness, cough, and dyspnea. As the disease progresses, symptoms become more manifest with dysphagia, wheezing, stridor, and recurrent upper respiratory infections. In rare instances, the disease will progress to upper airway obstruction with respiratory compromise. Presentation in children is usually delayed, mainly due to a low clinical suspicion of disease, since symptoms overlap with other common disease entities of childhood (such as bronchitis and asthma). Most juvenile patients are diagnosed by the age of 5 [18]. Up to 30 % of children and 16 % of adults will develop extralaryngeal disease extension of the disease

Fig. 10.1 a and **b** Extensive
circumferential involvement
of the trachea with recurrent
respiratory papillomatosis.
Note characteristic
mulberry-type texture of the
polypoid lesions

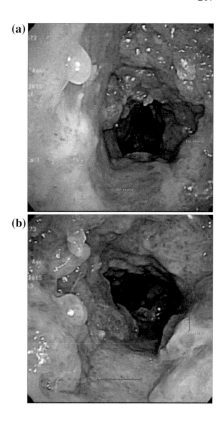

(a)

(b)

[19]. Extralaryngeal sites include esophagus, trachea, and lower respiratory tract. Clinical course is highly variable; some patients will present with a rapid progression of symptoms, whereas others will have a slower progression with some even achieving spontaneous regression of lesions. Presentation in adults is not as well documented as in children, though a similar occult onset with highly variable progression is thought to mimic that of children. Progression to the lower respiratory tract occurs in approximately 20 % of adults [19] and may occur more commonly in children (Fig. 10.1). Laryngoscopy and/or bronchoscopy remains the most confirmatory test for the condition. The papillomas exhibit a characteristic mulberry texture or a bunch of grapes like appearance. Pulmonary spread of RRP can occur; when it does, it can be identified as non-calcified nodules with central cavitation on radiographic imaging (Fig. 10.2). This manifestation of RRP is the most aggressive of the extralaryngeal presentations.

Disease severity is sometimes labeled "aggressive" as defined by distal spread, need for tracheostomy, four surgical operations annually, or >10 surgeries in total. Aggressive disease is seen more often in juveniles, especially in an earlier age of onset. HPV-11 is seen more often in aggressive disease, especially in adults [20]. Though overwhelmingly thought to be a benign disease, malignant transformation into squamous cell carcinoma has been reported albeit rare, accounting for less than

Fig. 10.2 Chest X-ray
revealing multiple
non-calcified pulmonary
nodules, some of them are
cavitating

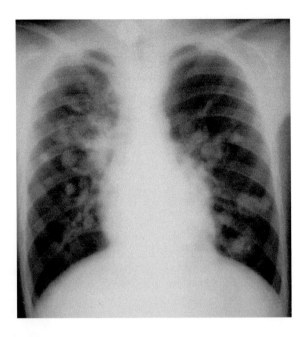

1 % of all clinical cases [21]. Mortality from RRP is low, approximately 1–2 %, and occurs primarily due to progressive airway obstruction, malignant transformation, and progressive pulmonary parenchymal disease [19].

Treatment

The main therapy goal is to relieve airway obstruction. This includes avoiding long-term complications such as subglottic and glottic stenosis or web formation leading to airway stenosis [22]. As many patients have vocal cords involvement, voice preservation is also of utmost importance. Therefore, surgical resection of papillomatous lesions remains the mainstay of therapy for RRP. However, there is no "cure" for RRP, and no single surgical modality has consistently been shown to "eradicate" RRP. True cures may only be achieved with adjuvant therapy [23].

Surgical Management

Over the past decade, the microdebrider appears to have surpassed the CO_2 laser as the debulking modality of choice in the US and Europe based on the ENT literature [19, 24]. The frequency of different modalities for the treatment/palliation of the more distal airway disease often treated by pulmonologists and thoracic surgeons is unknown.

Microdebrider

The microdebrider consists of a disposable blade which is a hollow metal tube with a port for suction. It cuts tissue with simultaneous removal of the debris from the airway. Blades of various sizes and configurations are available. A hand piece connected to wall suction tubing controls the blade via an electrically powered motor. Finally, a console controls the hand piece via a foot pedal which allows the operator to determine the speed and the direction of rotation of the blade. The tip of the blade is slightly angulated, which may permit leaving the underlying native tissue undisturbed. Because it is a nonthermal technique, there is no risk of thermal injury to surrounding tissue. In addition, the operator does not have to worry about the amount of O_2 delivered and the risk of airway fire. On the other hand, it can only be used with rigid bronchoscopy or suspension laryngoscopy because the hollow metal tube is not flexible. Limited evidence has shown the microdebrider to provide greater improvements in voice quality and shorter procedure times, and it appears to be more cost-effective when compared to carbon dioxide laser [25–28].

Carbon Dioxide (CO_2) Laser

The CO_2 is the most commonly used thermal ablation technique for RRP in the larynx. It has an emission wavelength of 10,600 nm and converts light to thermal energy being absorbed by intracellular water. In expert hands, it is a very precise tool. The CO_2 laser vaporizes RRP lesions while cauterizing tissue surfaces thus minimizing bleeding. A single-center retrospective study of 244 RRP patients treated with CO_2 laser every 2 months reported "remission" (no visible RP 2 months after last procedure) in 37 %, "clearance" (lack of clinically apparent disease for 3 years post last treatment) in 6 %, and "cure" (lack of recurrence 5 years after last removal) in 17 % [29]. The ideal frequency of which this therapy should be performed has not been determined. One of the main criticisms surrounding CO_2 is the "diffuse" thermal damage to papillomas surrounding tissue [30]. This could lead to scarring of adjacent areas with its inherent complications and perhaps spread of viral particles to unaffected areas [22]. Also, active viral genomic DNA has been found in the laser smoke or "plume" which can be a source of infection to the operator and assistants [31–33].

Other Thermal Ablation Techniques

A number of other techniques have been investigated. Pulse dye laser treatment has been performed in an office setting in patients with upper airway RRP with very good tolerance [34], but this may not apply to patients with more distal disease.

Also in patients with upper airway disease, the 532-nm potassium titanyl phosphate (KTP) laser has been shown to provide 90 % or greater disease regression in 80 % of patients when the procedure was performed under general anesthesia [35] and at least 75 % regression in 62 % of patients when performed in an office-based setting without general anesthesia [36].

Photodynamic therapy (PDT) is another ablation technique that has been investigated. A Cochrane review from 2014 selected a single trial with a total of 23 participants to provide a recommendation on the use of PDT for RRP [37]. This study randomized patients requiring treatment with CO_2 laser or microdebrider at least three times per year to receive a single PDT dose at 6 or 18 months after enrollment [38]. It is important to note that 17 patients were available for final analysis and only 15 actually received PDT. Marked improvement in laryngeal disease was noted over time but not in tracheal RRP. Laryngeal remission was reported in 5 out of 15 patients 12–15 months post-therapy. Recurrence treated with CO_2 laser was noted after this period in 4 patients that continued to be followed. One patient required intubation and eventual tracheotomy due to significant airway swelling. Based on current evidence, PDT cannot be recommended for the treatment of RRP outside of a clinical trial.

Very limited reports suggest that argon plasma coagulation may be another alternative for the treatment of RRP, especially of the lower airways [39, 40].

Adjuvant Therapy

Adjuvant treatment includes both local and systemic therapies. Adjuvant therapy is generally instituted in patients requiring surgical debulking every 2–3 months [41]. Other accepted indications include airway compromise and multiple sites of airway disease [41, 42].

Antivirals

Cidofovir

This is probably the most commonly used adjuvant therapy in RRP [19]. Cidofovir is an antiviral nucleoside analogue of deoxycytidine monophosphate and is currently approved by the US Food and Drug Administration for the treatment of AIDS-related cytomegalovirus retinitis. Therefore, it is used in an "off-label" fashion in the treatment of RRP. The majority of practitioners use a total dose of 20–40 mg per case in adults, typically in a concentration of 2.5–5 mg/ml [41]. Complete response rates have been reported to range between 56 and 82 % with mean relapse-free time between 10 and 49 months [43–48]. However, these data do not come from the only randomized study performed to date [49]. In this small study of 19 patients, individuals were randomized to have cidofovir or placebo injected into affected areas whenever surgical intervention was needed. Though significant improvement was noted at 2- and 12-month follow-ups, there was no difference between groups.

A major concern of the FDA with the use of cidofovir for RRP is the potential risk of malignant transformation based on animal studies [23]. However, a systematic review of 31 case series involving 188 patients noted dysplasia in 5 patients (2.7 %) [50]. A more recent review of 635 RRP patients of whom 275 received cidofovir demonstrated 4 cases of malignancies of the upper airway and trachea following the use of this drug versus 18 out of 360 individuals that did not receive it [51]. No statistically significant difference was noted between groups, though.

Individual case reports have shown that inhaled cidofovir may also be effective [52, 53].

Acyclovir

Small uncontrolled studies have suggested a benefit with the use of acyclovir [54–56]. However, because the mechanism of action of acyclovir would not explain its efficacy against HPV, it is possible the improvement is due to herpes coinfections [57].

Ribavarin

A limited number of cases using ribavarin demonstrated an increase in the interval between surgical managements of RRP [58, 59]. The lack of control limits the evidence to recommend this drug for routine use.

Interferon and Other Immunogenic Drugs

Interferon-α, an immunoregulation drug, was once the most widely used adjuvant therapy for RRP. However, over the past 10–15 years, very few studies evaluating this drug in RRP have been published suggesting its use is in significant decline. Earlier well-designed studies demonstrated a lower growth rate in patients receiving interferon in addition to surgical treatment when compared to individuals treated with surgical therapy alone [60, 61]. However, the initial response did not appear to be sustained [60]. The more recent studies suggest patients with HPV-6 tend to respond better to interferon compared to patients with HPV-11 [62, 63]. Though interferon is generally well tolerated, more than 50 % of patients have at least one side effect [64]. The main adverse reactions include fever, chills, arthralgias and myalgias, and headache.

Recently, granulocyte–monocyte colony-stimulating factor (GM-CSF) and pegylated interferon alpha 2a (Peg-IFNα-2a) demonstrated a decrease in the number of surgical interventions in a small number of patients [65]. Though promising, the lack of control precludes further recommendation on the use of this regimen at this time.

Bevacizumab

The epithelium from papillomas of patients with RRP has been shown to have strong expression of vascular endothelial growth factor (VEGF)-A as well as expression of VEGF receptor (VEGFR) VEGFR-1 and VEGFR-2 messenger RNAs in the underlying vascular endothelial cells [66]. Based on these findings, small non-controlled studies utilizing both intralesional bevacizumab and intravenous bevacizumab in patients with RRP have been performed [67–69]. All these studies demonstrated a decrease in the frequency of surgical procedures in most patients. The IV systemic option may be beneficial in patients with poorly accessible papilloma lesions [69].

Epidermal Growth Factor Receptor (EGFR) Inhibitors

Respiratory papillomas overexpress EGFR when compared with normal laryngeal epithelium [70, 71]. A total of 6 patients treated with these drugs have been reported in the English literature. In one case report, a teenager was treated with gefitinib, a tyrosine kinase inhibitor [72]. There was significant decrease in the papilloma growth and number of surgical procedures. In another case report, a man requiring frequent surgical debridements was treated with a combination of erlotinib (another tyrosine kinase inhibitor) and celecoxib with remarkable clinical response [73]. In a case series with 4 patients, 3 individuals who received panitumumab (a fully human monoclonal antibody specific to the epidermal growth factor receptor) also demonstrated a significant decrease in the number of surgical procedures and one demonstrated complete response [74]. The fourth patient on this study received gefitinib also with great response after failing other therapies. It is important to note that 3 patients who responded to panitumumab were previously treated with erlotinib and celecoxib (2 cases) and erlotinib, interferon, and gefitinib (1 case) without response. In cancer, EGFR tyrosine kinase inhibitors have been shown to provide a response in some patients with certain tumor mutations, whereas panitumumab might be effective in tumors that overexpress EGFR. Since no sensitizing EGFR mutation has been identified in papillomas to date, the use of panitumumab makes more sense over EGFR tyrosine kinase inhibitors. In addition, these drugs cannot be recommended for routine use until larger studies are performed.

Cyclooxygenase (COX)-2 Inhibitors

Papillomas have been shown to overexpress COX-2 through different pathways [75, 76]. Treatment of these cells with celecoxib suppressed proliferation and induced apoptosis [75]. A celecoxib multicentered, randomized, double-blind placebo controlled study funded by the US National Institutes of Health is currently underway.

Measles–Mumps–Rubella (MMR) Vaccine

A small single-center investigation of 26 patients with RRP randomized 13 patients to surgical treatment followed by coating of the excised lesion base with MMR and the other half to surgical therapy alone [77]. There was no statistically significant difference in the recurrence-free remission between groups.

Indole-3-Carbinol

Indole-3-carbinol (I3C) is derived from the hydrolysis of glucobrassicin, a compound found in cruciferous vegetables such as broccoli, Brussels sprouts, cabbage, and cauliflower. It is an FDA-approved nutritional supplement. In animal study, inhibition of estrogen metabolism using I3C reduced the formation of HPV-induced papilloma tumors in a significant number of mice [78]. In a prospective open-label study, 33 patients with RRP were eligible for long-term follow-up. Eleven (33 %) patients experienced remission of papillomatous growth and did not require repeat surgical treatment after being placed on I3C, 10 (30 %) patients had a required less frequent surgery, and 12 patients (36 %) had no clinical response. As per multiple other studies, the lack of a control arm begs for additional investigation before I3C can be recommended on a routine basis.

Zinc

Zinc-deficient subjects appear to be more susceptible infections [79–81]. A single case report demonstrated significant improvement of RRP after correcting the patient's zinc deficiency [82].

Retinoids

Metabolites and analogues of vitamin A have been reported to have antiproliferative effects on epithelial tissues [83]. Case reports/series and pilot studies with the use of 13-cis-retinoic acid have been reported with mixed results [83–86]. Again, the limited data do not allow any firm recommendation on its use in RRP.

Propranolol

It has been hypothesized this drug downregulates VEGF [87]. The role of VEGF in RRP has been discussed previously. Maturo et al. investigated the use of propranolol in 3 children with RRP. One had no response and two demonstrated a significant decrease in the number of surgical procedures compared to previous year [87].

Gastroesophageal Reflux (GERD)

Some believe GERD may trigger proliferation or spread of papilloma disease [8]. A number of reports suggest treating GERD decreases the frequency of surgical treatment [88–90] and the risk of web formation [91].

HPV Vaccines

A prospective single-arm study with 11 patients with aggressive RRP receiving a quadrivalent vaccine against HPV types 6, 11,16, and 18 demonstrated a mean interval between surgical procedures of 271.2 days before the vaccination and 537.4 days after [92]. A retrospective study in 13 patients with recurrent disease after intralesional cidofovir who received the quadrivalent vaccine demonstrated no recurrence during a 1-year follow-up in 85 % of the subjects [93]. The two patients who were noted to have recurrence after the first vaccine dose failed to demonstrate any recurrence one year after the third dose of the vaccine. This possible therapeutic effect of vaccination against HPV has also been shown in much larger samples in women with high-grade cervical dysplasia [94].

Summary

RRP is a rare disease, but has a characteristic appearance that should be identified since specific therapy is available, and progressive/untreated disease can have significant morbidity. RRP is separated into both juvenile and adult forms, though clinical manifestations seem to be similar. HPV types 6 and 11 account for over 95 % of RRP cases. Though early disease seems limited to the laryngeal area, progression to the lower respiratory tract is not uncommon, especially in adults. Early symptoms are non-specific consisting mainly of cough and hoarseness, and progression of disease can lead to wheezing, dysphagia, and stridor. In patients with symptomatic lower respiratory tract disease (subglottic space and more distal), we typically treat with the microdebrider, argon plasma coagulation, local cidofovir injection, or any combination of these. We have been increasingly recommending HPV vaccination to our patients.

References

1. Goon P, Sonnex C, Jani P, Stanley M, Sudhoff H. Recurrent respiratory papillomatosis: an overview of current thinking and treatment. Eur Arch Otorhinolaryngol. 2008;265:147–51.
2. Ullmann E. On the etiology of the laryngeal papillomata. Acta Otolaryngol. 1923;5:317–34.
3. Mounts P, Shah KV, Kashima H. Viral etiology of juvenile- and adult-onset squamous papilloma of the larynx. Proc Natl Acad Sci. 1982;79:5425–29.
4. Dickens P, Srivastava G, Loke SL, Larkin S. Human papillomavirus 6, 11, and 16 in laryngeal papillomas. J Pathol. 1991;165:243–6.
5. Derkay CS, Darrow DH. Recurrent respiratory papillomatosis. Ann Otol Rhinol Laryngol. 2006;115:1–11.
6. Bonagura VR, Hatam L, DeVoti J, Zeng F, Steinberg BM. Recurrent respiratory papillomatosis: altered CD8$^+$ T-cell subsets and T_H1/T_H2 cytokine imbalance. Clin Immunol. 1999;93:302–11.
7. Rodman R, Mutasa S, Dupuis C, Spratt H, Underbrink M. Genetic dysregulation in recurrent respiratory papillomatosis. Laryngoscope. 2014;124:E320–5.
8. Venkatesan NN, Pine HS, Underbrink MP. Recurrent respiratory papillomatosis. Otolaryngol Clin North Am. 2012;45:671–94.
9. Oh ST, Longworth MS, Laimins LA. Roles of the E6 and E7 proteins in the life cycle of low-risk human papillomavirus type 11. J Virol. 2004;78:2620–6.
10. Lindeberg H, Elbrønd O. Laryngeal papillomas: the epidemiology in a Danish subpopulation 1965-1984. Clin Otolaryngol Allied Sci. 1990;15:125–31.
11. Omland T, Akre H, Vårdal M, Brøndbo K. Epidemiological aspects of recurrent respiratory papillomatosis: a population-based study. Laryngoscope. 2012;122:1595–99.
12. Cohn AM, Kos JT, Taber LH, Adam E. Recurring laryngeal papilloma. Am J Otolaryngol—Head Neck Med Sur. 1981;2:129–32.
13. Ruiz R, Achlatis S, Verma A, Born H, Kapadia F, Fang Y, Pitman M, Sulica L, Branski RC, Amin MR. Risk factors for adult-onset recurrent respiratory papillomatosis. Laryngoscope. 2014;124:2338–44.
14. Kashima HK, Shah F, Lyles A, Glackin R, Muhammad N, Turner L, Van Zandt S, Whitt S, Shah K. A comparison of risk factors in juvenile-onset and adult-onset recurrent respiratory papillomatosis. Laryngoscope. 1992;102:9–13.

15. Born H, Ruiz R, Verma A, Taliercio S, Achlatis S, Pitman M, Gandonu S, Bing R, Amin MR, Branski RC. Concurrent oral human papilloma virus infection in patients with recurrent respiratory papillomatosis: a preliminary study. Laryngoscope. 2014;124:2785–90.
16. Steinberg BM, Topp WC, Schneider PS, Abramson AL. Laryngeal papillomavirus infection during clinical remission. N Engl J Med. 1983;308:1261–4.
17. Best SR, Niparko KJ, Pai SI. Biology of human papillomavirus infection and immune therapy for HPV-related head and neck cancers. Otolaryngol Clin North Am. 2012;45:807–22.
18. Larson DA, Derkay CS. Epidemiology of recurrent respiratory papillomatosis. APMIS. 2010;118:450–4.
19. Schraff S, Derkay CS, Burke B, Lawson L. AMerican Society of Pediatric Otolaryngology Members' experience with recurrent respiratory papillomatosis and the use of adjuvant therapy. Arch Otolaryngol—Head Neck Sur. 2004;130:1039–42.
20. Omland T, Akre H, Lie KA, Jebsen P, Sandvik L, Brøndbo K. Risk factors for aggressive recurrent respiratory papillomatosis in adults and juveniles. PLoS One. 2014;9:e113584.
21. Cook JR, Hill DA, Humphrey PA, Pfeifer JD, El-Mofty SK. Squamous cell carcinoma arising in recurrent respiratory papillomatosis with pulmonary involvement: emerging common pattern of clinical features and human papillomavirus serotype association. Mod Pathol. 2000;13:914–8.
22. Derkay CS, Wiatrak B. Recurrent respiratory papillomatosis: a review. Laryngoscope. 2008;118:1236–47.
23. Taliercio S, Cespedes M, Born H, Ruiz R, Roof S, Amin M, Branski R. Adult-onset recurrent respiratory papillomatosis. a review of disease pathogenesis and implications for patient counseling. JAMA Otolaryngol Head Neck Surg. 2014.
24. Manickavasagam J, Wu K, Bateman ND. Treatment of paediatric laryngeal papillomas: web survey of British Association of Paediatric Otolaryngologists. J Laryngol Otol. 2013;127:917–21.
25. El-Bitar MAZG. Powered instrumentation in the treatment of recurrent respiratory papillomatosis: An alternative to the carbon dioxide laser. Arch Otolaryngol—Head Neck Surg. 2002;128:425–8.
26. Pasquale K, Wiatrak B, Woolley A, Lewis L. Microdebrider versus CO_2 laser removal of recurrent respiratory papillomas: a prospective analysis. Laryngoscope. 2003;113:139–43.
27. Patel N, Rowe M, Tunkel D. Treatment of recurrent respiratory papillomatosis in children with the microdebrider. Ann Otol Rhinol Laryngol. 2003;112:7–10.
28. Holler T, Allegro J, Chadha NK, Hawkes M, Harrison RV, Forte V, Campisi P. Voice outcomes following repeated surgical resection of laryngeal papillomata in children. Otolaryngol Head Neck Surg. 2009;141:522–6.
29. Dedo HH, Yu KCY. CO_2 laser treatment in 244 patients with respiratory papillomas. Laryngoscope. 2001;111:1639–44.
30. Alkotob ML, Budev MM, Mehta AC. Recurrent respiratory papillomatosis. J Bronchol. 2004;11:132–9.
31. Sawchuk WS, Weber PJ, Lowy DR, Dzubow LM. Infectious papillomavirus in the vapor of warts treated with carbon dioxide laser or electrocoagulation: detection and protection. J Am Acad Dermatol. 1989;21:41–9.
32. Hallmo P, Naess O. Laryngeal papillomatosis with human papillomavirus DNA contracted by a laser surgeon. Eur Arch Otorhinolaryngol. 1991;248:425–7.
33. Kashima HK, Kessis T, Mounts P, Shah K. Polymerase chain reaction identification of human papillomavirus DNA in CO_2 laser plume from recurrent respiratory papillomatosis. Otolaryngol Head Neck Surg. 1991;104:191–5.
34. Rees CJ, Halum SL, Wijewickrama RC, Koufman JA, Postma GN. Patient tolerance of in-office pulsed dye laser treatments to the upper aerodigestive tract. Otolaryngol Head Neck Surg. 2006;134:1023–7.
35. Burns JA, Zeitels SM, Akst LM, Broadhurst MS, Hillman RE, Anderson R. 532 nm pulsed potassium-titanyl-phosphate laser treatment of laryngeal papillomatosis under general anesthesia. Laryngoscope. 2007;117:1500–4.

36. Zeitels SM, Akst LM, Burns JA, Hillman RE, et al. Office-Based 532-nm pulsed KTP laser treatment of glottal papillomatosis and dysplasia. Ann Otol Rhinol Laryngol. 2006;115:679–85.
37. Lieder A, Khan MK, Lippert BM. Photodynamic therapy for recurrent respiratory papillomatosis. Cochrane Database Syst Rev. 2014;6:CD009810.
38. Shikowitz MJ, Abramson AL, Steinberg BM, et al. Clinical trial of photodynamic therapy with meso-tetra (hydroxyphenyl) chlorin for respiratory papillomatosis. Arch Otolaryngol—Head Neck Surg. 2005;131:99–105.
39. Bergler W, Hönig M, Götte K, Petroianu G, Hörmann K. Treatment of recurrent respiratory papillomatosis with argon plasma coagulation. J Laryngol Otol. 1997;111:381–4.
40. Wong JL, Tie ST, Lee J, Kannan SK, Ali MRR, Ibrahim A, Rahman JAA. A case of recurrent respiratory papillomatosis successfully removed via endoscopic argon plasma coagulation (APC) with no evidence of recurrence. Med J Malaysia. 2014;69:195–6.
41. Derkay CS, Volsky PG, Rosen CA, Pransky SM, McMurray JS, Chadha NK, Froehlich P. Current use of intralesional cidofovir for recurrent respiratory papillomatosis. Laryngoscope. 2013;123:705–12.
42. Derkay CS. Task force on recurrent respiratory papillomas: a preliminary report. Arch Otolaryngol—Head Neck Surg. 1995;121:1386–91.
43. Snoeck R, Wellens W, Desloovere C, Ranst MV, Naesens L, De Clercq E, Feenstra L. Treatment of severe laryngeal papillomatosis with intralesional injections of cidofovir (S)-1-(3-hydroxy-2-phosphonylmethoxypropyl)cytosine. J Med Virol. 1998;54:219–25.
44. Dikkers FG. Treatment of recurrent respiratory papillomatosis with microsurgery in combination with intralesional cidofovir—a prospective study. Eur Arch Otorhinolaryngol. 2006;263:440–3.
45. Naiman AN, Ayari S, Nicollas R, Landry G, Colombeau B, Froehlich P. Intermediate-term and long-term results after treatment by cidofovir and excision in juvenile laryngeal papillomatosis. Ann Otol Rhinol Laryngol. 2006;115:667–72.
46. Pudszuhn A, Welzel C, Bloching M, Neumann K. Intralesional Cidofovir application in recurrent laryngeal papillomatosis. Eur Arch Otorhinolaryngol. 2007;264:63–70.
47. Wierzbicka M, Jackowska J, Bartochowska A, Józefiak A, Szyfter W, Kędzia W. Effectiveness of cidofovir intralesional treatment in recurrent respiratory papillomatosis. Eur Arch Otorhinolaryngol. 2011;268:1305–11.
48. Graupp M, Gugatschka M, Kiesler K, Reckenzaun E, Hammer G, Friedrich G. Experience of 11 years use of cidofovir in recurrent respiratory papillomatosis. Eur Arch Otorhinolaryngol. 2013;270:641–6.
49. McMurray JS, Connor N, Ford CN. Cidofovir efficacy in recurrent respiratory papillomatosis: a randomized, double-blind, placebo-controlled study. Ann Otol Rhinol Laryngol. 2008;117:477–83.
50. Broekema FI, Dikkers FG. Side-effects of cidofovir in the treatment of recurrent respiratory papillomatosis. Eur Arch Otorhinolaryngol. 2008;265:871–9.
51. Tjon PG, Ilmarinen T, den Heuvel ER, Aaltonen LM, Andersen J, Brunings JW, Chirila M, Dietz A, Ferran Vilà F, Friedrich G, Gier HHW, Golusinski W, Graupp M, Hantzakos A, Horcasitas R, Jackowska J, Koelmel JC, Lawson G, Lindner F, Remacle M, Sittel C, Weichbold V, Wierzbicka M, Dikkers FG. Safety of intralesional cidofovir in patients with recurrent respiratory papillomatosis: an international retrospective study on 635 RRP patients. Eur. Arch. Oto-Rhino-Laryngol. 2013;270:1679–87.
52. Giles BL, Seifert B. CR12/339–Nebulized cidofovir for recurrent respiratory papillomatosis: a case report. Paediatr Respir Rev. 2006;7:S330.
53. Ksiazek J, Prager JD, Sun GH, Wood RE, Arjmand EM. Inhaled cidofovir as an adjuvant therapy for recurrent respiratory papillomatosis. Otolaryngol—Head Neck Surg. 2011;144:639–41.
54. Endres DR, Bauman NM, Burke D, Smith RJ. Acyclovir in the treatment of recurrent respiratory papillomatosis. A pilot study. Ann Otol Rhinol Laryngol. 1994;103:301–5.

55. Kiroğlu M, Cetik F, Soylu L, Abedi A, Aydoğan B, Akçali C, Kiroğlu F, Ozsahinoğlu C. Acyclovir in the treatment of recurrent respiratory papillomatosis: a preliminary report. Am J Otolaryngol. 1994;15:212–4.
56. Chaturvedi J, Sreenivas V, Hemanth V, Nandakumar R. Management of adult recurrent respiratory papillomatosis with oral acyclovir following micro laryngeal surgery: a case series. Ind J Otolaryngol Head Neck Surg. 2014;66:359–63.
57. Pou AM, Jordan JA, Barua P, Shoemaker DL, et al. Adult respiratory papillomatosis: Human papillomavirus type and viral coinfections as predictors of prognosis. Ann Otol Rhinol Laryngol. 1995;104:758–62.
58. McGlennen RC, Adams GL, Lewis CM, Faras AJ, Ostrow RS. Pilot trial of ribavirin for the treatment of laryngeal papillomatosis. Head Neck. 1993;15:504–12.
59. Balauff A, Sira J, Pearman K, McKiernan P, Buckels J, Kelly D. Successful ribavirin therapy for life-threatening laryngeal papillomatosis post liver transplantation. Pediatr Transplant 2001;5:142–4.
60. Healy GB, Gelber RD, Trowbridge AL, Grundfast KM, Ruben RJ, Price KN. Treatment of recurrent respiratory papillomatosis with human leukocyte interferon. N Engl J Med. 1988;319:401–7.
61. Leventhal BG, Kashima HK, Weck PW, et al. Randomized surgical adjuvant trial of interferon alfa-n1 in recurrent papillomatosis. Arch Otolaryngol—Head Neck Surg. 1988;114:1163–9.
62. Gerein V, Rastorguev E, Gerein J, Jecker P, Pfister H. Use of interferon-alpha in recurrent respiratory papillomatosis: 20-year follow-up. Ann Otol Rhinol Laryngol. 2005;114:463–71.
63. Szeps M, Dahlgren L, Aaltonen L, Öhd J, Kanter-Lewenshon L, Dahlstrand H, Munck-Wikland E, Grandér D, Dalianis T. Human papillomavirus, viral load and proliferation rate in recurrent respiratory papillomatosis in response to alpha interferon treatment. J Gen Virol. 2005;86:1695–702.
64. Nodarse-Cuní H, Iznaga-Marín N, Viera-Alvarez D, Rodríguez-Gómez H, et al. Interferon alpha-2b as adjuvant treatment of recurrent respiratory papillomatosis in Cuba: National Programme (1994–1999 report). J Laryngol Otol. 2004;118:681–7.
65. Suter-Montano T, Montaño E, Martínez C, Plascencia T, Sepulveda MT, Rodríguez M. Adult recurrent respirator papillomatosis: a new therapeutic approach with pegylated interferon alpha 2a (Peg-IFNα-2a) and GM-CSF. Otolaryngol Head Neck Surg. 2013;148:253–60.
66. Rahbar R, Vargas SO, Folkman J, McGill TJ, et al. role of vascular endothelial growth factor-A in recurrent respiratory papillomatosis. Ann Otol Rhinol Laryngol. 2005;114:289–95.
67. Rogers DJ, Ojha S, Maurer R, Hartnick CJ. Use of adjuvant intralesional bevacizumab for aggressive respiratory papillomatosis in children. JAMA Otolaryngol—Head Neck Surg. 2013;139:496–501.
68. Sidell DR, Nassar M, Cotton RT, Zeitels SM, de Alarcon A. High-dose sublesional bevacizumab (Avastin) for pediatric recurrent respiratory papillomatosis. Ann Otol Rhinol Laryngol. 2014;123:214–21.
69. Mohr M, Schliemann C, Biermann C, Schmidt L, Kessler T, Schmidt J, Wiebe K, Müller K, Hoffmann TK, Groll AH, Werner C, Kessler C, Wiewrodt R, Rudack C, Berdel WE. Rapid response to systemic bevacizumab therapy in recurrent respiratory papillomatosis. Oncol Lett. 2014;8:1912–8.
70. Vambutas A, Di Lorenzo TP, Steinberg BM. Laryngeal papilloma cells have high levels of epidermal growth factor receptor and respond to epidermal growth factor by a decrease in epithelial differentiation. Cancer Res. 1993;53:910–4.
71. Johnston D, Hall H, DiLorenzo TP, Steinberg BM. Elevation of the epidermal growth factor receptor and dependent signaling in human papillomavirus-infected laryngeal papillomas. Cancer Res. 1999;59:968–74.
72. Bostrom B, Sidman J, Marker S, Lander T, Drehner D. GEfitinib therapy for life-threatening laryngeal papillomatosis. Arch Otolaryngol—Head Neck Surg. 2005;131:64–7.
73. Limsukon A, Susanto I, Hoo GWS, Dubinett SM, Batra RK. Regression of recurrent respiratory papillomatosis with celecoxib and erlotinib combination therapy. Chest. 2009;136:924–6.

74. Moldan M, Bostrom B, Tibesar R, Lander T, Sidman J. Epidermal growth factor receptor inhibitor therapy for recurrent respiratory papillomatosis. F1000Res 2013;2:202.
75. Wu R, Abramson AL, Shikowitz MJ, Dannenberg AJ, Steinberg BM. Epidermal Growth Factor-2 expression mediated through phosphatidylinositol-3 kinase, not mitogen-activated protein/extracellular signal-regulated kinase kinase, in recurrent respiratory papillomas. Clin Cancer Res. 2005;11:6155–61.
76. Wu R, Abramson AL, Symons MH, Steinberg BM. Pak1 and Pak2 are activated in recurrent respiratory papillomas, contributing to one pathway of Rac1-mediated COX-2 expression. Int J Cancer. 2010;127:2230–7.
77. Lei J, Yu W, Yuexin L, Qi C, Xiumin S, Tianyu Z. Topical measles-mumps-rubella vaccine in the treatment of recurrent respiratory papillomatosis: results of a preliminary randomized, controlled trial. Ear Nose Throat J 2012;91:174–5.
78. Newfield L, Goldsmith A, Bradlow HL, Auborn K. Estrogen metabolism and human papillomavirus-induced tumors of the larynx: chemo-prophylaxis with indole-3-carbinol. Anticancer Res. 1993;13:337–41.
79. Bondestam M, Foucard T, Gebre-Medhin M. Subclinical trace element deficiency in children with undue susceptibility to infections. Acta Paediatr Scand. 1985;74:515–20.
80. Van Wouwe JP. Clinical and laboratory assessment of zinc deficiency in Dutch children. A review. Biol Trace Elem Res. 1995;49:211–25.
81. Bahl R, Bhandari N, Hambidge KM, Bhan MK. Plasma zinc as a predictor of diarrheal and respiratory morbidity in children in an urban slum setting. Am J Clin Nutr. 1998;68:414S–7S.
82. Bitar M, Baz R, Fuleihan N, Muallem M. Can zinc be an adjuvant therapy for juvenile onset recurrent respiratory papillomatosis? Int J Pediatr Otorhinolaryngol. 2007;71:1163–73.
83. Alberts DS, Coulthard SW, Meyskens FLJ. Regression of aggressive laryngeal papillomatosis with 13-cis-retinoic acid (accutane). J Biol Response Mod. 1986;5:124–8.
84. Bell R, Hong WK, Itri LM, McDonald G, Stuart Strong M. The use of cis-retinoic acid in recurrent respiratory papillomatosis of the larynx: A randomized pilot study. Am J Otolaryngol —Head Neck Med Surg 1988;9:161–164.
85. Lippman SM, Donovan DT, Frankenthaler RA, Weber RS, Earley CL, Hong WK, Goepfert H. 13-Cis-retinoic acid plus interferon-alpha 2a in recurrent respiratory papillomatosis. J Natl Cancer Inst. 1994;86:859–61.
86. Osborne C, LeBoeuf H, Jones DV, J. Isotretinoin in respiratory papillomatosis. Ann Intern Med 2000;132:1007.
87. Maturo S, Tse SM, Kinane TB, Hartnick CJ. Initial experience using propranolol as an adjunctive treatment in children with aggressive recurrent respiratory papillomatosis. Ann Otol Rhinol Laryngol 2011;120:17–20.
88. Borkowski G, Sommer P, Stark T, Sudhoff H, Luckhaupt H. Recurrent respiratory papillomatosis associated with gastroesophageal reflux disease in children. Eur Arch Otorhinolaryngol. 1999;256:370–2.
89. Harcourt JP, Worley G, Leighton SEJ. Cimetidine treatment for recurrent respiratory papillomatosis. Int J Pediatr Otorhinolaryngol. 1999;51:109–13.
90. McKenna M, Brodsky L. Extraesophageal acid reflux and recurrent respiratory papilloma in children. Int J Pediatr Otorhinolaryngol. 2005;69:597–605.
91. Holland BW, Koufman JA, Postma GN, McGuirt WF. Laryngopharyngeal reflux and laryngeal web formation in patients with pediatric recurrent respiratory papillomas. Laryngoscope. 2002;112:1926–9.
92. Hočevar-Boltežar I, Matičič M, Šereg-Bahar M, Gale N, Poljak M, Kocjan B, Žargi M. Human papilloma virus vaccination in patients with an aggressive course of recurrent respiratory papillomatosis. Eur Arch Otorhinolaryngol. 2014;271:3255–62.
93. Chirilă M, Bolboacă SD. Clinical efficiency of quadrivalent HPV (types 6/11/16/18) vaccine in patients with recurrent respiratory papillomatosis. Eur Arch Otorhinolaryngol. 2014;271:1135–42.
94. Kang WD, Choi HS, Kim SM. Is vaccination with quadrivalent HPV vaccine after loop electrosurgical excision procedure effective in preventing recurrence in patients with high-grade cervical intraepithelial neoplasia (CIN2-3)? Gynecol Oncol. 2013;130:264–8.

Chapter 11
Parasitic Diseases of the Lung

Danai Khemasuwan, Carol Farver and Atul C. Mehta

Introduction

Parasitic infection can be categorized into helminthic and protozoal infections. Although, there is a decreasing trend of parasitic infection worldwide due to improved socioeconomic conditions and better hygiene practices, the urbanization of the cities around the world, global climate changes, international traveling, and increasing numbers of immunocompromised individuals have expanded the population who is vulnerable to parasitic diseases [1]. The diagnosis of parasitic diseases of the respiratory system is relatively difficult because clinical manifestations and radiologic findings are non-specific. Therefore, high index of suspicion, travel history, and a detailed interrogation of personal hygiene are crucial for diagnosis of parasitic lung diseases. The helminthes can affect respiratory system in different phases of their life cycle. In this chapter, we discuss the clinical manifestations, radiographic, bronchoscopic and pathologic findings, and management of several helminthic and protozoal lung diseases. The term "pneumatodes" has been used to represent the group of parasites that affect airways and lungs. Some of the unique presentations of each parasite are also addressed which may be helpful to pulmonologist in managing these uncommon diseases (Tables 11.1 and 11.2).

D. Khemasuwan (✉)
Interventional Pulmonary and Critical Care Medicine, Intermoutain
Medical Center, Murray, UT, USA
e-mail: danai_md@hotmail.com

C. Farver
Department of Pathology, Cleveland Clinic, Cleveland, OH, USA

A.C. Mehta
Lerner College of Medicine, Buoncore Family Endowed Chair in Lung Transplantation,
Respiratory Institute, Cleveland Clinic, Cleveland, OH, USA
e-mail: Mehtaa1@ccf.org

A.C. Mehta
Pulmonary Medicine, Respiratory Institute, Cleveland Clinic, Cleveland, OH, USA

© Springer International Publishing Switzerland 2016   231
A.C. Mehta et al. (eds.), *Diseases of the Central Airways*,
Respiratory Medicine, DOI 10.1007/978-3-319-29830-6_11

Table 11.1 Key features of protozoal infections of lung

Protozoal parasites	Endemic area	Mode of transmission	Presentation	Bronchoscopic evaluation	Treatment
- Pulmonary amebiasis	Worldwide	Ingestion	Fever, right upper quadrant abdominal pain, lung abscess, hepatobronchial fistula	Surgical lung biopsy shows *E. histolytica* trophozoites	Metronidazole
- Pulmonary leishmaniasis	Asia, Africa, and Central and South America	Sand fly-borne infection	Pneumonitis, pleural effusion, mediastinal lymphadenopathy	Transbronchial needle biopsy of a mediastinal lymph node showing histiocytes containing *L. donovani* organisms.	Pentavalent antimonials, liposomal amphotericin B, and miltefosine
- Pulmonary malaria	Tropical and subtropical areas	Mosquito-borne infection	Fever, cough, acute respiratory distress syndrome (ARDS)	N/A	Intravenous artesunate and artemisinin
- Pulmonary babesiosis	North America	*Ixodes* tick-borne infection	Fever, drenching sweats, acute respiratory distress syndrome (ARDS)	N/A	A combination of atovaquone plus azithromycin or clindamycin plus quinine
- Pulmonary toxoplasmosis	Worldwide	Ingestion	Generalized lymphadenopathy, interstitial pneumonia, diffuse alveolar damage	Histologic examination of lung biopsy can identify *T. gondii* tachyzoites in necrotic area	Pyrimethamine and sulfadiazine

Table 11.2 Main features of parasitic diseases of lung

Parasite	Infective form	Endemic area	Mode of transmission	Pulmonary presentation	Bronchoscopic evaluation	Treatment
Nematodes						
Ascariasis (*Ascaris lumbricoides*)	Eggs and larva	Asia, Africa, and South America	Ingestion	Eosinophilic pneumonia, cough, wheezing, dyspnea	Presence of parasite in the airways	Mebendazole and albendazole
Hookworm (*Ancyclostoma duodenale*) (*Necator americanus*)	Larva	Tropical and subtropical areas	Skin penetration	Eosinophilic pneumonia, cough, wheezing, dyspnea, alveolar hemorrhage	Presence of hookworm in sputum, a marked eosinophil predominance from BAL	Mebendazole and albendazole
Strongyloidiasis (*Strongyloides stercoralis*)	Filariform larvae	Tropical and subtropical areas	Skin penetration	Eosinophilic pneumonia, cough, wheezing, dyspnea, hyperinfection syndrome	Bloody bronchoalveolar lavage (BAL) and presence of parasite from BAL under microscopic examination	Ivermectin and albendazole
Syngamosis (*Mammomonogamus laryngeus*)	Eggs or adult worms	Asia, Africa, and South America	Ingestion	Foreign body-like lesion in bronchus nocturnal cough	Presence of parasite in the airways	Removal via bronchoscopy
Dirofilariasis (*Dirofilaria immitis*)	Larva	Tropical and subtropical areas	Mosquito-borne infection	Cough, chest pain, fever, dyspnea, mild eosinophilia, and lung nodules	Surgical lung biopsy	None (self-limited)

(continued)

Table 11.2 (continued)

Parasite	Infective form	Endemic area	Mode of transmission	Pulmonary presentation	Bronchoscopic evaluation	Treatment
Tropical pulmonary eosinophilia (*Brugia malayi*) (*Wuchereria bancrofti*)	Larva	Tropical and subtropical areas (South and Southeast Asia)	Mosquito-borne infection	Eosinophilic pneumonia, cough, wheezing, dyspnea, restrictive pattern on spirometry, decreased diffusion lung capacity	BAL shows eosinophils more than 50 % of the total cells	Diethylcarbamazine (DEC)
Visceral larva migrans (*Toxocara canis*) (*Toxocara catis*)	Larva	Worldwide	Ingestion	Eosinophilic pneumonia, episodic wheezing	N/A	Diethylcarbamazine (DEC)
Trichinella infection (*Trichinella spiralis*)	Larva	Worldwide	Ingestion	Cough, pulmonary infiltrates, dyspnea is due to respiratory muscles involvement	N/A	Mebendazole
Trematodes						
Schistosomiasis (*Schistosoma* spp)	Cercarial larvae	East Asia, South America, sub-Saharan Africa	Skin penetration	Pulmonary hypertension, and Katayama fever	An eosinophil predominance from BAL in the absence of parasites	Praziquantel
Paragonimiasis (*Paragonimus* spp)	Metacercaria (infective larvae)	Southeast Asia, South America, Africa	Ingestion of infested crustaceans	Fever, cough, hemoptysis, chest pain, and pleural effusion	Bronchial stenosis due to mucosal edema and mucosal nodularity	Praziquantel and triclabendazole

(continued)

Table 11.2 (continued)

Parasite	Infective form	Endemic area	Mode of transmission	Pulmonary presentation	Bronchoscopic evaluation	Treatment
Cestodes						
Hydatid disease (*Echinococcus granulosus*)	Eggs	Worldwide (esp. Middle East)	Ingestion	Chest pain, cough, hemoptysis, pleural lesion, expectoration of cyst contents, and hypersensitivity reaction	Bronchoscopic examination reveals sac-like cyst in the airway	Surgical removal of cysts, followed by mebendazole and albendazole
Mesomycetozoea						
Rhinosporidiosis (*Rhinosporidium seeberi*)	Spores	South Asia	Ingestion of contaminated water	Strawberry-like, nasopharyngeal polyps, epistaxis, nasal congestion	Bronchoscopy revealed pinkish mulberry-like rhinosporidiosis mass in the airway	Therapeutic bronchoscopy and dapsone

Protozoal Parasites

Pulmonary Amebiasis

Entamoeba histolytica amebiasis occurs worldwide. Human becomes infected via feco-oral route by ingestion of mature *E. histolytica* cyst. Trophozoites invade the intestinal mucosa and enter the bloodstream which results in systemic infection. Invasive amebiasis is an emerging parasitic disease in human immunodeficiency virus (HIV)-infected patients [2]. Pleuropulmonary amebiasis occurs mainly by local extension from the amoebic liver abscess. Patients usually present with fever, right upper quadrant abdominal pain, chest pain, and cough. Lung abscess, hepatobronchial fistula, and pyopneumothorax can occur as complications from pleuropulmonary amebiasis. The radiographic findings are elevated right hemidiaphragm, hepatomegaly, and pleural effusion. Live trophozoites of *E. histolytica* can be found in sputum, pleural fluid, or lung biopsy. The presence of amoeba in the stool does not indicate active *E. histolytica* infection because there are two other non-pathologic *Entamoeba* species found in humans. A combination of serologic tests with detection of the parasite by antigen detection by polymerase chain reaction (PCR) is the most preferred approach to diagnosis [3]. Metronidazole is treatment of choice for invasive amoebiasis.

Pulmonary Leishmaniasis

Leishmania donovani is transmitted by various species of the sand fly and causes visceral leishmaniasis [4]. The endemic areas of leishmaniasis are Asia, Africa, and Central and South America. Pulmonary manifestations include pneumonitis, pleural effusion, and mediastinal lymphadenopathy [5]. Leishmania amastigotes can be found in the alveoli and mediastinal lymph node biopsy. Diagnosis of leishmaniasis is confirmed by the presence of the parasites in bone marrow aspirates or by the detection of PCR-amplified Leishmania. The treatment of choices includes pentavalent antimonials and liposomal amphotericin B. Oral miltefosine can also be used against visceral leishmaniasis [5].

Pulmonary Manifestations of Malaria

Plasmodium spp. are intra-erythrocytic protozoa, primarily transmitted by the Anopheles mosquito [6]. *Plasmodium falciparum* can cause cerebral malaria which may potentially fatal. The pulmonary manifestations range from dry cough to severe and rapidly fatal acute respiratory distress syndrome (ARDS). The gold standard for the diagnosis of malarial infection is microscopic examination of stained thick and thin blood smears. Radiographic findings include lobar consolidation, diffuse interstitial edema, and pleural effusion. Mitochondrial PCR detection of Plasmodium DNA in saliva and urine has been described. However, this technology needs further validation [7]. Intravenous artesunate and parenteral artemisinin derivatives are effective treatments against *P. falciparum* in humans [8].

Pulmonary Babesiosis

Babesiosis is caused by hemoprotozoan parasites, *Babesia microti*, and *B. divergens* [9]. Ixodes scapularis is a vector of babesiosis. The symptoms are fever, drenching sweats, loss of appetite, myalgia, and headache. Splenic infarction and spontaneous splenic rupture have been reported in acute babesiosis [10]. In severe case, ARDS can occur after a few days after initiation of medical therapy. Chest radiography reveals bilateral infiltrates with pulmonary edema. Diagnosis is made by examination of a Giemsa-stained thin blood smear which shows tetrads inside the red blood cells (maltese cross formation). The two major antibiotic regimens consist of a combination of clindamycin and quinine or atovaquone and azithromycin. These regimens are orally given for 7–10 days [11]. Atovaquone plus azithromycin is preferred therapy.

Pulmonary Toxoplasmosis

Toxoplasmosis is caused by the protozoan parasite, *Toxoplasma gondii*. Cats are primary hosts of *T. gondii* [12]. Humans become infected by ingestion of parasitic cyst-contaminated undercooked food. The symptoms of toxoplasmosis are myalgia and generalized lymphadenopathy. Pulmonary toxoplasmosis has been reported with increasing frequency in HIV-infected patients. Pulmonary manifestations include interstitial pneumonia, diffuse alveolar damage, or necrotizing pneumonia [13]. Diagnosis of toxoplasmosis is based on the detection of the bradyzoites of *T. gondii* in body tissue (Fig. 11.1). A real-time PCR-based assay in BAL fluid has been reported in HIV-positive patients. Toxoplasmosis can be treated with a combination of pyrimethamine and sulfadiazine for 3–4 weeks [14].

Fig. 11.1 Lung infected with
Toxoplasmosis gondii (*arrow*)
with diffuse alveolar damage
(DAD) (H&E stain, ×100)
(Courtesy of Danai
Khemasuwan, MD, MBA,
and Carol Farver, MD)

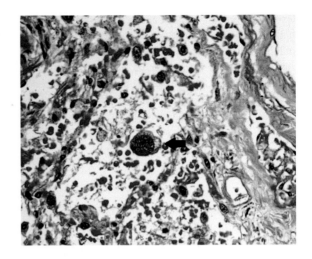

Helminthic Parasites

Nematodes (Roundworms)

Ascariasis

Ascaris lumbricoides is one of the most common parasitic infestations, affecting over a billion of the world's population causing more than thousand deaths annually [1]. *A. lumbricoides* is transmitted through the feco-oral route. Ascaris larvae migrate to the lungs via either the venules of the portal system or the lymphatic drainage. Larval ascariasis causes Löffler's syndrome, consisting of wheezing, pulmonary infiltrations, and a moderate eosinophilia [15]. The larvae can cause alveolar inflammation, necrosis, and hemorrhage. It is difficult to diagnose ascariasis infestation during its larvae phase. The sputum may show numerous eosinophils. However, stool examination usually yields negative results for eggs during larval stage because there is no reproducing adult ascaris in the host to produce eggs [16]. The diagnosis requires a high degree of suspicion. Occasionally, the diagnosis can be confirmed by identifying larvae in the sputum. Solitary pulmonary nodules (SPN) can also develop if the larva dies and evokes a granulomatous reaction [17]. Adult ascaris has been reported to cause airway obstruction in a child producing a complete lobar collapse [18]. Mechanical removal of ascaris through bronchoscopy is the management of choice. Mebendazole and albendazole are the most effective agents against ascariasis. The prognosis is excellent after eradication of ascariasis with anti-parasitic agents.

Ancylostomiasis (Hookworm Disease)

The common hookworms are *Ancylostoma duodenale* and *Necator americanus*. The latter is found in the parts of southern USA. Hookworm larvae enter human hosts via the skin, producing itching and local infection. *A. duodenale* larvae are also orally infective [19]. Hookworm infestation involves larval migration through the lungs via the bloodstream resulting in a hypersensitivity reaction. Patients usually present with transient eosinophilic pneumonia (Löffler's syndrome) [19]. Patients may ingest a large number of *A. duodenale* larvae and develop a condition known as Wakana disease. It is characterized by nausea, vomiting, dyspnea, cough, throat irritation, hoarseness, and eosinophilia [19]. Larval migration may also cause alveolar hemorrhage [20]. Similar to ascariasis, the diagnosis of a hookworm infestation during the larvae phase could be difficult. Computed tomography (CT) of the chest may reveal transient, migratory, patchy alveolar infiltrates [21]. Sputum examination may reveal occult blood, eosinophils, and, rarely, migrating larvae [22]. Bronchoscopic examination may reveal airway erythema and high eosinophil counts in bronchoalveolar lavage fluid (BALF) [23]. Patients can become profoundly anemic and malnourished. These manifestations may provide clinical clues to support the diagnosis. Anti-parasitic agents for hookworm are mebendazole and albendazole.

Strongyloidiasis

Strongyloides stercoralis is a common roundworm that is endemic throughout the tropical area, but also found worldwide in all climates. Infective filariform larvae can penetrate the skin and infect human hosts. The larvae migrate through the soft tissues and enter the lungs via the bloodstream. A majority of roundworms migrate up the bronchial tree to the pharynx and are swallowed, entering the gastrointestinal tract [24]. The larvae can reenter the circulatory system, returning to the lungs and causing autoinfection [24]. The life cycle of Strongyloides can be completed entirely within one host. The term "hyperinfection syndrome" describes the presentation of sepsis from enteric flora, mostly in immunocompromised patients [25]. The hallmarks of hyperinfection are exacerbation of gastrointestinal and pulmonary symptoms, and the detection of large number of larvae in stool and sputum [26]. Common pulmonary symptoms include wheezing, hoarseness, dyspnea, and hemoptysis. Chest X-ray usually demonstrates focal or bilateral interstitial infiltrates. Pleural effusions are present in 40 % of patients, and lung abscess is found in 15 % [27]. Diffuse alveolar hemorrhage is usually found in patients with disseminated strongyloidiasis. Adult respiratory distress syndrome (ARDS) may result as a reaction to the dead larvae. A massive migration of larvae through the intestinal wall can result in sepsis from gram-negative bacteria [26]. *Strongyloides* infestation can be potentially fatal if untreated.

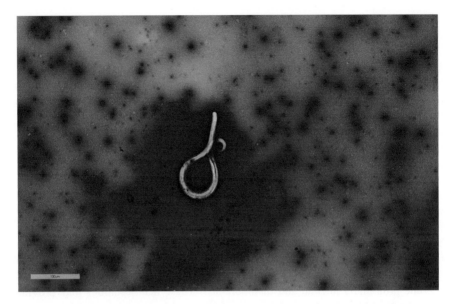

Fig. 11.2 Strongyloides larvae from BAL (H&E stain, 200×) (Courtesy of Danai Khemasuwan, MD, MBA, and Carol Farver, MD)

The diagnosis can be confirmed by the presence of larvae in the stool, duodenal aspirate, sputum, pleural fluid, BAL fluid, or lung biopsies (Figs. 11.2 and 11.3) [28]. The sensitivity of a stool exam for ova and larvae is 92 % when performed on three consecutive samples [29]. Enzyme-linked immunosorbent assay (ELISA)

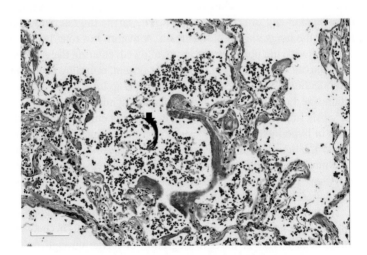

Fig. 11.3 Strongyloides larvae (*arrow*) present in alveolar space in lung with diffuse alveolar damage (DAD); (H&E stain, 400×) (Courtesy of Danai Khemasuwan, MD, MBA, and Carol Farver, MD)

measures IgG responses to the Strongyloides antigen. However, false-negative results can occur during acute infection as it takes 4–6 weeks to mount the immune response [30]. ELISA is sensitive but non-specific due to cross-reactivity with filarial infestations [28]. Oral ivermectin remains the treatment of choice for uncomplicated Strongyloides infection. In case of disseminated disease, a reduction of immunosuppressive therapy is recommended besides treatment with ivermectin [26, 31].

Syngamosis

Nematoda of the genus *Mammomonogamus* affect the respiratory tract of domestic mammals. Human is rarely become infested via respiratory tract. Most cases of human syngamosis are reported from tropical areas, including South America, the Caribbean, and Southeast Asia [32]. The life cycle is not completely known. Two hypotheses have been proposed in regard to its life cycle. One is that humans become infested via the ingestion of food or water contaminated with larvae or embryonated eggs. The larvae complete the life cycle in the pulmonary system, and the adult worms migrate to the central airways as the preferred site of infection [33]. An alternative hypothesis is that the patients are infected by the adult worms present in contaminated food or water. This mode of transmission is supported by its short incubation period (6–11 days) [34]. The diagnosis is usually made by flexible bronchoscopy or when the worms are expelled after vigorous coughing. The removal of parasites through bronchoscopy is sufficient to improve the symptoms. There are no studies to support the effectiveness of antihelminthic drugs. However, they may be considered as an adjunct in the treatment [34, 35].

Dirofilariasis

Dirofilaria immitis is the filarial nematode that primarily infects dogs. Humans are considered accidental hosts since *D. immitis* is not able to mature to an adult form. The endemic areas of dirofilariasis are Southern Europe, Asia, Australia, and America. *D. immitis* is transmitted to humans by mosquitoes harboring infective third-stage larvae. The larva travels to the right ventricle and develops into an immature adult worm. It is then swept into the pulmonary arteries. The worm dies as a result of the inflammatory response and evokes granuloma formation [36]. A majority of patients with pulmonary dirofilariasis are asymptomatic. However, some patients may develop cough, hemoptysis, chest pain, fever, dyspnea, and mild eosinophilia ∼5 %) [37]. A peripheral or a pleural-based SPN is a typical presentation. The nodule may show increased fluoro-deoxy-glucose (FDG) avidity on a positron emission tomography (PET) scan [38, 39] and is often confused with malignancy. Calcification occurs within only 10 % of these nodules. CT may show

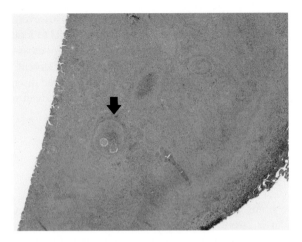

Fig. 11.4 A presence of Dirofilaria worms within pulmonary artery and causing pulmonary infarction (H&E stain, 27×) (Courtesy of Danai Khemasuwan, MD, MBA, and Carol Farver, MD)

a branch of pulmonary artery entering the nodule [40]. Serology has poor specificity due to cross-reactivity with other helminthes. The diagnosis is established by identifying the worm in the excised lung tissue (Figs. 11.4 and 11.5). In patients with high risk of cancer, these lung nodules may be confused with malignancy. Needle biopsy and brushings are usually non-diagnostic due to the small sample size. The condition is self-limiting and does not require any specific treatment [37].

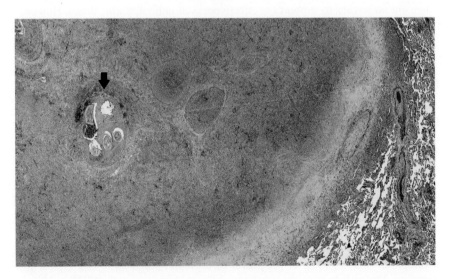

Fig. 11.5 Cross sections of a coiled Dirofilaria worms (*arrow*) within involved artery causing surrounding infarction of lung tissue. Note the smooth cuticle (Movat stain, 30×) (Courtesy of Danai Khemasuwan, MD, MBA, and Carol Farver, MD)

Tropical Pulmonary Eosinophilia

Tropical pulmonary eosinophilia (TPE) is a syndrome of immunologic reaction to microfilaria of the lymphatic-dwelling organisms *Brugia malayi* and *Wuchereria bancrofti*. It is a mosquito-borne infestation. The larvae reside in the lymphatics and develop into mature adult worms. The endemic areas of TPE are in the tropical and subtropical regions of South and Southeast Asia. Travelers from non-endemic areas are at risk of developing TPE because they do not have natural immunity against microfilaria compared with subjects living in endemic area. The microfilariae are released into the circulation and may be trapped in the pulmonary circulation [41]. Trapped microfilariae demonstrate a strong immunogenicity and trigger anti-microfilarial antibodies, resulting in asthma-like symptoms. The hallmark of TPE is a high absolute eosinophil count (5000–80,000/mm^3) [42]. The radiologic features include reticulonodular opacities predominantly in the middle and the lower lung zones, miliary mottling, and predominant hila with increased vascular markings at the bases [43]. Chest CT may demonstrate bronchiectasis, air trapping, calcification, and mediastinal lymphadenopathy [44]. Pulmonary functions indicate a restrictive defect with mild airway obstruction [42]. BAL fluid may contain numerous eosinophils. Occasionally, microfilaria can be identified on brushings or biopsies [45]. The chronic phase of TPE may lead to progressive and irreversible pulmonary fibrosis [41].

The standard treatment for TPE is diethylcarbamazine (DEC). Patients usually show improvement within 3 weeks. However, many patients may be left with a mild form of interstitial lung disease and diffusion impairment on pulmonary function tests [46]. Concomitant use of corticosteroid may have a role in TPE. However, a clinical trial is required to determine the proper dose and duration of DEC therapy.

Toxocariasis

Toxocara canis and *Toxocara cati* are roundworms that primarily affect the dog and cat, respectively. These roundworms are common parasites that cause visceral larva migrans and eosinophilic lung disease in humans. Toxocariasis is transmitted to humans via ingestion of food that is contaminated with parasite eggs. The larvae can migrate throughout the host's body, including the lungs [5]. The pathologic manifestations of visceral larva migrans are due to a hypersensitivity response to the migrating larvae. Visceral larva migrans can present with fever, cough, wheezing, seizures, and anemia. Examination features include general lymph node enlargement, hepatomegaly, and splenomegaly. Leukocytosis and severe eosinophilia are demonstrated in a peripheral smear. Chest X-ray reveals pulmonary infiltrates with hilar and mediastinal lymphadenopathy. Bilateral pleural effusion can occur [47]. Non-cavitating pulmonary nodules have also been reported [48]. The diagnosis of toxocariasis is established by an ELISA for the larval antigens [49]. The treatment of choice is DEC; however, DEC may exacerbate the inflammatory reactions due to killing of larvae. Thus, it is advised to use corticosteroid along with DEC to ease the inflammatory response [5].

Trichinella Infection

Trichinella spiralis is the most common Trichinella species that infects humans. Trichinella is a food-borne disease from undercooked pork containing larval trichinellae. In addition to the pork meat, wild animals such as bear meat may also contain *T. spiralis* [50]. The larvae migrate and reside in the gastrointestinal tract until they develop into an adult form. Fertilized female worms release first-stage larvae into the bloodstream and the lymphatics [51]. Pulmonary involvement, although uncommon, produces shortness of breath and pulmonary infiltrates. Dyspnea is due to parasitic invasion of the diaphragm and the accessory respiratory muscles [39]. The diagnosis is confirmed by muscle biopsy, which may demonstrate *T. spiralis* larvae. An ELISA using anti-*Trichinella* IgG antibodies can confirm the diagnosis in humans [52]. A 2-week course of mebendazole with analgesics and corticosteroids is the recommended treatment [51].

Trematodes (Flatworms)

Schistosomiasis

Five schistosomes species cause disease in humans: *Haematobium, Mansoni, Japonicum, Intercalatum, and Mekongi* [21]. The endemic area for *S. haematobium* and *S. mansoni* are sub-Saharan Africa and South America, and for *S. japonicum*, Far East [21]. Schistosomiasis is the second most common cause of mortality among parasitic infections after malaria worldwide [1]. *S. haematobium* resides in the urinary bladder, while *S. mansoni* and *S. japonicum* reside in the mesenteric beds [5]. Humans become infested through the skin from a contact with fresh water containing *Schistosomal* cercaria (infective larva). After the cercariae have penetrated the skin, they migrate to the lung and the liver. There are several case reports of acute schistosomiasis (Katayama fever) among travelers with history of swimming in Lake Malawi and rafting in sub-Saharan Africa [53].

In acute schistosomiasis, patients present with dyspnea, wheezing, dry cough, abdominal pain, hepatosplenomegaly, myalgia, and eosinophilia [54]. Patients experience shortness of breath due to an immunologic reaction to antigens released by the worms. The level of circulating immune complexes correlates with symptoms and with the intensity of infection.

In chronic schistosomiasis, embolization of the eggs in the portal system causes periportal fibrosis and portal hypertension. Pulmonary involvement can occur as a result of the systemic migration of parasitic eggs from the portal system. The eggs trigger an inflammatory response that leads to pulmonary artery hypertension and subsequent development of cor pulmonale in 2–6 % of patients [55]. Apoptosis of the endothelial cells in the pulmonary vasculature plays a role in the pathogenesis of schistosomal-associated cor pulmonale [56]. Chest X-ray and CT may show diffuse reticulonodular pattern or ground-glass opacities [57]. In the acute phase, BALF may reveal eosinophilia in the absence of parasites. The diagnosis is confirmed by microscopic examination of stool and urine or by rectal biopsy. However, the sensitivity of these tests is low for an early infection. ELISA can be used as a screening test and is confirmed by enzyme-linked immunoelectrotransfer blot. These tests become positive within 2 weeks after the infestation. Schistosomal ova can be found in the lung biopsy specimen.

Acute schistosomiasis is treated with praziquantel. The treatment is repeated within several weeks since it has no antihelminthic effect on the juvenile stages of the parasites [58]. Acute pneumonitis can be observed 2 weeks after the treatment, which is believed to be related to lung embolization of adult worms from the pelvic veins [59]. Patients with schistosomal-associated pulmonary arterial hypertension (PAH) can be treated with PAH-specific therapy along with anti-parasitic medications [59].

Paragonimiasis

Paragonimus species, including *westermani*, cause paragonimiasis that usually involves the lungs. Infection of *paragonimus* species is geographically distributed in Southeast Asia, African, and South America. The mode of transmission is ingestion of the metacercaria (infective larvae) from undercooked crustaceans. Undercooked meat of crab-eating mammals (wild boars and rat) can infect humans as indirect route of transmission [60]. The larvae penetrate the intestinal wall, migrating through the diaphragm and the pleura, into the bronchioles [61]. The eggs are produced by the mature adult worms which are expelled in the sputum or swallowed and passed with the stool. Typically acute symptoms include fever, chest pain, and chronic cough with hemoptysis [62]. Pleural effusion and pneumothorax may be the first manifestation during the migration of the juvenile worms through the pleura. Chest X-ray demonstrates patchy infiltrates, nodular opacities, pleural effusion, and fluid-filled cysts with ring shadows [5]. Chest CT may reveal a band-like opacity abutting the visceral pleura (worm migration tracks), bronchial wall thickening, and centrilobular nodules. Bronchoscopic examination may reveal airway narrowing from mucosal edema [63]. Lung biopsy may show chronic eosinophilic inflammation. The diagnosis is confirmed by the presence of eggs or larvae in the sputum sample or BALF. The pleural fluid, when present, is an exudate with eosinophilia, mostly sterile, without the presence of any organisms

[64]. Eosinophilia and elevated serum IgE levels are observed in more than 80 % of infected patients [5]. Serological tests with ELISA and a direct fluorescent antibody (DFA) are highly sensitive and specific for establishing the diagnosis [65]. Praziquantel and triclabendazole are the treatments of choice with a high cure rate of 90 and 98.5 %, respectively [5].

Cestodes

Echinococcosis

Echinococcus granulosus and *E. multilocularis* are the parasite species that cause hydatid disease in humans. *E. granulosus* is endemic in sheep-herding areas of the Mediterranean, Eastern Europe, the Middle East, and Australia. An estimated 65 million individuals in these areas are infected [1]. Humans become accidental hosts either by direct contact with the primary hosts (usually dogs) or by the ingestion of food contaminated with feces containing parasite eggs [5]. The larvae reach the bloodstream and lymphatic circulation of intestines and migrate to the liver which is the main habitat in human host. Two different presentations of echinococcosis are as follows: (a) cystic hydatidosis and (b) alveolar echinococcosis.

In most cases, lung hydatidosis is a single cyst (72–82 %). An echinococcal infection becomes symptomatic after 5–15 years, secondary to local compression or dysfunction of the affected organ. Pulmonary cysts expand at a slower rate of 1–5 cm per year than liver cysts, and calcification of the cyst is less common [66]. Pulmonary symptoms from the intact cyst include cough, fever, dyspnea, and chest pain. The cyst may rupture into a bronchus and cause hemoptysis and/or expectoration of cystic fluid containing parasitic components (hydatoptysis) which is considered a pathognomonic finding of cyst rupture [67]. The patients may present with hydropneumothorax or empyema. Occasionally, a ruptured cyst can cause an anaphylactic-like reaction and pneumonia [21]. Cystic hydatidosis is diagnosed by chest radiography which demonstrates a well-defined homogenous fluid-filled round opacity. Ruptured cysts may demonstrate an empty cavity, but it is more usual to have characteristic features such as air crescent, pneumocyst, and floating membrane ("water lily sign") (Fig. 11.6) on radiologic examination [68]. The "meniscus" or "crescent" sign and Cumbo's sign (onion peel) have also been described. Thoracic ultrasonography may be useful to confirm the cystic structure, demonstrating the characteristic double-contour (pericyst and parasitic membrane endocyst) of intact cysts. Daughter cysts are also occasionally observed in pulmonary hydatidosis [68]. Bronchoscopic examination reveals sac-like cysts in the airway (Fig. 11.7). Bronchoscopic extraction of the hydatid cyst is possible; however, there is a risk of cyst rupture. Therefore, it should be considered on a case-by-case basis. Serological tests are more sensitive in patients with liver

Fig. 11.6 Water lily sign (CT scan obtained at level of right middle lobe shows ruptured hydatid cyst. After rupture and discharge of cyst fluid into pleural cavity, endocyst collapses, sediments, and floats in remaining fluid at bottom of original cyst) (Courtesy by Farid Rashidi, MD)

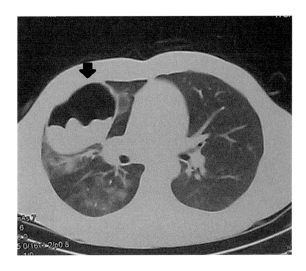

Fig. 11.7 Protruded hydatid cyst from left lower lob (LLL) bronchus (Courtesy by Farid Rashidi, MD)

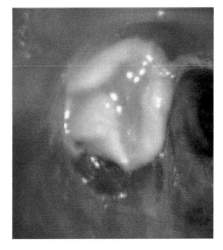

involvement (80–94 %) than with lung hydatidosis (65 %) [5]. Hydatid cyst rupture can increase sensitivity of serological tests to be more than 90 % [67]. Surgical resection of the cysts is the main treatment of pulmonary hydatidosis and aims to remove the intact hydatid cyst and treat associated parenchymal and bronchial disease. The principle of surgery is to preserve as much as lung tissue as possible. Lung parenchyma around a hydatid cyst is often affected by the lesion and may show chronic congestion, hemorrhage, and interstitial pneumonia. These inflammatory changes in the lung tissue often resolve after surgery [69]. Spillage of hydatid fluid must be avoided to prevent secondary hydatidosis. After complete removal of hydatid cyst, the cavity needs to be irrigated with hypertonic saline solution and it is obliterated with separate purse-string sutures. Surgical specimens may reveal echinococcus cyst fragments (Figs. 11.8 and 11.9).

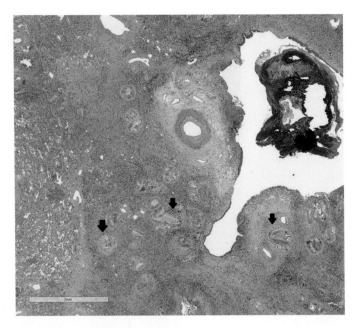

Fig. 11.8 Echinococcus cyst fragments in lung biopsy. The *arrows* highlight the collapsed chitinous layer of a death hydatid cyst. (H&E stain, ×15) (Courtesy of Danai Khemasuwan, MD, MBA, and Carol Farver, MD)

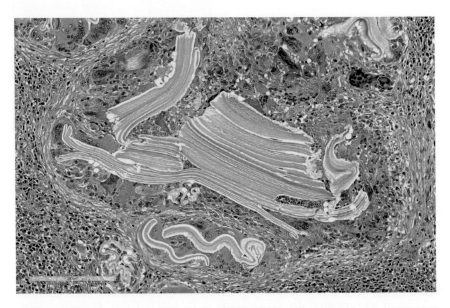

Fig. 11.9 Echinococcus cyst fragments in lung biopsy. The fragmented echinococcus cyst with collapse chitinous layer resides within granulomatous reaction. (H&E stain, ×180) (Courtesy of Danai Khemasuwan, MD, MBA, and Carol Farver, MD)

Medical therapy may have a role in poor surgical candidates and when there is intra-operative spillage of fluid from hydatid cyst. Antihelminthic agents, such as mebendazole or albendazole, have shown only 25–34 % cure rates [70]. The disadvantage of antihelminthic therapy is that it may weaken the cyst wall and increases the risk of spontaneous rupture. In addition, if the parasite dies due to the drug, the cyst membrane may remain within the cavity and lead to secondary complications, including infections [71]. Percutaneous treatment by puncture, aspiration, injection, and re-aspiration (PAIR) has rarely been used in pulmonary cysts because of the risk of anaphylactic shock, pneumothorax, pleural spillage, and bronchopleural fistulae [72].

Pulmonary alveolar echinococcosis is a rare but severe and potentially fatal form of echinococcosis. This form is restricted to the Northern Hemisphere. The liver is the first target for the parasite, with a long, silent incubation period. Pulmonary involvement results from either dissemination or the direct extension of the hepatic echinococcosis with intrathoracic rupture through the diaphragm into the bronchial tree, pleural cavity, or mediastinum. Chest X-ray or CT may aid in the diagnosis. ELISA and indirect hemagglutination assay are available and offer early detection in endemic areas. Radical resection of localized lesions is the only curative treatment yet and is rarely possible in invasive and disseminated disease. Mebendazole and albendazole can be used, but the required treatment duration needs is a minimum of 2 years after the radical surgery [73].

Mesomycetozoea

Rhinosporidiosis

Rhinosporidiosis is a chronic granulomatous infectious disease caused by *Rhinosporidium seeberi*. Recent molecular studies have categorized class Mesomycetozoea at the border of animal–fungal kingdom [74]. The infection is endemic in South Asia [75]. Patients usually presents with polypoidal lesions which are friable and have a high risk of bleeding during resection and high tendency of recurrence. The common sites of presentation are nose and nasopharynx. However, lesions can involve tracheobronchial tree which may lead to partial or complete airway obstruction [76]. There are only three case reports of bronchial involvement which all of them are reported from South Asia. CT is the preferred imaging technique since it offers details of the extension of disease. Bronchoscopic management plays a major role in bronchial involvement of rhinosporidiosis. The mass can completely cauterized with bronchoscopic snare and excised mass can be removed by the basket. Microscopic examination of the resected specimen demonstrated bronchial subepithelium with sporangia filled with small round endospores. The bleeding can be controlled by cauterization. Dapsone is the only medication found to arrest the maturation of the sporangia, but the lesion may recur after months or years [77]. Thus, follow-up bronchoscopy is recommended to monitor early signs of recurrence.

Conclusion

Global warming, international travel, and immigration has changed the old paradigm of natural distribution of helminthic and protozoal infestations which have been dominant mainly in the tropical and subtropical areas. In addition, the increasing use of immunosuppressive drugs and increasing organ transplantations also result in resurgence of parasitic lung infections worldwide. Therefore, it is important for pulmonologists to recognize the epidemiology, life cycles, clinical presentation, laboratory diagnosis, and treatments of these "pneumatodes" in order to make the proper management in these patients.

References

1. Martínez S, Restrepo CS, Carrillo JA, et al. Thoracic manifestations of tropical parasitic infections: a pictorial review. Radiographics. 2005;25(1):135–55.
2. Hsu MS, Hsieh SM, Chen MY, et al. Association between amebic liver abscess and human immunodeficiency virus infection in Taiwanese subjects. BMC Infect Dis. 2008;8:48.
3. Tanyuksel M, Petri WA Jr. Laboratory diagnosis of amoebiasis. Clin Microbiol Rev. 2003;16:713–29.
4. Piscopo TV, Mallia AC. Leishmaniasis. Postgrad Med J. 2006;82:649–57.
5. Vijayan VK. Parasitic lung infections. Curr Opin Pulm Med. 2009;15:274–82.
6. World Health Organization. Estimated burden of malaria in 2006. In: World malaria report 2008. Geneva (Switzerland): WHO; 2008. p 9–15.
7. Ghayour Najafabadi Z, Oormazdi H, Akhlaghi L, et al. Mitochondrial PCR-based malaria detection in saliva and urine of symptomatic patients. Trans R Soc Trop Med Hyg. 2014 Apr 25. (Epub ahead of print).
8. Rosenthal PJ. Artesunate for the treatment of severe falciparum malaria. N Engl J Med. 2008;358:1829–36.
9. Vannier E, Gewurz BE, Krause PJ. Human babesiosis. Infect Dis Clin North Am. 2008;22:469–88.
10. Florescu D, Sordilo PP, Glyptis A, et al. Splenic infarction in human babesiosis: two cases and discussion. Clin Infect Dis. 2008;46:e8–11.
11. Krause PJ. Babesiosis diagnosis and treatment. Vector Borne Zoonotic Dis. 2003;3:45–51.
12. Dodds EM. Toxoplasmosis. Curr Opin Opthalmol. 2006;17:557–61.
13. Petersen E, Edvinsson B, Lundgren B, et al. Diagnosis of pulmonary infection with Toxoplasma gondii in immunocompromised HIV-positive patients by real-time PCR. Eur J Clin Microbiol Infect Dis. 2006;25:401–4.
14. Martinez-Giron R, Estiban JG, Ribas A, et al. Protozoa in respiratory pathology: a review. Eur Respir J. 2008;32:1354–70.
15. Gelpi AP, Mustafa A. Ascaris pneumonia. Am J Med. 1968;44:377–89.
16. Butts C, Hnderson SO. Ascariasis. Top Emerg Med. 2003;25:38–43.

17. Osborne DP, Brown RB, Dimmette RM. Solitary pulmonary nodule due to *Ascaris lumbrocoides*. Chest. 1961;40:308–10.
18. Lapid O, Kreiger Y, Berstein T, et al. Airway obstruction by *Ascaris* roundworm in a burned child. Burns. 1999;25:673–5.
19. Hotez PJ, Brooker S, Bethony JM, et al. Hookworm infection. N Engl Med. 2004;35:799–807.
20. Sarinas PS, Chitkara RK. Ascariasis and hookworm. Semin Respir Infect. 1997;12:130–7.
21. Kuzucu A. Parasitic diseases of the respiratory tract. Curr Opin Pulm Med. 2006;12:212–21.
22. Beigel Y, Greenberg Z, Ostfeld I. Clinical problem-solving. Letting the patient off the hook. N Engl J Med. 2000;342(22):1658–61.
23. Maxwell C, Hussain R, Nutman TB, et al. The clinical and immunologic responses of normal human volunteers to low dose hookworm (*Necator americanus*) infection. Am J Trop Med Hyg. 1987;37:126–34.
24. Keiser PB, Nutman TB. Strongyloides stercoralis in the immunocompromised population. Clin Microbiol Rev. 2004;17:208–17.
25. Namisato S, Motomura K, Haranaga S, et al. Pulmonary strongyloides in a patient receiving prednisolone therapy. Int med. 2004;43:731–6.
26. Mejia R, Nutman TB. Screening, prevention, and treatment for hyperinfection syndrome and disseminated infections caused by *Strongyloides stercoralis*. Curr Opin Infect Dis. 2012;25:458–63.
27. Woodring JH, Halfhill H, Berger R, et al. Clinical and imaging features of pulmonary strongyloidiasis. South Med J. 1996;89:10–8.
28. Saddiqui AA, Berk SL. Diagnosis of *Strongyloides sterocoralis* infection. Clin Infect Dis. 2001;33:1040–7.
29. Cartwright CP. Utility of multiple stool specimen ova and parasite examinations in a high prevalence setting. J Clin Mocrobiol. 1999;37:2408–11.
30. Krolewiecki AJ, Ramanathan R, Fink V, et al. Improved diagnosis of *Strongyloides sterocoralis* using recombinant antigen-based serologies in a community-wide study in northern Argentina. Clin Vaccine Immunol. 2010;17:1624–30.
31. Suputtamongkol Y, Premasathian N, Bhumimuang K, et al. Efficacy and safety of single and double doses of ivermectin versus 7-day high dose albendazole for chronic *Strongyloidiasis*. PLoS Negl Trop Dis. 2011;5:e1044.
32. Kim HY, Lee SM, Joo JE, et al. Human syngamosis: the first case in Korea. Thorax. 1998;53:717–8.
33. Severo LC, Conci LMA, Camargo JJP, et al. Syngamosis: two new Brazilian cases and evidence of a possible pulmonary cycle. Trans R Soc Trop Med Hyg. 1988;82:467–8.
34. Weinstein L, Molovi A. Syngamus laryngeus infection (syngamosis) with chronic cough. Ann Intern Med. 1971;74:577–80.
35. de Lara Tde A, Barbosa MA, de Oliveira MR, et al. Human syngamosis. Two cases of chronic cough caused by *Mammomonogamus laryngeus*. Chest. 1993;103:264–5.
36. Theis JH. Public health aspects of dirofilariasis in the United States. Vet Parasitol. 2005;133:157–80.
37. de Campos JR, Barbas CS, Filomeno LT, et al. Human pulmonary dirofilariasis: analysis of 24 cases from Sao Paulo Brazil. Chest. 1997;112:729–33.
38. Oshiro Y, Murayama S, Sunagawa U, et al. Pulmonary dirofilariasis: computed tomography findings and correlation with pathologic features. J Comput Assist Tomogr. 2004;28:796–800.
39. Moore W, Franceschi D. PET findings in pulmonary dirofilariasis. J Thorac Imaging. 2005;20:305–6.
40. Chitkara RK, Sarinas PS. Dirofilaria, visceral larva migrans, and tropical pulmonary eosinophilia. Semin Respir Infect. 1997;12:138–48.
41. Bogglid AK, Keystone JS, Kain KC. Tropical pulmonary eosinophilia: a case series in a setting of nonendemicity. Clin Infect Dis. 2004;39:1123–8.
42. Vijayan VK. Immunopathogenesis and treatment of eosinophilic lung diseases in the tropics. In: Sharma OP, editor. Lung biology in health and disease: tropical lung disease. 2nd ed. New York: Taylor & Francis; 2006. p. 195–239.

43. Savani DM, Sharma OP. Eosinophilic lung disease in the tropics. Clin Chest Med. 2002;23:377–96.
44. Sandhu M, Mukhopadhyay S, Sharma SK. Tropical pulmonary eosinophilia: a comparative evaluation of plain chest radiography and computed tomography. Australas Radiol. 1996;40:32–7.
45. Ottesen EA, Nutman TB. Tropical pulmonary eosinophilia. Annu Rev Med. 1992;43:417–24.
46. Vijayan VK, Rao KV, Sankaran K, et al. Tropical eosinophilia: clinical and physiological response to diethylcarbamazine. Resp Med. 1991;85:17–20.
47. Figueiredo SD, Taddei JA, Menezes JJ, et al. Clinical-epidemiological study of toxocariasis in a pediatric population. J Pedistr (Rio J). 2005;81:126–32.
48. Sane AC, Barber BA. Pulmonary nodules due to *Toxocara canis* infection in an immunocompetent adult. South Med J. 1997;90:78–9.
49. Sespommier D. Toxocariasis: clinical aspects, epidemiology, medical ecology, and molecular aspects. Clin Microbiol Rev. 2003;16:265–72.
50. Harbottle JE, English DK, Schultz MG. Trichinosis in bears in northeastern United States. HSMHA Health Rep. 1971;86(5):473–6.
51. Bruschi F, Murrell K. Trichinellosis. In: Guerrant R, Walker DH, Weller PF, editors. Tropical infectious disease: principles, pathogens and practice, vol. 2. Philadelphia: Churchill Livingstone; 1999. p. 917–25.
52. Gomez-Moreales MA, Ludovisis A, Amati M, et al. Validation of an ELISA for the diagnosis of human trichinellosis. Clin Vaccine Immunol. 2008;15:1723–9.
53. Cooke GS, Lalvani A, Gleeson FV, et al. Acute pulmonary schistosomiasis in travelers returning from lake Malawi, sub-Saharan Africa. Clin Infect Dis. 1999;29:836–9.
54. Bottieau E, Clerinx J, de Vega MR, et al. Imported Katayama fever: clinical and biological features at presentation and during treatment. J Infect (in press).
55. Schwartz E. Pulmonary schistosomiasis. Clin Chest Med. 2002;23:433–43.
56. Simonneau G, Robbins IM, Beghetti M, et al. Updated clinical classification of pulmonary hypertension. J Am Coll Cardiol. 2009;541(suppl):S43–54.
57. Salama M, El-Kholy G, El-Haleem SA, et al. Serum soluble fas in patients with schistosomal cor pulmonale. Respiration. 2003;70:574–8.
58. Shu-Hua X. Development of antischistosomal drugs in China, with particular consideration to praziquantel and artemisinis. Acta Trop. 2005;96:153–67.
59. Sersar SI, Elnahas HA, Saleh AB, et al. Pulmonary parasitosis: applied clinical and therapeutic issues. Heart Lung Circ. 2006;15:24–9.
60. Meehan AM, Virk A, Swanson K, et al. Severe pleuropulmonary paragonimiasis 8 years after emigration from a region of endemicity. Clin Infect Dis. 2002;35(1):87–90.
61. Nakamura-Uchiyama F, Mukae H, Nawa Y. Paragonimiasis: a Japanese perspective. Clin Chest Med. 2002;23:409–20.
62. Velez ID, Ortega JE, Velasquez LE. Paragonimiasis: a view from Columbia. Clin Chest Med. 2002;23:421–31.
63. Jeon K, Song JU, Um SW, et al. Bronchoscopic findings of pulmonary paragonimiasis. Tuberc Respir Dis. 2009;67:512–6.
64. Mukae H, Taniguchi H, Matsumoto N, et al. Clinicoradiologic features of pleuropulmonary *Paragonimus westermani* on Kyusyu island Japan. Chest. 2001;120:514–20.
65. Lee JS, Lee J, Kim SH, et al. Molecular cloning and characterization of a major egg antigen in *Paragonimus westermani* and its use in ELISA for the immunodiagnosis of paragonimiasis. Parasitol Res. 2007;100:677–81.
66. Morar R, Feldman C. Pulmonary echinococcosis. Eur Respir J. 2003;21:1069–77.
67. Saygi A, Oztek I, Güder M, et al. Value of fibreoptic bronchoscopy in the diagnosis of complicated pulmonary unilocular cystic hydatidosis. Eur Respir J. 1997;10(4):811–4.
68. Pedosa I, Saiz A, Arrazola J, et al. Hydatid disease: radiologic and pathologic features and complications. Radiographics. 2000;20:795–817.
69. Sakamoto T, Gutierre C. Pulmonary complications of cystic echinococosis in children in Uruguay. Pathol Int. 2005;55:497–503.

70. Wen H, Yang WG. Public heath important of cystic echinococcosis in China. Acta Trop. 1997;67:133–45.
71. Kesmiri M, Baharvahdat H, Fattahi SH, et al. Albendazole versus placebo in treatment of echinococcosis. Trans Royal Soc Trop Med Hyg. 2001;95:190–4.
72. Junghanss T, Menezes Da Silva A, Horton J, et al. Clinical management of cystic echinococcosis: state of the art, problems and perspectives. Am J Trop Med Hyg. 2008;79:301–11.
73. Eckert J, Deplazes P. Biological, epidemiological, and clinical aspects of echinococcosis, a zoonosis of increasing concern. Clin Microbiol Rev. 2004;17:107–35.
74. Silva V, Pereira CN, Ajello L, et al. Molecular evidence for multiple host-specific strains in the genus *Rhinosporidium*. J Pathol Microbiol. 2007;50:718–21.
75. Fredricks DN, Jolly JA, Lepp PW, et al. *Rhinosporidum seeberi*: a human pathogen from novel group of aquatic protistan parasites. Emerg Infect Dis. 2000;6:273–82.
76. Banjara H, Panda RK, Daharwal AV, et al. Bronchial rhinosporidiosis: an unusual presentation. Lung India. 2012; 29: 173–5.
77. Job A, Venkateswaran S, Mathan M, et al. Medical therapy of rhinosporidiosis with dapsone. J Laryngol Otol. 1993;107:809–12.

Chapter 12
Tracheal Tumors

Debabrata Bandyopadhyay, Yaser Abu El-Sameed and Atul C. Mehta

Introduction

Primary tracheal tumors are rare. The majority of tracheal tumors in adults are malignant in nature with squamous cell carcinoma and adenoid cystic carcinoma being the two most common variants. Because of their non-specific presenting symptoms, a misdiagnosis or delayed diagnosis is not infrequent. In general, the prognosis is unfavorable for malignant lesions. Surgical resection, when possible, remains the best treatment option and is associated with good long-term outcome. Notwithstanding the recent technical advances, the tracheal surgery is still underemployed—suggesting that a more focused and aggressive approach is the need of the hour to manage these tumors. In this chapter, we discuss different types of tracheal tumors including their epidemiology, histology, clinical evaluation,

---

Declaration All authors had access to the manuscript and contributed equally to the writing of the manuscript.

D. Bandyopadhyay
Department of Thoracic Medicine, Geisinger Medical Center, Danville, PA, USA

Y.A. El-Sameed (✉)
Respiratory Institute, Cleveland Clinic Abu Dhabi, Karama Street, Abu Dhabi
United Arab Emirates
e-mail: AbuElSY@ClevelandClinicAbuDhabi.ae

A.C. Mehta
Lerner College of Medicine, Buoncore Family Endowed Chair in Lung Transplantation, Respiratory Institute, Cleveland Clinic, Cleveland, OH, USA
e-mail: Mehtaa1@ccf.org

A.C. Mehta
Pulmonary Medicine, Respiratory Institute, Cleveland Clinic, Cleveland, OH, USA

© Springer International Publishing Switzerland 2016
A.C. Mehta et al. (eds.), *Diseases of the Central Airways*,
Respiratory Medicine, DOI 10.1007/978-3-319-29830-6_12

management, and prognosis. The management section includes available different modalities of treatment including surgery, radiotherapy, and chemotherapy. We also discuss the role of therapeutic bronchoscopy in the management of such tumors.

Epidemiology

Primary tracheal tumors are uncommon, accounting for less than 0.1 % of all body tumors. The epidemiological analysis from Finland reported average annual incidence rate of tracheal carcinoma to be one per one million inhabitants between the years 1967 and 1985, with a male-to-female ratio of 7 to 3. There was a significant increase of disease burden with increasing age except for the age-group 70–79 years. Smoking was an important risk factor, at least among males [1]. Danish cancer registry reported 109 cases of primary tracheal cancers among 5.3 million inhabitants between the years 1978 and 1995, again with male predominance. In this series, the average age at diagnosis was 67 years, and majority of patients presented with stage IV disease [2]. The Netherlands Cancer Registry reported annual incidence of tracheal cancer at 0.142 per 100,000 populations between the years 1989 and 2002. Of the 308 reported cases, 72 % were men and the mean age at the time of diagnosis was 64 years [3].

Extraction of the primary tracheal malignancy cases from a major US population-based cancer registry—the Surveillance, Epidemiology, and End Results (SEER) database for the time period of 1988–2000 reveals 92 cases with mean age at presentation 59 years and an equal sex distribution. Forty-nine cases (53 %) presented with stage III or stage IV disease [4]. An epidemiological study [5] in the Korean population evaluated patients with primary tracheal tumors between the years 1989 and 2006, and only 37 tumors (14 benign, 23 malignant) were encountered at a tertiary referral center.

Characterization of Tracheal Tumors

Approximately 90 % of all tracheal tumors are malignant in adults in contrast to only 10–30 % in children [1–3, 6]. The squamous intraepithelial neoplasia (SIN) is a premalignant lesion comprising of various grades of dysplasia that can be seen in the trachea. There is a strong correlation of these lesions to smoking, but no convincing evidence of association with human papilloma virus exists [7].

Among the malignant neoplasms, squamous cell carcinoma (SCC) and adenoid cystic carcinoma (ACC) account for nearly 67 % of all cases. In the Danish registry, 63 % of the cancers were SCCs and only seven percent were ACCs [2]. Once again, SCC was the most common tumor type (41) followed by ACC (19) of 308 cases of tracheal tumors reported from the Netherlands [3]. The SCC was the predominant

(a)   (b)

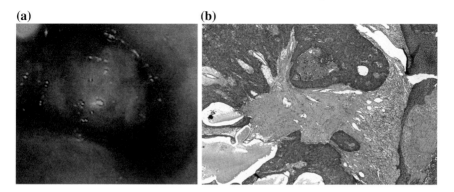

Fig. 12.1 a Large metastatic thymic carcinoma involving the trachea. **b** Histopathological examination confirming the thymic carcinoma. H&E, X 200. Reprinted from Choudhary et al. [94]. With permission from Wolters Kluwer Health

histology type (46 %) followed by ACC (26 %) in a US-based study [6]. The remaining malignant neoplasms are of either epithelial or mesenchymal origin [8, 9]. In one retrospective study of 360 patients with tracheal tumors, 11 had carcinoid tumors, 14 mucoepidermoid tumors (MECs), 13 sarcomas, 15 non-squamous bronchogenic carcinomas, 2 lymphomas, and 1 melanoma [10].

In addition to the tumors originating from the trachea, contiguous spread or secondary deposits can metastasize to the trachea from adjacent primaries in the thyroid, esophagus, larynx, thymus, and lung (Fig. 12.1) [11, 12]. Other sources of distant tracheal metastasis include colon, breast, and renal carcinomas and malignant melanoma [13, 14].

The other less common primary neoplasms of trachea belong to a diverse spectrum of benign and malignant histology, former being less frequent. Significant among them include squamous cell papilloma, hemangioma, lipoma, hamartoma, mucous gland adenoma, leiomyoma, granular cell tumor (GCT), chondroma, chondroblastoma, chondrosarcoma, Ewing's sarcoma, fibrous histiocytoma, pleomorphic adenoma, oncocytic adenoma, neurogenic tumors such as schwannoma, plexiform neurofibroma, and paraganglioma, fibrosarcoma, lymphoma, primary small cell cancer of trachea, epithelial–myoepithelial carcinoma, and inflammatory myofibroblastic tumor. Cases of glomus tumor involving the airway have been reported as well [8, 15–19]. Lymphomas and squamous cell papillomas involving the airways have been discussed in the separate chapters in this monograph.

Differential diagnosis of tracheal tumor should also include secondary lesions from renal cell, colon, breast, and esophageal carcinomas and melanoma, in a proper clinical setting.

Table 12.1 describes the common benign and malignant tracheal tumors.

Table 12.1 Common tracheal tumors

Tumors originating surface epithelium
1. Benign
Squamous cell papilloma
Papillomatosis
Adenoma
2. Malignant
Squamous cell carcinoma
Adenoid cystic carcinoma
Adenocarcinoma
Large cell undifferentiated carcinoma
Epithelial–myoepithelial carcinoma
3. Neuroendocrine tumor
Carcinoid tumor
Large cell neuroendocrine tumor
Primary small cell cancer
Tumors originating from mesenchymal tissue
1. Benign
Fibroma
Fibrous histiocytoma
Hemangioma
Glomus tumor
Paraganglioma
Leiomyoma
Schwann cell tumor
Neurofibroma
Chondroma
Chondroblastoma
Granular cell tumor
2. Malignant
Soft tissue sarcoma
Chondrosarcoma
Lymphoma
3. Undetermined
Inflammatory myofibroblastic tumor

Adapted from [15]. With the permission from Elsevier

Squamous Cell Carcinoma (SCC)

Primary SCC of the trachea is the most common tracheal tumor [2–6]. Macroscopically, these tumors grow as polypoid and frequently ulcerative mass projecting into the airways. Histologically, these tumors show a well-defined squamous differentiation of cells with or without keratinization [5].

Majority of SCC patients are male, presenting in sixth or seventh decade. There is a strong correlation with current and past smoking [20]. The most frequent presenting symptoms include dyspnea (55 %), hemoptysis (49 %), cough (42 %), and hoarseness (35 %) [6]. Stridor has also been reported. Unlike other variants, the SCC of trachea is diagnosed early, because hemoptysis is more common [15]. On radiological examination, these tumors can be either intraluminal, infiltrative, or exophytic [21].

Fig. 12.2 Squamous cell
carcinoma of the trachea:
Note the
exophytic/cauliflower-type
appearance of the lesion

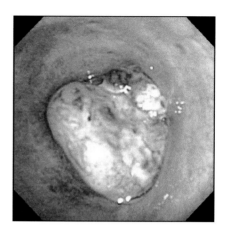

Bronchoscopic evaluation reveals that the majority of SCCs are bulky and obstructive
in nature (Fig. 12.2) [22]. Consequently, majority of these lesions cause airway
obstruction and thereafter tend to develop extraluminal invasion [21, 22].

The available data support surgical resection followed by radiotherapy as the best
possible treatment modality for SCC [23, 24]. The lymph node involvement or presence of disease at resection margins appears to have an adverse effect on overall
outcome of SCC [23]. In all population-based studies, SCC exhibited poorer survival
compared to other tracheal tumors [2–7]. It is due to the fact that SCC metastasizes early
to the lymph nodes and mostly presents at an advanced stage [25, 26]. Bronchoscopic
interventions can provide significant palliation to unresectable patients [27, 28].

Adenoid Cystic Carcinoma (ACC)

ACC (Fig. 12.3) of the trachea is relatively uncommon, and it differs in its natural
history and treatment modalities from SCC [29, 30]. The course of tracheal ACC is

Fig. 12.3 Adenoid cystic
carcinoma of the trachea—a
large submucosal mass
involving the axis of the
trachea in a young female,
never smoked. Reprinted
from Chua et al. [95]. With
permission from Wolters
Kluwer Health

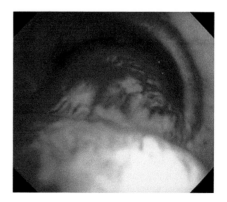

more indolent in nature [31, 32]. In many patients, its progression is slow enough to be mistaken for a benign tumor, but occasionally it presents with metastasis due to high-grade malignancy [33, 34]. The reported sites of distant metastasis include brain, long bones, liver, kidney, skin, and abdomen via hematogenous spread, in which case survival is often less than two years [30, 35, 36]. Lymph node spread is infrequent with ACC. Microscopically, the tumors typically are long, cylindrical structures lined by small cuboidal cells with deeply eosinophilic cores of basement-membrane-like material [35]. These cylinder-like structures account for the previous categorization of this tumor as "cylindroma." The eosinophilic cores stain positive with periodic acid–Schiff indicating the presence of mucinous material.

It is found in men and women equally, and mean age at presentation is 45 years [37]. ACC commonly presents with wheezing, cough, or stridor, but hemoptysis is rare. As a result, the tumors may get misdiagnosed as asthma or chronic bronchitis [15, 21]. These tumors often produce mass effect on the adjacent mediastinal structures rather than directly invading it. Study has shown that ACC of the upper airway is often locally invasive to the wall, still amenable to resection. Both, incomplete and when possible complete resection, have been shown to produce acceptable long-term outcome in patients with ACC [37]. Unlike SCC, long periods of remission can be obtained with radiotherapy alone [32]. However, surgical resection, followed by radiotherapy, provides the best length of survival for ACC patients [23, 38].

Mucoepidermoid Carcinoma (MEC)

Primary mucoepidermoid carcinoma (MEC) of the tracheobronchial tree is an uncommon tumor [39]. It arises from the submucosal glands and typically appears as a central endoluminal growth (Fig. 12.4) [39]. MEC is predominantly bland or

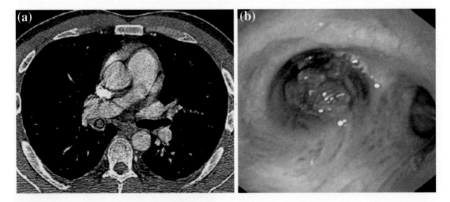

Fig. 12.4 Mucoepidermoid carcinoma. **a** CT scan of the chest revealing a lobulated mass involving right main bronchus (RMB). **b** Large, irregular, broad-based, friable, ulcerating vascular tumor mass in the RMB

cystic tumors with occasional mucin-secreting goblet cells and indeterminate cells [40]. These tumors are classified as low grade or high grade, on the basis of mitotic activity, cellular necrosis, and nuclear pleomorphism [41]. Low-grade tumors rarely spread to regional lymph nodes, while high-grade tumors frequently do so in addition to distant metastasis [42]. Therefore, the high-grade tumors are often unresectable, and outcome, even after radiotherapy, is poor [43]. Overall, patients with MEC have a better survival than patients with ACC.

The median age at diagnosis for patients with primary tracheobronchial MEC is 28 (7–73) years [44]. It is the most common malignant tracheobronchial tumor in younger individuals. No association with cigarette smoking has been noted [44]. Majority of the patients are treated with resection. Repeated surgical resection may be required for recurrence [45].

Carcinoid Tumors

Typical and atypical carcinoids (TC and AC) belong to neuroendocrine tumor (NET) group [46]. Carcinoid syndrome due to systemic release of vasoactive substance serotonin is observed in only 1–5 % of cases of tracheal carcinoid tumors [47]. Cytologically, this tumor consists of bland polygonal cells with round or oval nuclei, arranged in a distinct trabecular fashion. Gradation of the tumor is based on the number of mitotic figures present per high-power field (HPF) [46]. Bronchoscopically carcinoid tumors appear as rounded well-vascularized lesions, so caution is advised when performing biopsy (Fig. 12.5a–c) [48].

Common clinical presentations include recurrent respiratory tract infection, cough, and chest pain, or alternatively, it may remain completely asymptomatic. The average age of presentation is mid-40s, and 5- or 10-year survival is excellent, particularly in TC [47]. Prognosis is better after surgical resection. However, recurrence of tumor, particularly in cases of ACs, can occur [49]. Bronchoscopic resection of carcinoid tumor has been performed in inoperable or recurrent cases and in cases of typical carcinoid presenting as a pedunculated endobronchial lesion [50].

Octreotide, a somatostatin analog, has been used to manage symptoms of carcinoid syndrome [51]. The benefit of chemotherapy is not well established. Combination regimes such as 5FU and streptozotocin or dacarbazine are judged to be an option in cases with metastatic spread [52]. Everolimus, an inhibitor of the mammalian target of rapamycin (mTOR), has also been used in combination with octreotide in the management of NET causing carcinoid syndrome [53]. Other promising newer agents include vascular endothelial growth factor (VEGF) receptor inhibitor bevacizumab and interferon alpha-2b [54].

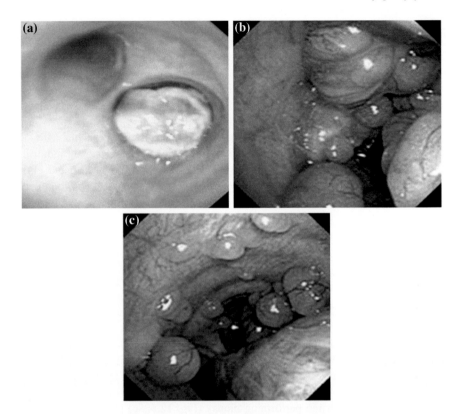

Fig. 12.5 a Typical carcinoid tumor involving the right main bronchus. **b, c** Multiple atypical carcinoid tumorlets involving the trachea. Note the smooth, vascular, pedunculated nature of the lesion

Mucous Gland Adenoma (Mucinous Cystadenoma)

Benign adenomas arising from bronchial mucous glands are extremely rare, arising from the submucosal seromucous glands and ducts of proximal airways [55]. They present as a solitary, well-circumscribed, multicystic, predominately exophytic tumors, mostly located in the middle and lower-third of trachea [56]. The tumors are rich in mucins and are immunopositive for epithelial markers. The age at presentation ranges from 25 to 67 years. Mucous gland adenoma needs to be distinguished from low-grade malignant tumors of the airways, especially low-grade MEC. The complete resection is curative [55, 56].

Rare Tracheal Neoplasms

Tracheal hamartomas are benign lesions, composed of cartilage, bones, fats, smooth muscles, and connective tissues. Chronic inflammatory and squamous metaplasia often covers the outer layer, so bronchoscopic biopsy can be deceptive at times. They are common in elderly population and in males. They appear as exophytic, sessile, or polypoid mass with CT imaging showing fat attenuation [57]. Bronchoscopic resection with argon photocoagulation, electrocautery snare, and cryotherapy is safe and effective in removing these lesions [58].

Tracheal lipoma (Fig. 12.6) arises from subcutaneous fatty tissue in middle-aged males. Spindle cell lipoma has been more commonly described. They are usually slow-growing tumor, often presenting as obstructive airway diseases [59].

Primary neurogenic tumor is extremely uncommon, and more cases of **schwannoma** have been reported than neurofibroma. However, trachea is the most common site for primary pulmonary neurofibroma [60]. They are usually benign tumor and can be an element of von Recklinghausen's disease [61]. Recurrence has occurred after bronchoscopic resection but none after surgical resection (Fig. 12.7a–b).

Glomus tumor or glomangiomyoma is a soft tissue tumor of hands and feet, which rarely occurs in the tracheal tree. These are small, well-circumscribed benign lesions composed of glomus cells, blood vessels, and smooth muscle cells although cases of suspected malignant glomus tumor of trachea have also been described (Figs. 12.8 and 12.9) [19, 62].

Tracheal granular cell tumors are largely benign tumors, most commonly seen in women. Histologically, this tumor is composed of spindle cells with eosinophil and positive for S100 staining. More commonly, they are an asymptomatic, incidental finding. Either surgical or interventional bronchoscopic resection is curative, but recurrence can occur (Fig. 12.10a, b) [63].

Primary tracheal lymphomas include both Hodgkin's variety and non-Hodgkin's variety. Few cases of mucosa-associated lymphoid tissue (MALT) lymphoma have been described. They are potentially treatable and have a good prognosis [57].

Tracheal chondrosarcomas are rare extraosseous cartilaginous tumor, which appear as exophytic growth (Fig. 12.11) [64]. It can occur after incomplete resection or malignant transformation of chondroma. Tracheal chondrosarcoma can also be seen in Maffucci syndrome [65].

Primary epithelial–myoepithelial tumors (EMCa) of trachea are low-grade malignant tumors, metastasize to lymph node early, and are known to mimic sarcoidosis. They can give rise to hypercalcemia, and lymph node biopsy can demonstrate non-caseating granuloma as well [66].

The inflammatory myofibroblastic tumors (IMT), which most commonly occur in lungs, have also been recognized in trachea. It is a low-grade malignant neoplasm of unknown origin. It is composed of myofibroblastic spindle cells along with inflammatory infiltrates such as plasma cells, lymphocytes, and eosinophils. Approximately, half of the tumors are positive for anaplastic lymphoma kinase

Fig. 12.6 a CT scan of the
chest revealing an exophytic
mass involving the
mid-trachea. The density of
the mass lesion is similar to
that of subcutaneous fat,
suggesting diagnosis of
endobronchial lipoma. **b**,
c Cut surface of the in vivo
lesion exhibiting lipomatous
nature of the lesion. Reprinted
from Swigris et al. [96]. With
permission from Wolters
Kluwer Health

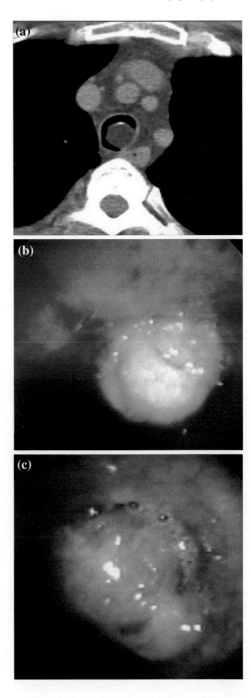

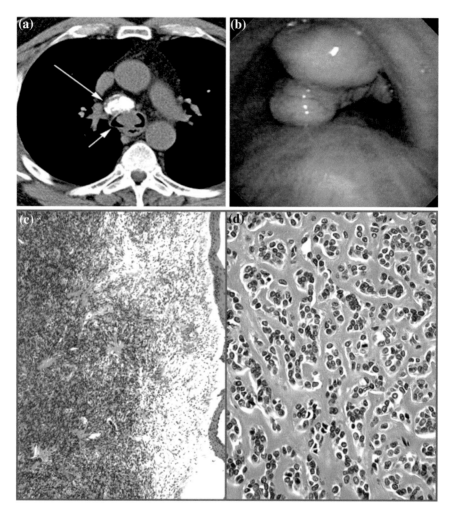

Fig. 12.7 a, b Endobronchial schwannoma involving the trachea. Note extraluminal calcified component of the lesion. **c** The tumor underlying the tracheal mucosa has a cellular spindle cell appearance. **d** The high-power field also exhibits a more epithelioid appearance of the tumor cells with mitosis. Reprinted from Shah et al. [97]. With permission from Elsevier

(ALK) gene rearrangement. Clinically, it often simulates resistant asthma leading to respiratory failure and rarely causes hemoptysis. In addition to surgical resection, newer biologic agent crizotinib has shown initial promise (Fig. 12.12) [67].

Irrespective of histology and malignant potential, the majority of these benign tumors of trachea are resectable at diagnosis, either bronchoscopically or surgically with reconstruction [8].

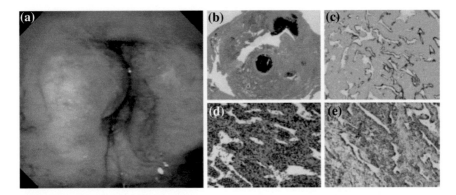

Fig. 12.8 **a** Glomus tumor (glomangiomyoma) exhibiting a smooth surface, *yellowish* in color, soft and fluctuant, and partially obstructing glottic chink. **b** A circumscribed tumor was completely surrounded by a fibrous pseudocapsule (hematoxylin and eosin [H&E] stain). **d** Presence of vascular channels with smooth muscle cells (H&E stain). **c, e** CD34 antibody-stained endothelial cells (*right upper*) and smooth muscle actin antibody-stained smooth muscle cells (*right lower*). Reprinted from Usuda et al. [98]. With permission from Wolters Kluwer Health

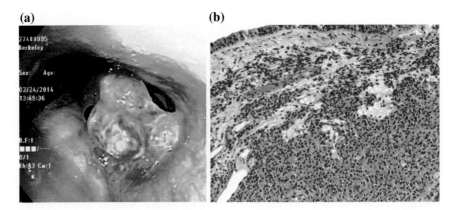

Fig. 12.9 Glomus tumor. **a** Bronchoscopic appearance of the glomus tumor. **b** Pathology of glomus tumor located at mucosal surface; note the sheets of smooth muscle cells (×200 magnification)

Evaluations

Clinical Features

As stated earlier, missed and delayed diagnosis is not uncommon in tracheal tumors due to non-specific and often asthma-mimicking symptoms [25]. This is more likely in cases of slowly growing benign tumors. Majority of tracheal tumors occur in

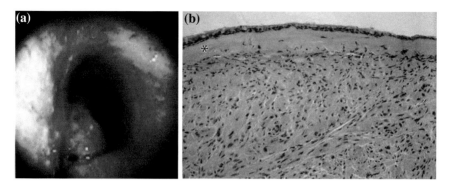

Fig. 12.10 **a** Exophytic growth of granular cell tumor inside trachea with submucosal infiltration into tracheal wall. **b** Granular tumor cells are spindle-shaped cells with abundant granular cytoplasm. Reprinted from Chan et al. [99]. With permission from Wolters Kluwer Health

Fig. 12.11 Primary chondrosarcoma of the trachea—a large, exophytic, lobulated, vascular mass arising from the anterior wall of trachea. Note the islands of pale tissue, which were hard in consistency on forceps palpation. Reprinted from Alkotob et al. [100]. With permission from Wolters Kluwer Health

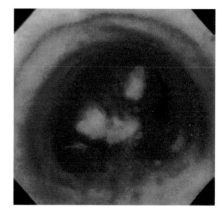

lower one-third of the trachea. Most patients are current or former smokers; the strongest association is with SCC. Dyspnea is the most common symptom in benign and hemoptysis in malignant tumors [8]. Because of their rapid growth and onset of hemoptysis, malignant tumors are often diagnosed earlier than benign tumors [14]. By the time a patient with tracheal tumor develops dyspnea, more than 75 % of the airway circumference is already obstructed [6, 25].

Other symptoms include chronic cough, wheezing, or stridor [6, 68]. Patients may present with recurrent episodes of pneumonia or atelectasis. Acute respiratory failure from complete occlusion of the airway is rare, but carries a high mortality rate. The presenting complaints in a series of 74 patients with primary tracheal tumors were dyspnea (55 %), hemoptysis (48 %), cough (42 %), and hoarseness (35 %) [6]. Persistent and progressive local disease can cause complications such as fatal hemorrhage, tracheoesophageal fistula, tracheal necrosis, and tracheal stenosis [30, 69].

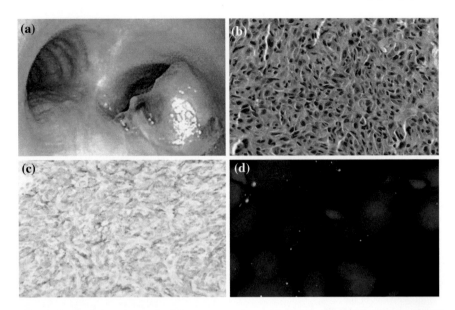

Fig. 12.12 Inflammatory myofibroblastoma. **a** A large lobulated partially obstructing tracheal mass. **b** Cytologically bland spindle cells (*red arrow*) and inflammatory cells (mostly lymphocytes). **c** Immunohistochemical stain for ALK (D5F3 clone)—ALK stains the cytoplasm (*arrow*), and *blue* are the nuclei. **d** Dual-color FISH for ALK mutation—the *green* (centromere) and *red* (telomere) dots together with *yellow* center are non-mutated ALK-containing chromosomes, and the mutated chromosome has the *red* and *green* dots separated. Courtesy of Tanmay Panchabhai, MD

The presentation also varies depending on the type of the tumors. The SCC usually manifests as a rapid onset tumor with hemoptysis and obstructive symptoms. It has a tendency for the early involvement of lymph nodes and development of distant metastasis. In contrast, ACC is a tumor with slower growth, consequently diagnosed late. It tends to extend over a long distance in the submucosa [70]. It can also spread to regional lymph nodes, but less often than SCC.

A TNM classification has been proposed for tracheal tumor (illustrated in Table 12.2), which helps to predict survival among the patients with malignant lesions [6, 15].

Pulmonary Function Tests

Spirometry and flow volume loop can offer a clue to the presence of tracheal tumor. In variable extrathoracic obstruction, peak inspiratory flow (PIF) will be predominantly reduced. In fixed extrathoracic obstruction, both PIF and peak expiratory flow (PEF) are reduced. The variable intrathoracic obstruction, on the other hand, is characterized by decreased PEF and preserved PIF [15].

Table 12.2 Proposed TNM classification of tracheal tumor

T—Tumor stage	
Tx	Tumor cannot be assessed
TIS	Tumor without any invasion
T1	Tumor limited to mucosa
T1a	T1 with tumor size <3 cm
T1b	T1 with tumor size ≥3 cm
T2	Tumor invading cartilage or adventitia
T3	Tumor invading tracheal wall or larynx
T4	Tumor invading carina or main bronchus
T5	Tumor invading other mediastinal structure
N—Nodal stage	
Nx	Lymph node cannot be assessed
N0	No Lymph node metastasis
N1	Lymph node positive—upper paratracheal, prevascular, retrotracheal lymph node
N2	Lymph node positive—lower paratracheal, subaortic, and upper mediastinal lymph nodes
M—Metastasis	
Mx	Metastasis cannot be assessed
M0	No metastasis
M1	Metastasis to lymph node beyond N1 and N2
M2	Distant metastasis

Adapted from [15]. With the permission from Elsevier

Radiology

The initial investigation for patients with tracheal tumors is usually chest roentgen-ogram because of shortness of breath or wheeze [71]. However, less than half of the tracheal tumors are actually diagnosed using this imaging modality [72]. Findings on chest radiographs include tracheal narrowing, abnormal calcifications, postobstruc-tive atelectasis, or pneumonia. The lateral view of the chest often displays lesion obstructing the tracheal column better than the posteroanterior view (Fig. 12.13).

Computed tomography (CT) scan is the imaging of choice for diagnosis of tra-cheal tumor [72]. It may show a tracheal mass, and the radiological appearance of the tumors can be classified as intraluminal (exophytic), infiltrative, extrinsic, or mixed forms [13]. The intraluminal variety leads to irregular narrowing of tracheal lumen. The infiltrative form of tracheal tumor characteristically involves posterior wall of trachea differentiating it from many tracheal lesions mimicking tumor infiltration. The CT scan is an excellent tool for detecting and determining extent of disease as well as in evaluating airways distal to the obstruction. However, it often fails to clearly delineate tumor relationship with mucosa or submucosa [20]. The newer software algorithms that allow three-dimensional evaluation of the airways may show the specific pattern. The utility of magnetic resonance imaging is unclear, but it has been reported in ACC [73]. The optical coherence tomography has the ability to

Fig. 12.13 Lateral view of
the chest X-ray revealing a
large endotracheal mass that
was not recognized on the
posteroanterior view

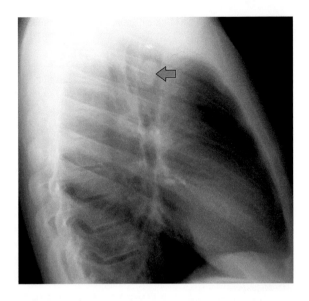

delineate microstructures such as the epithelium, mucosa, cartilage, and glands [21].
However, presently its role is confined to experimental studies and has limited
application in clinical practice.

Bronchoscopy

Bronchoscopy with appropriate sampling remains the gold standard to establish the
definitive diagnosis of tracheal tumors. It can also clarify whether airway
obstruction is intrinsic, extrinsic, or combined. Bronchoscopy may demonstrate a
single polypoid lesion, sessile or pedunculated, multiple "cauliflower-like" exophytic tumor [20]. The infiltrative tumor appears as a circumferential thickening
involving the posterior wall. Bronchoscopy can also reveal tracheal wall collapse by
an extrinsic tumor. Endobronchial ultrasound of the trachea may distinguish
between compression and infiltration of the trachea by an extrinsic mass [73]. The
endoscopic ultrasound (EUS) can be utilized when a CT scan or bronchoscopy
suggests posterior tumor wall invasion by an extrinsic lesion.

Management

The epidemiological studies from different countries suggest a diagnostic dilemma
leading to delayed diagnosis. As a result, many cases are often unresectable by the
time the diagnosis is confirmed. The surgical resection is regarded as the only
curative option.

Surgery

Surgery, when possible, remains the treatment of choice for primary tracheal tumor [37, 38]. Unfortunately, the available data indicate that many patients who met the criteria for surgical resection did not receive surgery [25]. In the Danish registry, majority of the patients received radiotherapy as single treatment and only nine patients were offered surgery [2]. The report from the Netherlands showed that surgical treatment led to good survival, yet it was only used in 12 % of patients, while 53 % received radiation therapy [3]. In the SEER [5] database from the USA, 34 % did not undergo surgery, while it has the potential to cure all patients with benign and low-grade malignant tumors [15]. Therefore, surgical resection should be assiduously considered as the treatment of choice for benign and malignant tracheal tumors and patients be referred to appropriate centers at the earliest, whenever possible [23].

The decision to resect a tracheal tumor depends on many factors such as general health of the patient, site of the tumor, tumor histology, and length of trachea that would remain postresection [15]. Modern surgical techniques for tracheal resection such as laryngotracheal, tracheal, or carinal reconstruction and different tracheal mobilization techniques would allow resection in more than half of the cases [74, 75]. However, it involves careful patient evaluation, preservation of tracheal blood supply during the surgery, and accepting risk of unclear margin [15, 74].

Complications of tracheal surgery include tracheal restenosis, anastomotic dehiscence, anterior spinal cord ischemia, and fistula formation [76, 77]. In a series of 147 post-tracheal or carinal resection patients, six developed restenosis, but all underwent re-resection successfully [23]. Other reported complications are subcutaneous emphysema, granulation tissue formation, bilateral pneumonia, cardiac arrhythmia, pneumomediastinum, mediastinitis, and neck hematoma [25]. One important determinant of complications following tracheal resection is the extent of resection [78, 79]. Conservative surgery, when appropriate, has a lower complication rate than more extensive resections [80, 81].

The postoperative mortality from tracheal surgery can be significant, approaching to 10 % in one study [9]. It correlated with the length of the resection, the type of resection, the need for a laryngeal release, and the histological type of the cancer. Another retrospective analysis noted overall postoperative mortality of 7 % for the surgeries performed between 1962 and 2002, but it had improved with each passing decade from 21 to 3 % [38].

Radiotherapy

Radiation therapy has an important role in the management of certain types of tracheal tumors. Patients with unresectable tumor have a poor outcome in general, irrespective of radiotherapy treatment. However, those who received radiation had a better survival, suggesting that primary radiotherapy in inoperable cases may represent a viable treatment option [69]. Current evidences indicate that radiotherapy should be offered to all patients following surgical resection.

The impact of radiation therapy in patients with resectable and unresectable primary malignant tracheal tumor has been studied [82]. Patients, who received radiotherapy, had a significantly better overall survival and lower cumulative incidence of death from tracheal cancer. Treatment with radiotherapy was associated with improved survival, particularly in patients with squamous cell histology, regional extension of disease, and even those who did not undergo resection. Nevertheless, the epidemiology data suggest that the tracheal tumors treated with radiotherapy alone had a poor survival, in general [2].

Chemotherapy

Cisplatin-based chemotherapy has been studied in the management of metastatic SCC of the trachea. At present, the role of chemotherapy is limited. It is generally reserved for the palliative treatment of symptomatic, locally recurrent or metastatic disease that is not amenable to further surgery or radiotherapy [15].

Combination Therapy

Some reports describe the utility of combination of chemotherapy and radiotherapy in the treatment of unresectable patients. Radiation therapy with concurrent carboplatin and paclitaxel, or nedaplatin and 5-fluorouracil might be an effective treatment option for an advanced ACC [83].

In one analysis of resected SCC, outcome of patients treated with concurrent postoperative chemotherapy (cisplatin) and radiotherapy was compared to that with postoperative radiotherapy alone. There was a significant improvement in local and regional disease control as well as disease-free survival in the combined treatment group. However, the combined modality was also associated with a substantial increase in adverse side effects [84].

Data from the USA suggest that those with surgery and adjuvant radiotherapy have a better disease-specific and overall survival compared to those treated with radiotherapy with or without associated chemotherapy. Although patients undergoing surgery and receiving radiotherapy did better than those undergoing surgery alone, the difference was not significant. Similar results have been reported with combined radiotherapy and surgery in the management of ACC [85]. The 5- and 10-year absolute survival and local disease control were significantly better in the combined surgery and radiation therapy.

Bronchoscopic Intervention

Bronchoscopic interventions have a significant role in the management of tracheal tumors [14, 24]. However, malignant tumors often invade into and beyond the airway wall. Therefore, bronchoscopic treatment of endobronchial tumors does not always guarantee the complete resection of the tumor [86, 87]. The main role of bronchoscopic tumor ablation should be palliative in patients who are not surgical candidates or as a bridge to restore airway patency in preparation for definitive surgery [15, 21].

The experience with Ultraflex metallic stent insertion for palliation of benign and malignant upper airway obstructions suggests improvement in breathlessness, an increase of mean FEV_1 of 0.88 and 0.28 l in benign and malignant obstructions, respectively, and a mean peak expiratory flow rate increment by 109 and 97 l/min, respectively [88]. Twenty-nine percent were alive at three years, although survival was disproportionately higher in benign obstruction [88]. However, another study using Montgomery T-tube in patients in malignant stenosis for palliation yielded a disappointing result [89]. The short (<30 days) and intermediate (>30 days) risks of tracheobronchial stents in patients with malignant airway disease included tumor ingrowth, excessive granulation tissue formation, stent migration, and restenosis. The majority of complications occurred after 30 days that often required further interventions such as bronchoscopic laser debridement, dilation, and stent removal [90].

The endotracheal tumors can be resected bronchoscopically using either Nd-YAG (neodymium–yttrium, aluminum, garnet) or Nd-YAP (neodymium–yttrium, aluminum perovskite) laser resection, argon plasma coagulation, electrocoagulation, cryotherapy, or photodynamic therapy to keep airways patent with palliative intent [90]. The endobronchial brachytherapy alone or as a boost for primary radiotherapy holds promise in patients with either non-resectable primary tumor or in recurrence of tumor [91]. Local control was achieved in all cases at the time of subsequent first bronchoscopic evaluation. Emergent bronchoscopic interventions through a rigid bronchoscope immediately resolved acute dyspnea and respiratory failure related to malignant airway obstruction, liberating them from mechanical ventilation in majority of the patients, in one study. Furthermore, those who underwent additional definitive therapy survived even longer than otherwise [27].

Future Strategies

The rapid expansion of technology has offered newer treatment options for patients with tracheal tumors. Ongoing research suggests that tracheal allogenic transplantation may become available as a new treatment modality [28]. The first clinical transplantation of the tracheobronchial airway with a stem-cell-seeded bioartificial nanocomposite was reported in 2011 in a patient with recurrent primary cancer of the distal trachea and main bronchus [92]. After complete tumor resection, the airway was replaced with a tailored bioartificial nanocomposite previously seeded with autologous bone marrow mononuclear cells. There were no major complications, and the patient was asymptomatic and tumor-free five months after the transplantation. The bioartificial nanocomposite showed patent anastomoses lined with a vascularized neomucosa and was partly covered by nearly healthy epithelium.

Other novel treatments including composite autografts and allografts, chimeric autografts and allografts, tissue-engineered grafts, prosthetic scaffolds, and the use of free-tissue vascularized carriers hold future promise [93]. The tracheal replacement with fresh aortic allografts in two patients with chemotherapy- and radiotherapy-resistant tumor MEC and ACC has been reported. The aortic allografts in both the patients showed the development of respiratory epithelium one year after the surgery [93].

Prognosis

Many studies demonstrate that staging tracheal cancer with a TNM-based classification (see Table 12.2) helps to predict survival [4, 6, 15]. The overall survival rate in the Danish registry was 32, 20, and 13 % at 1, 2, and 5 years, respectively [2]. The median survival in tracheal tumor was 10 months with 1-, 5-, and 10-year survival rates at 43, 15, and 6 %, respectively, in the Netherlands [3]. The important factors predicting outcome included early diagnosis, tumor histology, and treatment options such as definitive surgery [24]. The 5-year survival rate was 50 % in tumor-resected patients but with radiotherapy alone was only 6 % in the Danish population [2]. In general, the outlook after complete surgical resection is good and a 5-year survival rate ranges between 39 and 79 %, and the 10-year survival rate between 18 and 51 % [3]. In the SEER database, there was a significant improvement in survival for patients who underwent any type of surgery than who did not; the overall 5-year survival rate was 27 %. Patients with localized disease had a better outcome with a 5-year survival rate of 46 % than patients with regional or distant disease. Among those with localized disease, the 5-year survival rate was 24 % for SCC versus 90 % for ACC [22]. The prognosis of patients with ACC was significantly better because of their predominantly local growth pattern. In contrast, SCCs had worse outcomes than any other histological type, with a 5-year overall survival only 13 % [22].

Geissert and colleagues noted 5- and 10-year survival rates in resected ACC 52 and 29 % (unresectable 33 and 10 %) and in resected SCC 39 and 18 % (unresectable 7.3 and 4.9 %) [38]. The favorable outcome of both SCC and ACC following surgical resection showed a significant association with completeness of resection, negative airway margins, and adenoid cystic histology, but not with tumor length, lymph node status, or type of resection [38].

In contrast, the outcome analysis in the USA revealed no significant difference between combination of surgery and radiotherapy than surgery alone. Patients with ACC had better rates of disease-specific and overall survival than other lesions. The 5-year disease-specific mortality was 73 % and all-cause mortality 79 % [6]. Another retrospective multicenter study from 26 centers noted 5- and 10-year survival rates at 47 and 36 %, respectively; the survival was significantly higher with complete resections than with incomplete resections and postoperative radiotherapy [9].

Conclusion

In conclusion, primary tracheal tumors are uncommon malignancies of the airways, and in adult population, majority are malignant. The presenting symptoms are often ambiguous; consequently, definitive diagnosis does get delayed impacting the prognosis. Early diagnosis and appropriate selection of patients for histologically complete resection are paramount toward improving outcome for primary tracheal tumors.

References

1. Manninen MP, Antila PJ, Pukander JS, Karma PH. Occurrence of tracheal carcinoma in Finland. Acta Otolaryngol. 1991;111(6):1162–9.
2. Licht PB, Friis S, Pettersson G. Tracheal cancer in Denmark: a nationwide study. Eur J Cardiothorac Surg. 2001;19(3):339–45.
3. Honings J, van Dijck JAAM, Verhagen AFTM, van der Heijden HFM, Marres HAM. Incidence and treatment of tracheal cancer: a nationwide study in the Netherlands. Ann Surg Oncol. 2007;14(2):968–76.
4. Bhattacharyya N. Contemporary staging and prognosis for primary tracheal malignancies: a population-based analysis. Otolaryngol Head Neck Surg. 2004;131(5):639–42.
5. Ahn Y, Chang H, Lim YS, Hah JH, Kwon TK, Sung MW, Kim KH. Primary tracheal tumors: review of 37 cases. J Thorac Oncol. 2009;4(5):635–8.
6. Webb BD, Walsh GL, Roberts DB, Sturgis EM. Primary tracheal malignant neoplasms: the University of Texas MD Anderson Cancer Center experience. J Am Coll Surg. 2006;202 (2):237–46.
7. Junker K. Pathology of tracheal tumors. Thorac Surg Clin. 2014;24(1):7–11.
8. Gaissert HA, Grillo HC, Shadmehr MB, Wright CD, Gokhale M, Wain JC, Mathisen DJ. Uncommon primary tracheal tumors. Ann Thorac Surg. 2006;82(1):268–73.
9. Regnard JF, Fourquier P, Levasseur P. Results and prognostic factors in resections of primary tracheal tumors: a multicenter retrospective study. J Thorac Cardiovasc Surg. 1996;111(4):808–14 The French Society of Cardiovascular Surgery.
10. Miller DL, Allen MS. Rare pulmonary neoplasms. Mayo Clin Proc. 1993;68(5):492–8.
11. Goldstein J. Primary carcinoma of the trachea: report of two cases. S Med J. 1977;70(4):434–6.
12. Morency G, Chalaoui J, Samson L, Sylvestre J. Malignant neoplasms of the trachea. Can Assoc Radiol J. 1989;40(4):198–200.

13. Li W, Ellerbroek NA, Libshitz HI. Primary malignant tumors of the trachea. A radiologic and clinical study. Cancer. 1990;66(5):894–9.
14. Grillo HC. Reconstruction of the trachea after resection for neoplasm. Head Neck Surg. 1981;4(1):2–8.
15. Macchiarini P. Primary tracheal tumours. Lancet Oncol. 2006;7(1):83–91.
16. Stevic R, Milenkovic B, Stojsic J, Pesut D, Ercegovac M, Jovanovic D. Clinical and radiological manifestations of primary tracheobronchial tumours: a single centre experience. Ann Acad Med Singapore. 2012;41(5):205–11.
17. He J, Xu X, Chen M, et al. Novel method to repair tracheal defect by pectoralis major myocutaneous flap. Ann Thorac Surg. 2009;88(1):288–91.
18. Choi IH, Song DH, Kim J, Han J. Two cases of glomus tumor arising in large airway: well organized radiologic, macroscopic and microscopic findings. Tuberc Respir Dis. 2014;76 (1):34–7.
19. Norder E, Kynyk J, Schmitt AC, Gauhar U, Islam S. Glomus tumor of the trachea. J Bronchol Interv Pulmonol. 2012;19(3):220–3.
20. Jamjoom L, Obusez EC, Kirsch J, Gildea T, Mohammed TL. Computed tomography correlation of airway disease with bronchoscopy—part II: tracheal neoplasms. Curr Prob Diagn Radiol. 2014;43(5):278–84.
21. Herth F, Ernst A, Schulz M, Becker H. Endobronchial ultrasound reliably differentiates between airway infiltration and compression by tumor. Chest. 2003;123(2):458–62.
22. Howard DJ, Haribhakti VV. Primary tumours of the trachea: analysis of clinical features and treatment results. J Laryngol Otol. 1994;108(3):230–2.
23. Grillo HC, Mathisen DJ. Primary tracheal tumors: treatment and results. Ann Thorac Surg. 1990;49(1):69–77.
24. Gaissert HA. Primary tracheal tumors. Chest Surg Clin N Am. 2003;13(2):247–56.
25. Honings J, Gaissert HA, Verhagen AF, van Dijck JA, van der Heijden HF, van Die L, Bussink J, Kaanders JH, Marres HA. Undertreatment of tracheal carcinoma: multidisciplinary audit of epidemiologic data. Ann Surg Oncol. 2009;16(2):246–53.
26. Urdaneta AI, Yu JB, Wilson LD. Population based cancer registry analysis of primary tracheal carcinoma. Am J Clin Oncol. 2011;34(1):32–7.
27. Colt HG, Harrell JH. Therapeutic rigid bronchoscopy allows level of care changes in patients with acute respiratory failure from central airways obstruction. Chest. 1997;112(1):202–6.
28. Delaere PR. Tracheal transplantation. Curr Opin Pulm Med. 2012;18(4):313–20.
29. Albers E, Lawrie T, Harrell JH, Yi ES. Tracheobronchial adenoid cystic carcinoma: a clinicopathologic study of 14 cases. Chest. 2004;125(3):1160–5.
30. Kim KH, Sung MW, Chung PS, Rhee CS, Park CI, Kim WH. Adenoid cystic carcinoma of the head and neck. Arch Otolaryngol Head Neck Surg. 1994;120(7):721–6.
31. Allen MS. Malignant tracheal tumors. Mayo Clin Proc. 1993;68(7):680–4.
32. Fields JN, Rigaud G, Emami BN. Primary tumors of the trachea. Results of radiation therapy. Cancer. 1989;63(12):2429–33.
33. Grillo HC. Management of tracheal tumors. Am J Surg. 1982;143(6):697–700.
34. Perelman MI, Koroleva N, Birjukov J, Goudovsky L. Primary tracheal tumors. Semin Thorac Cardiovasc Surg. 1996;8(4):400–2.
35. Moran CA, Suster S, Koss MN. Primary adenoid cystic carcinoma of the lung. A clinicopathologic and immunohistochemical study of 16 cases. Cancer. 1994;73(5): 1390–7.
36. Spiro RH, Huvos AG. Stage means more than grade in adenoid cystic carcinoma. Am J Surg. 1992;164(6):623–8.
37. Maziak DE, Todd TR, Keshavjee SH, Winton TL, Van Nostrand P, Pearson FG. Adenoid cystic carcinoma of the airway: thirty-two-year experience. J Thorac Cardiovasc Surg. 1996;112(6):1522–32.
38. Gaissert HA, Grillo HC, Shadmehr MB, Wright CD, Gokhale M, Wain JC, Mathisen DJ. Long-term survival after resection of primary adenoid cystic and squamous cell carcinoma of the trachea and carina. Ann Thorac Surg. 2004;78(6):1889–97.

39. Kim TS, Lee KS, Han J, Im JG, Seo JB, Kim JS, Kim HY, Han SW. Mucoepidermoid carcinoma of the tracheobronchial tree: radiographic and CT findings in 12 patients. Radiology. 1999;212(3):643–8.
40. Brandwein MS, Ivanov K, Wallace DI, et al. Mucoepidermoid carcinoma: a clinicopathologic study of 80 patients with special reference to histological grading. Am J Surg Pathol. 2001;25(7):835–45.
41. Heitmiller RF, Mathisen DJ, Ferry JA, Mark EJ, Grillo HC. Mucoepidermoid lung tumors. Ann Thorac Surg. 1989;47(3):394–9.
42. Barsky SH, Martin SE, Matthews M, Gazdar A, Costa JC. "Low grade" mucoepidermoid carcinoma of the bronchus with "high grade" biological behavior. Cancer. 1983;51(8):1505–9.
43. Abdennadher M, Rivera C, Gibault L, Fabre E, Pricopi C, Arame A, Foucault C, Dujon A, Le Pimpec BF, Riquet M. Mucoepidermoid tracheo-bronchial tumors in adulthood. A series of 22 cases. Rev Pneumol Clin. 2015;71(1):27–36.
44. Chin C-H, Huang C-C, Lin M-C, Chao T-Y, Liu S-F. Prognostic factors of tracheobronchial mucoepidermoid carcinoma—15 years experience. Respirology. 2008;13(2):275–80.
45. Song Z, Liu Z, Wang J, Zhu H, Zhang Y. Primary tracheobronchial mucoepidermoid carcinoma—a retrospective study of 32 patients. World J Surg Oncol. 2013;11:62.
46. Tsuta K, Raso MG, Kalhor N, Liu DD, Wistuba II, Moran CA. Histologic features of low-and intermediate-grade neuroendocrine carcinoma (typical and atypical carcinoid tumors) of the lung. Lung Cancer. 2011;71(1):34–41.
47. Morandi U, Casali C, Rossi G. Bronchial typical carcinoid tumors. Semin Thorac Cardiovasc Surg. 2006;18(3):191–8.
48. Machuca TN, Cardoso PFG, Camargo SM, Signori L, Andrade CF, Moreira ALS, da Silva Moreira J, Felicetti JC, Camargo JJ. Surgical treatment of bronchial carcinoid tumors: a single-center experience. Lung Cancer. 2010;70(2):158–62.
49. Ducrocq X, Thomas P, Massard G, Barsotti P, Giudicelli R, Fuentes P, Wihlm JM. Bronchial carcinoid tumors. Ann Thorac Surg. 1998;65(5):1410–4.
50. Brokx HAP, Risse EK, Paul MA, Grünberg K, Golding RP, Kunst PW, Eerenberg JP, van Mourik JC, Postmus PE, Mooi WJ, Sutedja TG. Initial bronchoscopic treatment for patients with intraluminal bronchial carcinoids. J Thorac Cardiovasc Surg. 2007;133(4):973–8.
51. Filosso PL, Ruffini E, Oliaro A, Papalia E, Donati G, Rena O. Long-term survival of atypical bronchial carcinoids with liver metastases, treated with octreotide. Eur J Cardiothorac Surg. 2002;21(5):913–7.
52. Sun W, Lipsitz S, Catalano P, Mailliard JA, Haller DG. Phase II/III study of doxorubicin with fluorouracil compared with streptozocin with fluorouracil or dacarbazine in the treatment of advanced carcinoid tumors: Eastern Cooperative Oncology Group Study E1281. J Clin Oncol. 2005;23(22):4897–904.
53. Pavel ME, Hainsworth JD, Baudin E, et al. Everolimus plus octreotide long-acting repeatable for the treatment of advanced neuroendocrine tumours associated with carcinoid syndrome (RADIANT-2): a randomised, placebo-controlled, phase 3 study. Lancet. 2011;378 (9808):2005–12.
54. Yao JC, Phan A, Hoff PM, Chen HX, Charnsangavej C, Yeung SC, Hess K, Ng C, Abbruzzese JL, Ajani JA. Targeting vascular endothelial growth factor in advanced carcinoid tumor: a random assignment phase II study of depot octreotide with bevacizumab or pegylated interferon alpha-2b. J Clin Oncol. 2008;26(8):1316–23.
55. Ferguson CJ, Cleeland JA. Mucous gland adenoma of the trachea: case report and literature review. J Thorac Cardiovasc Surg. 1988;95(2):347–50.
56. England DM, Hochholzer L. Truly benign "bronchial adenoma". Report of 10 cases of mucous gland adenoma with immunohistochemical and ultrastructural findings. Am J Surg Pathol. 1995;19(8):887–99.
57. Wu CC, Shepard JA. Tracheal and airway neoplasms. Semin Roentgenol. 2013;48(4):354–64.
58. Wang JW, Huang M, Zha WJ, Zhou LF, Qi X, Wang H. Flexible bronchoscopic intervention for endobronchial hamartoma. Zhonghua Jie He He Hu Xi Za Zhi. 2013;36(12):963–7.

59. Swigris JJ, Coulter TD, Mehta AC. Endobronchial lipoma. J Bronchol Interv Pulmonol. 1999;6(4):277–9.
60. Srivali N, Boland JM, Ryu JH. Endobroncheal neurofibroma. QJM. Advanced access 25 Oct 2015.
61. Khan S, Lenox R, Mehta AC. Endobronchial neurofibromas. J Bronchol Interv Pulmonol. 1995;2:143–4.
62. Huang C, Liu QF, Chen XM, Li L, Han ZJ, Zhou XY, Liu L, Li SQ. A malignant glomus tumor in the upper trachea. Ann Thorac Surg. 2015;99(5):1812–4.
63. van der Maten J, Blaauwgeers JL, Sutedja TG, Kwa HB, Postmus PE, Wagenaar SS. Granular cell tumors of the tracheobronchial tree. J Thorac Cardiovasc Surg. 2003;126 (3):740–3.
64. Alkotob LM, Miller R, Mehta AC. Primary endobronchial chondrosarcoma. J Bronchol Interv Pulmonol. 2001;8:110–1.
65. Wagnetz U, Patsios D, Darling G, Las Heras F, Hwang D. Tracheal chondrosarcoma—a rare complication in Maffucci syndrome. Br J Radiol. 2009;82(981):e178–81.
66. Dong H, Tatsuno BK, Betancourt J, Oh SS. Tracheal epithelial-myoepithelial carcinoma associated with sarcoid-like reaction: a case report. Respir Med Case Rep. 2014;14:34–6.
67. Pecoraro Y, Diso D, Anile M, Russo E, Patella M, Venuta F. Primary inflammatory myofibroblastic tumor of the trachea. Respirol Case Rep. 2014;2(4):147–9.
68. Cai C, Jiang RC, Li ZB, et al. Two-stage tracheal reconstruction of primary tracheal non-Hodgkin lymphoma with nitinol mesh stent and cervical myocutaneous flap. Ann Thorac Surg. 2008;85(3):e17–9.
69. Li Z, Tang P, Xu Z. Experience of diagnosis and treatment for primary cervical tracheal tumors. Zhonghua Er Bi Yan Hou Tou Jing Wai Ke Za Zhi. 2006;41(3):208–10.
70. Spizarny DL, Shepard JA, McLoud TC, Grillo HC, Dedrick CG. CT of adenoid cystic carcinoma of the trachea. Am J Roentgenol. 1986;146(6):1129–32.
71. Weber AL, Grillo HC. Tracheal tumors. A radiological, clinical, and pathological evaluation of 84 cases. Radiol Clin North Am. 1978;16(2):227–46.
72. Jo ETV, Morehead RS. Hemoptysis and dyspnea in a 67-year-old man with a normal chest radiograph. Chest. 1999;116(3):803–7.
73. Akata S, Ohkubo Y, Park J, et al. Multiplanar reconstruction MR image of primary adenoid cystic carcinoma of the central airway: (MPR of central airway adenoid cystic carcinoma). Clin Imaging. 2001;25(5):332–6.
74. Hoerbelt R, Padberg W. Primary tracheal tumors of the neck and mediastinum: resection and reconstruction procedures. Chirurg. 2011;82(2):125–33.
75. Wolf M, Shapira Y, Talmi YP, Novikov I, Kronenberg J, Yellin A. Laryngotracheal anastomosis: primary and revised procedures. Laryngoscope. 2001;11:622–7.
76. Lanuti M, Mathisen DJ. Management of complications of tracheal surgery. Chest Surg Clin N Am. 2003;13(2):385–97.
77. Denlinger CE. A balanced perspective for management of tracheal salivary gland-type carcinomas. J Thorac Cardiovasc Surg. 2010;140(2):394.
78. De Perrot M, Fadel E, Mercier O, Mussot S, Chapelier A, Dartevelle P. Long-term results after carinal resection for carcinoma: does the benefit warrant the risk? J Thorac Cardiovasc Surg. 2006;131(1):81–9.
79. Mitchell JD, Mathisen DJ, Wright CD, et al. Clinical experience with carinal resection. J Thorac Cardiovasc Surg. 1999;117(1):39–53.
80. Lowe JE, Bridgman AH, Sabiston DC. The role of bronchoplastic procedures in the surgical management of benign and malignant pulmonary lesions. J Thorac Cardiovasc Surg. 1982;83 (2):227–34.
81. Breyer RH, Dainauskas JR, Jensik RJ, Faber LP. Mucoepidermoid carcinoma of the trachea and bronchus: the case for conservative resection. Ann Thorac Surg. 1980;29(3):197–204.
82. Xie L, Fan M, Sheets NC, Chen RC, Jiang G-L, Marks LB. The use of radiation therapy appears to improve outcome in patients with malignant primary tracheal tumors: a SEER-based analysis. Int J Radiat Oncol Biol Phys. 2012;84(2):464–70.

83. Suzuki T. What is the best management strategy for adenoid cystic carcinoma of the trachea? Ann Thorac Cardiovasc Surg. 2011;17(6):535–8.
84. Cooper JS, Pajak TF, Forastiere AA, et al. Postoperative concurrent radiotherapy and chemotherapy for high-risk squamous-cell carcinoma of the head and neck. N Engl J Med. 2004;350(19):1937–44.
85. Mendenhall WM, Morris CG, Amdur RJ, Werning JW, Hinerman RW, Villaret DB. Radiotherapy alone or combined with surgery for adenoid cystic carcinoma of the head and neck. Head Neck. 2004;26(2):154–62.
86. Okada S, Yamauchi H, Ishimori S, Satoh S, Sugawara H, Tanaba Y. Endoscopic surgery with a flexible bronchoscope and argon plasma coagulation for tracheobronchial tumors. J Thorac Cardiovasc Surg. 2001;121(1):180–2.
87. Shah H, Garbe L, Nussbaum E, Dumon JF, Chiodera PL, Cavaliere S. Benign tumors of the tracheobronchial tree. Endoscopic characteristics and role of laser resection. Chest. 1995;107 (6):1744–51.
88. Husain SA, Finch D, Ahmed M, Morgan A, Hetzel MR. Long-term follow-up of ultraflex metallic stents in benign and malignant central airway obstruction. Ann Thorac Surg. 2007;83(4):1251–6.
89. Pereszlenyi A, Igaz M, Majer I, Harustiak S. Role of endotracheal stenting in tracheal reconstruction surgery—retrospective analysis. Eur J Cardiothorac Surg. 2004;25(6):1059–64.
90. Cavaliere S, Venuta F, Foccoli P, Toninelli C, La Face B. Endoscopic treatment of malignant airway obstructions in 2,008 patients. Chest. 1996;110(6):1536–42.
91. de Carvalho HA, Figueiredo V, Pedreira WL, Aisen S. High dose-rate brachytherapy as a treatment option in primary tracheal tumors. Clinics (Sao Paulo). 2005; 60(4):299–304.
92. Jungebluth P, Alici E, Baiguera S, Le Blanc K, Blomberg P, Bozóky B, Crowley C, Einarsson O, Grinnemo KH, Gudbjartsson T, Le Guyader S, Henriksson G, Hermanson O, Juto JE, Leidner B, Lilja T, Liska J, Luedde T, Lundin V, Moll G, Nilsson B, Roderburg C, Strömblad S, Sutlu T, Teixeira AI, Watz E, Seifalian A, Macchiarini P. Tracheobronchial transplantation with a stem-cell-seeded bioartificial nanocomposite: a proof-of-concept study. Lancet. 2011;378(9808):1997–2004.
93. Rich JT, Gullane PJ. Current concepts in tracheal reconstruction. Curr Opin Otolaryngol Head Neck Surg. 2012;20(4):246–53.
94. Choudhary C et al. Metastatic endotracheal and endobronchial thymic carcinoma. J Bronchol Interv Pulmonol. 2007;14:264–266.
95. Chua A-P, Joshi M, Mehta AC. Bronchial mucoepidermoid carcinoma. J Bronchol Interv Pulmonol. 2009;16(1):39–40.
96. Swigris J, Coulter T, Mehta A. Endobronchial lipoma. J Bronchol Interv Pulmonol. 1999; 6 (4):277–279.
97. Shah SS, Karnak D, Shah SN, Biscotti C, Murthy S, Mehta AC. Clinical-pathologic conference in thoracic surgery: a malignant peripheral nerve sheath tumor of the trachea. J Thorac Cardiovasc Surg. 2006; 132(6):1455–9.
98. Usuda K, Gildea T, Lorenz R. Laryngeal glomangiomyoma. J Bronchol Interv Pulmonol. 2005; 12(2):102–103.
99. Chan C-C, Farver C, Mehta AC. Granular cell tumor of the trachea. J Bronchol Interv Pulmonol. 1997; 4:52–53.
100. Alkotob L, Miller R, Mehta AC. Primary endobronchial chondrosarcoma. J Bronchol Interv Pulmonol. 2001; 8(2):110–111.

Chapter 13
Lymphomas of the Large Airways

Hardeep S. Rai and Andrea Valeria Arrossi

Introduction

Lymphomas occurring in the airways and/or pulmonary parenchyma can present as either primary or secondary. There are no universally accepted criteria for diagnosing a lymphoma as primary in the lung; however, traditionally, it has been defined as a lymphoma that presents as one or more pulmonary lesions with no clinical, pathologic, or radiographic evidence of lymphoma elsewhere in the past, at present, or for 3 months after presentation [1–3]. Secondary lung involvement may occur either from hematogenous spread, or contiguous involvement from affected hilar or mediastinal lymph nodes.

Primary pulmonary/airway lymphomas are rare, and their pathologic distinction from other more common lung neoplasms or even benign lymphoid proliferations may be challenging. Immunohistochemical stains using specific monoclonal antibodies are necessary to determine clonality and to identify specific cell surface antigens that will help in the classification of the neoplasm. Other ancillary tests including flow cytometry and/or molecular studies for the detection of immunoglobulin gene or T cell gamma or beta receptor gene rearrangements constitute additional diagnostic techniques that are very helpful, especially in small biopsies.

H.S. Rai (✉)
Respiratory Institute, Cleveland Clinic, 9500 Euclid Avenue, A-90, Cleveland,
OH 44195, USA
e-mail: raih@ccf.org

A.V. Arrossi
Anatomic Pathology, Cleveland Clinic, 9500 Euclid Avenue, A-90, Cleveland,
OH 44195, USA

© Springer International Publishing Switzerland 2016   281
A.C. Mehta et al. (eds.), *Diseases of the Central Airways*,
Respiratory Medicine, DOI 10.1007/978-3-319-29830-6_13

An overview and classification of primary pulmonary/airway lymphoproliferative disorders will be discussed in the following sections, and a practical diagnostic
approach including imaging studies and histopathologic diagnosis will be
presented.

Historical Background

The presence of bronchial-associated lymphoid tissue (BALT) and its relationship
to the lymphoid system in general and mucosal immunity were first described by
Bienenstock et al. in 1973 [4]. Lymphoid tissue is generally absent or inconspic-
uous in the adult lung, except in pathologic states [5, 6]. When present, it is usually
seen as small collections of lymphocytes along the lymphatic routes, especially
bronchovascular bundles, lobular septa, and pleura. Lymphoid tissue along the
airways is part of the specialized, more diffuse immunologic compartment of
mucosa-associated lymphoid tissue (MALT) that has the ability to combat pathogens at mucosal sites. In the lung, this lymphoid tissue is referred to as
bronchial-associated lymphoid tissue (BALT). BALT shares morphologic features
of MALT at other sites and displays the same reactions, such as reactive hyperplasia
and immunoblastic proliferation, and constitutes the origin of most primary
pulmonary/airway lymphomas, which are marginal zone B cell lymphomas. In the
early literature, the term "pseudolymphoma" has been employed in many cases to
denote the more favorable prognosis of primary malignant lymphomas of the lung
in comparison with lymphomas at other sites [1, 7, 8]. Though the concept of
pseudolymphoma has been maintained over the years, it was not until the introduction of immunocytochemical techniques that polytypic (polyclonal) reactive
lymphoid proliferations could be separated from monotypic (monoclonal) neoplastic lesions, and this opened the starting point to resolve the debate whether
lymphoid lesions in the lung represented true lymphomas or pseudolymphomas
[2, 3, 9–15]. Furthermore, the subsequent advent of molecular genetic techniques
allowed the identification of a broader and more specific clinical and pathological
spectrum of lymphoproliferative disorders.

Incidence

Secondary involvement of the lung by nodal lymphoproliferative disorders is much
more frequent (25–40 %) than primary pulmonary lymphomas, which are rare and
represent 3–7 % of extranodal non-Hodgkin's lymphoma [16–18]. The age peak
incidence is in the sixth decade. Individuals younger than 30 years of age are rarely
affected. Both females and males are more or less equally affected [2, 9, 14, 17–26].
Lymphomas involving primarily the large airways, especially the trachea, are
extremely rare [27–30].

Extranodal marginal B cell lymphoma is the most common type of primary pulmonary/airway lymphoma, comprising approximately 75 % of the cases [3, 17, 19, 20, 23, 24, 31]. The second most common malignant lymphoid proliferation is diffuse large B cell lymphoma [23]. Other less common types include lymphomatoid granulomatosis, anaplastic large cell lymphoma, and lymphoproliferative disorders associated with an immunocompromised state. Primary pulmonary Hodgkin's lymphomas are extremely rare.

Etiology

MALT lymphomas comprise a heterogeneous group of small B cell lymphomas characterized by lymphocytes that show morphologic and functional similarities to the non-neoplastic marginal zone B cells that surround germinal centers. Extranodal MALT lymphoma, the most frequent type of lymphoproliferative disorder primary to the lung and airways, is frequently associated with chronic inflammation and persistent antigen stimulation, as demonstrated originally in the gastric MALT lymphomas following infection with Helicobacter pylori [32]. In the lung, MALT lymphomas have been associated with chronic immune-mediated diseases such as Sjögren syndrome, rheumatoid arthritis, or immunodeficiency disorders [21, 33, 34].

Clinical Features

Primary pulmonary lymphomas are in the majority of the cases low-grade MALT lymphomas that are asymptomatic in over 50 % of the cases [2, 9, 14, 19, 21]. They can be incidentally discovered through chest imaging performed as part of a routine health examination of an asymptomatic patient [14, 19], when symptomatic patients present with non-specific respiratory symptoms such as cough, dyspnea, and chest pain [21, 24]. Contrarily, lymphomas involving the large airways, whether as primary endobronchial lesions, or spread from a parenchymal process, manifest often with symptoms of airway obstruction, such as cough, wheezing, and hemoptysis [35]. These symptoms may be manifested also in cases of lymphomas involving primarily the lung parenchyma that exert extrinsic compression on the airways. Wheezing may also be present in patients with lymphomatous infiltration of small airways [35]. Systemic symptoms such as fevers and weight loss ("B" symptoms) rarely occur [21].

Laboratory Investigations

Serum protein electrophoresis abnormalities may be present in patients with primary pulmonary lymphoma. Monoclonal gammopathy (predominantly IgM) is found in the majority of the cases (20–60 %), especially in MALT lymphomas with plasmacytic differentiation [3, 19, 21].

Imaging

Primary pulmonary MALT lymphomas share similar radiologic appearance as the secondary pulmonary/airway involvement by other forms of thoracic lymphomas [36]. The most frequent computed tomography (CT) finding of pulmonary parenchymal MALT lymphomas is single or multiple pulmonary nodules or masses or mass-like areas of consolidation that tend to show a peribronchovascular distribution (Fig. 13.1) [37]. Air bronchograms within areas of consolidation in addition to the presence of multiple pulmonary nodules on CT scans are commonly associated findings (Fig. 13.2). The presence of a halo of marginal ground glass shadowing around pulmonary nodules or masses in some patients and the presence of discrete patches of ground glass opacities in others have been described on high-resolution CT.

Few reports of lymphoma involving the tracheobronchial tree as the only site of involvement have been published. Three main radiological patterns have been described: (1) solitary intraluminal polypoid lesion with or without secondary obstructive changes in the lung periphery, (2) multiple round-shaped nodular protrusions less than 5 mm, and (3) a diffuse and smooth wall thickening pattern

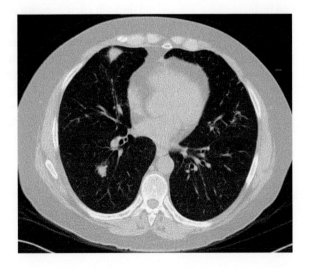

Fig. 13.1 Low-grade B cell extranodal marginal zone MALT lymphoma presenting as multiple nodular opacities in a 57-year-old female

Fig. 13.2 Irregularly
marginated 2.5 cm mass in
superior segment of the right
lower lobe with a
bronchiectatic air
bronchogram. Extranodal
marginal zone B cell
lymphoma of MALT

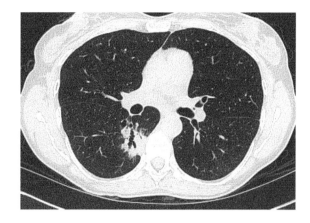

[38–41]. Secondary radiological findings may include post-obstructive lobar atelectasis, lobular air trapping, and post-obstructive bronchopneumonia [38].

Differential radiologic diagnoses of lymphomas primarily involving the large airways include other large airway diseases, neoplastic and non-neoplastic, such as relapsing polychondritis, tracheobronchopathia osteochondroplastica, tracheobronchial amyloidosis, granulomatosis with polyangiitis, tracheobronchitis associated with inflammatory bowel disease, and salivary gland neoplasms and bronchogenic carcinomas. Relapsing polychondritis, a rare autoimmune disorder, may present with diffuse or localized laryngotracheobronchial involvement manifesting as airway wall thickening and airway stenosis. Airway malacia or airway wall calcifications, present in 10–50 % of cases [42], may be a distinctive feature from airway lymphoma. Tracheobronchopathia osteochondroplastica shows multiple submucosal nodules with osteocartilaginous cores projecting into the lumen. The disease characteristically spares the posterior membrane, predominantly involving the distal trachea and proximal primary bronchi [43]. Tracheobronchial amyloidosis reveals luminal surface irregularity, focal circumferential wall thickening and, in many cases, widespread dense mural calcifications largely sparing the posterior tracheal membrane [44]. In patients with granulomatosis with polyangiitis (GPA), the principal CT findings include subglottic stenosis, circumferential mucosal thickening, irregularity, and ulceration of the tracheobronchial walls [43, 45]. Large airway involvement in inflammatory bowel diseases manifests radiologically mainly as upper airway stenosis (subglottic) and bronchiectasis [46]. Tracheal salivary gland neoplasms, most commonly adenoid cystic carcinomas, usually show an intraluminal mass of soft tissue density with occasional extension through the tracheal wall on CT [47].

Fluoro 2-deoxyglucose positron emission tomography (FDG-PET) has been used for the staging, evaluation, and management of lymphomas; however, its value in the evaluation of extranodal MZL has been unclear. The clinical utility in staging and management was suggested in a recent study of patients with histologically confirmed MALT lymphomas, since 80 % of 42 patients had FDG-PET avid lesions and were at higher stage than the patients with negative scans [48].

Fig. 13.3 Diffuse large B cell
lymphoma presenting as a
large non-obstructing,
infiltrative, friable, and
granular lesion involving the
distal trachea and main carina

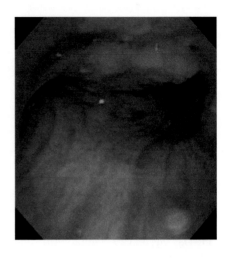

Flexible Bronchoscopy

In individuals with clinically apparent systemic lymphoma that secondarily
involves the large airways, the most common endoscopic pattern is characterized by
the presence of diffuse submucosal nodules [49–52]. In primary endobronchial
lymphoma, however, the bronchoscopic findings correlate with the three patterns of
radiologic presentation described above: (1) solitary intraluminal polypoid lesion,
(2) multiple round-shaped nodular protrusions less than 5 mm, and (3) a diffuse and
smooth wall thickening pattern causing narrowing of the lumen (Fig. 13.3) [38, 40].

Lymphomas involving primarily the lung parenchyma that contiguously spread
to the airways involve bronchial mucosa with variable degrees of tumor necrosis
and can show cobblestone appearance, submucosal nodules or submucosal masses
visible at each division of the bronchial tree, at the sites of bronchus-associated
lymphoid tissue [52]. Extrinsic airway compression without direct involvement of
the airway can also be visualized endoscopically.

Pathology

This section refers to the pathology of the two most common types of lymphoma
involving the airways, marginal zone B cell lymphomas of MALT type and diffuse
large B cell lymphoma. Other types of lymphoma involve primarily the lung parenchyma with no or little involvement of the large airways, or have rarely been
reported, mainly as case reports. These include lymphomatoid granulomatosis,
post-transplant lymphoproliferative disorders, anaplastic large cell lymphoma, and
rare cases of NK/T cell lymphomas. Primary pulmonary Hodgkin's lymphoma is
extremely rare in the lung.

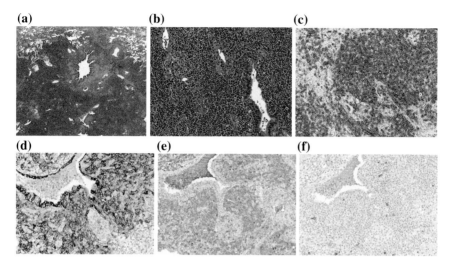

Fig. 13.4 Low-grade MALT lymphoma with plasmacytic differentiation involving the lung and airways, **a** (Hematoxylin and Eosin 1×) showing infiltration by small lymphocytes with lymphoepithelial lesions, **b** (Hematoxylin and Eosin 20×). The lymphocytes express B cell markers, **c** (CD20 20×), plasma cell markers, **d** (CD138 20×) and show kappa light chain restriction, **e** (Kappa 20×), while negative for lambda, **f** (Lambda 20×)

Pulmonary/airway MALT lymphomas show similar histologic characteristics to their counterpart in other extranodal sites. There are dense infiltrates of small B cell lymphocytes, and sometimes, they may show monocytoid B cell or, less commonly in the lung, plasmacytic differentiation. The monoclonal proliferation is admixed with polyclonal B and T cells. Reactive lymphoid follicles with germinal centers surround or are interspersed with the neoplastic lymphocytes. The lymphoid follicles can be very prominent and obscure the malignant process leading to diagnostic problems. Epithelial infiltration by neoplastic lymphocytes, so-called lymphoepithelial lesions, is common (Fig. 13.4). MALT lymphomas share the morphology and biology of marginal zone B cells, which are post-germinal center lymphocytes with memory functions that migrate from lymphoid tissues to extranodal sites where they can rapidly become antibody-producing plasma cells after antigenic stimulation. The marginal zone B phenotype can be demonstrated with immunohistochemistry, as the neoplastic lymphoid cells express B cell markers such as CD79, CD20, and CD43 [2, 3, 21, 24, 31]. There is usually expression of surface IgM, and less commonly IgG or IgA, whereas CD5, CD10, CD23, and IgD are negative. Immunohistochemistry or in situ hybridization may demonstrate Ig heavy or light chain restriction, and PCR may detect clonal IGH rearrangements; however, false-negative results can occur given the frequent patchiness of the monotypic areas. As in gastric and bowel MALT lymphomas, the chromosomal translocation t(11;18) (q21;q21) producing a fusion of the MALT1 and API2 genes constitutes the most frequent translocation encountered in pulmonary MALT

Fig. 13.5 Microphotograph of an endobronchial biopsy of primary tracheal large B cell lymphoma, hematoxylin and eosin, low magnification (2×) and medium magnification (20×), *left lower inlet* and CD 20 medium magnification (20×), *right lower inlet*. The picture shows squamous (*asterisk*) (metaplastic) lined mucosa with infiltration by large lymphoid cells (*double asterisk*) immunoreactive to B cell marker CD20

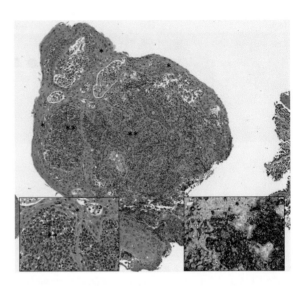

lymphomas (31–50 %) [32, 53–56] A subset of cases (6–10 %) show t(14;18) (q32; q21) or t(1;14)(p22;q32) translocations [57].

The second most common type of pulmonary lymphomas is diffuse large B cell lymphoma that can occur de novo or in the setting of malignant transformation of a low-grade marginal zone B cell lymphoma of MALT type. Histologically, they show a diffuse proliferation of large lymphoid cells with atypical high-grade nuclei that express pan-B cell antigens CD20, CD79a, and CD43 (Fig. 13.5) with variable CD10, bcl6, and bcl2 expression. Areas of necrosis and vascular infiltration may be seen [1, 3, 19–21, 23, 24, 31].

Diagnosis

The diagnosis of lymphoma involving the lung and/or airways requires tissue sampling through surgical samples or endobronchial, transbronchial, or transthoracic biopsy material. Selection of the diagnostic modality depends on the location and size of the pulmonary lesions, patient's comorbid conditions, functional status, and personal preferences. Flexible bronchoscopy with transbronchial biopsy and bronchoalveolar lavage for flow cytometry plays a significant role in the diagnosis of primary lymphoma of the lung. For lymphomas involving predominantly lung parenchyma, more invasive procedures are needed, such as image-guided transthoracic needle biopsy or surgical lung biopsy with either video assisted thoracoscopy (VATS), or open thoracotomy.

The histologic differential diagnoses depend on the type of the lymphoproliferative disorder being considered. Low-grade MALT lymphoma shows infiltration by mostly small lymphocytes usually with the presence of reactive lymphoid follicles with germinal centers and should be differentiated from reactive processes such as follicular bronchiolitis and follicular hyperplasia. If a parenchymal lesion is being evaluated, lymphocytic interstitial pneumonia may have a similar appearance. The ultimate diagnosis relies on the demonstration of a clonal proliferation with the use of immunohistochemical stains and/or molecular techniques, including in situ hybridization or PCR. On the other hand, diffuse large B cell lymphomas are high-grade lesions that should be differentiated from other high-grade malignant neoplasms such as carcinoma or melanoma. Using immunohistochemical stains, the expression of the leukocyte common antigen (LCA/CD45) can be demonstrated in lymphoid proliferations. Carcinomas express cytokeratin antigens and are negative for LCA/CD45. Melanomas are immunoreactive to S-100 protein and other melanocytic markers such as HMB-45, SOX-10, or MART-1 and negative for cytokeratins and LCA/CD45.

Flow cytometry analysis for the detection of clonal proliferations in the fluid obtained during a bronchoalveolar lavage constitutes a relatively noninvasive alternative and promising diagnostic tool in patients who are at high risk for more invasive procedures such as endobronchial and transbronchial biopsies, either due to advanced age, other comorbidities, and poor functional status. It has been shown that the detection of a B cell clonal population on bronchoalveolar lavage fluid is associated with a histologic diagnosis of pulmonary non-Hodgkin's lymphoma, with a specificity of 97 %, positive predictive value of 82 %, and negative predictive value of 95 % [58].

Treatment

Management choices for primary pulmonary lymphomas are based on histology, stage, biologic characteristics, patient's comorbidities, and performance status.

While surgery is usually only used for diagnostic purposes for lymphomas in general, it plays an important role in the treatment of localized pulmonary lymphomas [59]. Complete surgical resection is associated with an excellent long-term (10-year) survival of almost 90 % [60]. Other considerations include radiation, chemotherapy, and rituximab [20, 21, 24–26, 61, 62].

Prognosis

Primary pulmonary MALT lymphomas have an indolent course and a favorable prognosis [24], with an overall 5-year survival of over 60 % [3, 19–21, 23, 24, 60, 62] and a recurrence rate of up to 46 % [2, 3, 10]. Pulmonary recurrences are either within the ipsilateral lung or in both lungs. Extrapulmonary recurrent disease occurs mainly in lymph nodes; however skin, bone marrow, or visceral organs could be affected [2, 3, 25]. The median time to recurrence is 6–7 years, but late recurrences were reported up to 14 years [3, 21, 24, 26]. The prognostic factors affecting survival are not well defined [20, 21]. A subset of low-grade MALT lymphomas progress to diffuse large B cell lymphomas, which confer a worse prognosis [3].

Summary and Recommendations

Lymphoproliferative disorders can either involve the lungs and/or airways primarily, by hematogenous spread or by contiguous invasion from intrathoracic sites of nodal lymphoma. Primary pulmonary lymphomas are rare. The most frequent type of lymphoma involving primarily the lungs and airways is low-grade marginal zone B cell lymphoma of MALT type, usually associated with chronic persistent inflammatory conditions with persistent antigen stimulation such as Sjogren's syndrome or other autoimmune processes, or immunodeficiency disorders. Patients are usually asymptomatic, and the lymphoma is found during workup for the evaluation of other unrelated conditions. When symptoms are present, they vary according to the pattern of the disease. Cough, dyspnea, and chest pain are associated with pulmonary parenchymal lesions, and symptoms of airway obstruction are associated with lesions involving the airways. Pulmonary MALT lymphomas manifest on CT scans of the chest as single or multiple pulmonary nodules. Bronchoscopically, three main patterns can be seen in lymphomas involving the airways, including a solitary intraluminal polypoid lesion, multiple round-shaped nodular protrusions, or a diffuse and smooth wall thickening pattern, occasionally causing luminal narrowing. The diagnosis relies on the microscopic examination of tissue samples. The histologic differential diagnosis for low-grade MALT lymphoma is mainly reactive lymphoid hyperplasia, and the demonstration of a clonal proliferation through immunohistochemical stains and/or cytogenetic studies is essential for the diagnosis of lymphoma. Flow cytometry analysis of the bronchoalveolar fluid may constitute an aid in detecting a clonal proliferation in patients who are not eligible for other more invasive tissue-sampling procedures. The differential diagnoses of high-grade lesions such as diffuse large B cell lymphoma include other high-grade non-lymphoid malignant neoplasms such as carcinoma or melanoma, and immunohistochemical stains are useful to determine the lymphoid immunophenotype and classification of the lymphoproliferative disease. Treatment of primary pulmonary/airway lymphomas varies depending on histologic grade, patient's comorbidities, and performance status. Surgery and/or radiation is considered for localized lesions, and chemotherapy and rituximab constitute alternate treatment options, especially in patients with diffuse lesions. The long-term outcome of pulmonary lymphomas is favorable. Recurrences may occur in about 50 % of the cases, and the time to the recurrence may be as long as 14 years after presentation. Therefore, long-term follow-up is recommended.

References

1. Saltzstein SL. Pulmonary malignant lymphomas and pseudolymphomas: Classification, therapy, and prognosis. Cancer. 1963;16:928–55.
2. L'Hoste RJ Jr, Filippa DA, Lieberman PH, Bretsky S. Primary pulmonary lymphomas. A clinicopathologic analysis of 36 cases. Cancer. 1984;54(7):1397–406.
3. Li G, Hansmann ML, Zwingers T, Lennert K. Primary lymphomas of the lung: Morphological, immunohistochemical and clinical features. Histopathology. 1990;16 (6):519–31.
4. Bienenstock J, Johnston N, Perey DY. Bronchial lymphoid tissue. II. functional characterisitics. Lab Invest. 1973;28(6):693–8.
5. Pabst R, Gehrke I. Is the bronchus-associated lymphoid tissue (BALT) an integral structure of the lung in normal mammals, including humans? Am J Respir Cell Mol Biol. 1990;3(2): 131–135.
6. Tschernig T, Pabst R. Bronchus-associated lymphoid tissue (BALT) is not present in the normal adult lung but in different diseases. Pathobiology. 2000;68(1):1–8.
7. Julsrud PR, Brown LR, Li CY. Rosenow EC,3rd, Crowe JK. Pulmonary processes of mature-appearing lymphocytes: Pseudolymphoma, well-differentiated lymphocytic lymphoma, and lymphocytic interstitial pneumonitis. Radiology. 1978;127(2):289–96.
8. Hutchinson WB, Friedenberg MJ, Saltzstein S. Primary pulmonary pseudolymphoma. Radiology. 1964;82:48–56.
9. Herbert A, Wright DH, Isaacson PG, Smith JL. Primary malignant lymphoma of the lung: Histopathologic and immunologic evaluation of nine cases. Hum Pathol. 1984;15(5):415–22.
10. Koss MN, Hochholzer L, Nichols PW, Wehunt WD, Lazarus AA. Primary non-hodgkin's lymphoma and pseudolymphoma of lung: A study of 161 patients. Hum Pathol. 1983;14 (12):1024–38.
11. Colby TV, Carrington CB. Lymphoreticular tumors and infiltrates of the lung. Pathol Annu. 1983;18(Pt 1):27–70.
12. Colby TV, Carrington CB. Pulmonary lymphomas: Current concepts. Hum Pathol. 1983;14 (10):884–7.
13. Addis BJ, Hyjek E, Isaacson PG. Primary pulmonary lymphoma: A re-appraisal of its histogenesis and its relationship to pseudolymphoma and lymphoid interstitial pneumonia. Histopathology. 1988;13(1):1–17.
14. Kennedy JL, Nathwani BN, Burke JS, Hill LR, Rappaport H. Pulmonary lymphomas and other pulmonary lymphoid lesions. A clinicopathologic and immunologic study of 64 patients. Cancer. 1985;56(3):539–52.
15. Weiss LM, Yousem SA, Warnke RA. Non-hodgkin's lymphomas of the lung. A study of 19 cases emphasizing the utility of frozen section immunologic studies in differential diagnosis. Am J Surg Pathol. 1985;9(7):480–90.
16. Freeman C, Berg JW, Cutler SJ. Occurrence and prognosis of extranodal lymphomas. Cancer. 1972;29(1):252–60.
17. Cadranel J, Wislez M, Antoine M. Primary pulmonary lymphoma. Eur Respir J. 2002;20 (3):750–62.
18. Khalil MO, Morton LM, Devesa SS, et al. Incidence of marginal zone lymphoma in the united states, 2001–2009 with a focus on primary anatomic site. Br J Haematol. 2014;165(1):67–77.
19. Cordier JF, Chailleux E, Lauque D, et al. Primary pulmonary lymphomas. A clinical study of 70 cases in nonimmunocompromised patients. Chest. 1993;103(1):201–8.
20. Ferraro P, Trastek VF, Adlakha H, Deschamps C, Allen MS, Pairolero PC. Primary non-hodgkin's lymphoma of the lung. Ann Thorac Surg. 2000;69(4):993–7.
21. Kurtin PJ, Myers JL, Adlakha H, et al. Pathologic and clinical features of primary pulmonary extranodal marginal zone B-cell lymphoma of MALT type. Am J Surg Pathol. 2001;25 (8):997–1008.

22. Zinzani PL, Tani M, Gabriele A, et al. Extranodal marginal zone B-cell lymphoma of MALT-type of the lung: single-center experience with 12 patients. Leuk Lymphoma. 2003;44 (5):821–4.
23. Kim JH, Lee SH, Park J, et al. Primary pulmonary non-hodgkin's lymphoma. Jpn J Clin Oncol. 2004;34(9):510–4.
24. Graham BB, Mathisen DJ, Mark EJ, Takvorian RW. Primary pulmonary lymphoma. Ann Thorac Surg. 2005;80(4):1248–53.
25. Arkenau HT, Gordon C, Cunningham D, Norman A, Wotherspoon A, Chau I. Mucosa associated lymphoid tissue lymphoma of the lung: The royal marsden hospital experience. Leuk Lymphoma. 2007;48(3):547–50.
26. Xu HY, Jin T, Li RY, Ni YM, Zhou JY, Wen XH. Diagnosis and treatment of pulmonary mucosa-associated lymphoid tissue lymphoma. Chin Med J (Engl). 2007;120(8):648–51.
27. Kaplan MA, Pettit CL, Zukerberg LR, Harris NL. Primary lymphoma of the trachea with morphologic and immunophenotypic characteristics of low-grade B-cell lymphoma of mucosa-associated lymphoid tissue. Am J Surg Pathol. 1992;16(1):71–5.
28. Fidias P, Wright C, Harris NL, Urba W, Grossbard ML. Primary tracheal non-hodgkin's lymphoma. A case report and review of the literature. Cancer. 1996;77(11):2332–8.
29. Okubo K, Miyamoto N, Komaki C. Primary mucosa-associated lymphoid tissue (MALT) lymphoma of the trachea: A case of surgical resection and long term survival. Thorax. 2005;60 (1):82–3.
30. Kang JY, Park HJ, Lee KY, et al. Extranodal marginal zone lymphoma occurring along the trachea and central airway. Yonsei Med J. 2008;49(5):860–3.
31. Fiche M, Caprons F, Berger F, et al. Primary pulmonary non-hodgkin's lymphomas. Histopathology. 1995;26(6):529–37.
32. Isaacson PG. Update on MALT lymphomas. Best Pract Res Clin Haematol. 2005; 18(1):57–68.
33. Nicholson AG, Wotherspoon AC, Jones AL, Sheppard MN, Isaacson PG, Corrin B. Pulmonary B-cell non-hodgkin's lymphoma associated with autoimmune disorders: a clinicopathological review of six cases. Eur Respir J. 1996;9(10):2022–5.
34. Mhawech P, Krishnan B, Shahab I. Primary pulmonary mucosa-associated lymphoid tissue lymphoma with associated fungal ball in a patient with human immunodeficiency virus infection. Arch Pathol Lab Med. 2000;124(10):1506–9.
35. Rose RM, Grigas D, Strattemeir E, Harris NL, Linggood RM. Endobronchial involvement with non-hodgkin's lymphoma. A clinical-radiologic analysis. Cancer. 1986;57(9):1750–5.
36. Lewis ER, Caskey CI, Fishman EK. Lymphoma of the lung: CT findings in 31 patients. AJR Am J Roentgenol. 1991;156(4):711–4.
37. King LJ, Padley SP, Wotherspoon AC, Nicholson AG. Pulmonary MALT lymphoma: imaging findings in 24 cases. Eur Radiol. 2000;10(12):1932–8.
38. Yoon RG, Kim MY, Song JW, Chae EJ, Choi CM, Jang S. Primary endobronchial marginal zone B-cell lymphoma of bronchus-associated lymphoid tissue: CT findings in 7 patients. Korean J Radiol. 2013;14(2):366–74.
39. Nakajima T, Yasufuku K, Sekine Y, Yoshida S, Yoshino I. Mucosa-associated lymphoid tissue lymphoma of the left mainstem bronchus. Ann Thorac Surg. 2011;91(4):1281–3.
40. Ujita M, Sato H, Yamaguchi M, Toba K, Kobayashi H. Extranodal marginal zone lymphoma of mucosa-associated lymphoid tissue of the central bronchi. J Thorac Imaging. 2014;29(6): W91–3.
41. Meka M, Mirtcheva RT, Fishman D, Ghesani M. Type two or localized endobronchial non-hodgkin lymphoma. Clin Nucl Med. 2009;34(10):656–8.
42. Lin ZQ, Xu JR, Chen JJ, Hua XL, Zhang KB, Guan YJ. Pulmonary CT findings in relapsing polychondritis. Acta Radiol. 2010;51(5):522–6.
43. Prince JS, Duhamel DR, Levin DL, Harrell JH, Friedman PJ. Nonneoplastic lesions of the tracheobronchial wall: radiologic findings with bronchoscopic correlation. Radiographics. 2002;22(1):Spec No:S215–30.

44. O'Regan A, Fenlon HM, Beamis JF,Jr, Steele MP, Skinner M, Berk JL. Tracheobronchial amyloidosis. the boston university experience from 1984 to 1999. Medicine (Baltimore). 2000;79(2):69–79.
45. Marchiori E, Pozes AS, Souza Junior AS, et al. Diffuse abnormalities of the trachea: computed tomography findings. J Bras Pneumol. 2008;34(1):47–54.
46. Camus P, Piard F, Ashcroft T, Gal AA, Colby TV. The lung in inflammatory bowel disease. Medicine (Baltimore). 1993;72(3):151–83.
47. Spizarny DL, Shepard JA, McLoud TC, Grillo HC, Dedrick CG. CT of adenoid cystic carcinoma of the trachea. AJR Am J Roentgenol. 1986;146(6):1129–32.
48. Beal KP, Yeung HW, Yahalom J. FDG-PET scanning for detection and staging of extranodal marginal zone lymphomas of the MALT type: A report of 42 cases. Ann Oncol. 2005;16 (3):473–80.
49. Balikian JP, Herman PG. Non-hodgkin lymphoma of the lungs. Radiology. 1979; 132(3):569–76.
50. Banks DE, Castellan RM, Hendrick DJ. Lymphocytic lymphoma recurring in multiple endobronchial sites. Thorax. 1980;35(10):796–7.
51. Kilgore TL, Chasen MH. Endobronchial non-hodgkin's lymphoma. Chest. 1983;84(1):58–61.
52. Gallagher CJ, Knowles GK, Habeshaw JA, Green M, Malpas JS, Lister TA. Early involvement of the bronchi in patients with malignant lymphoma. Br J Cancer. 1983;48 (6):777–81.
53. Auer IA, Gascoyne RD, Connors JM, et al. T(11;18)(q21;q21) is the most common translocation in MALT lymphomas. Ann Oncol. 1997;8(10):979–85.
54. Ott G, Katzenberger T, Greiner A, et al. The t(11;18)(q21;q21) chromosome translocation is a frequent and specific aberration in low-grade but not high-grade malignant non-hodgkin's lymphomas of the mucosa-associated lymphoid tissue (MALT-) type. Cancer Res. 1997;57 (18):3944–8.
55. Ye H, Liu H, Attygalle A, et al. Variable frequencies of t(11;18)(q21;q21) in MALT lymphomas of different sites: significant association with CagA strains of H pylori in gastric MALT lymphoma. Blood. 2003;102(3):1012–8.
56. Okabe M, Inagaki H, Ohshima K, et al. API2-MALT1 fusion defines a distinctive clinicopathologic subtype in pulmonary extranodal marginal zone B-cell lymphoma of mucosa-associated lymphoid tissue. Am J Pathol. 2003;162(4):1113–22.
57. Streubel B, Simonitsch-Klupp I, Mullauer L, et al. Variable frequencies of MALT lymphoma-associated genetic aberrations in MALT lymphomas of different sites. Leukemia. 2004;18(10):1722–6.
58. Zompi S, Couderc LJ, Cadranel J, et al. Clonality analysis of alveolar B lymphocytes contributes to the diagnostic strategy in clinical suspicion of pulmonary lymphoma. Blood. 2004;103(8):3208–15.
59. Sammassimo S, Pruneri G, Andreola G, et al. A retrospective international study on primary extranodal marginal zone lymphoma of the lung (BALT lymphoma) on behalf of international extranodal lymphoma study group (IELSG). Hematol Oncol. 2015.
60. Eynden V, Fadel E, de Perrot M, de Montpreville V, Mussot S, Dartevelle P. Role of surgery in the treatment of primary pulmonary B-cell lymphoma. Ann Thorac Surg. 2007;83(1):236.
61. Huang J, Lin T, Li ZM, Xu R, Huang H, Jiang W. Primary pulmonary non-hodgkin's lymphoma: A retrospective analysis of 29 cases in a chinese population. Am J Hematol. 2010;85(7):523–5.
62. Stefanovic A, Morgensztern D, Fong T, Lossos IS. Pulmonary marginal zone lymphoma: a single centre experience and review of the SEER database. Leuk Lymphoma. 2008;49 (7):1311–20.

Chapter 14
Diffuse Idiopathic Pulmonary Neuroendocrine Cell Hyperplasia

Tathagat Narula, Carol Farver and Atul C. Mehta

Introduction

Neuroendocrine cells are specialized epithelial cells with the ability to synthesize, store, and release various peptides and amines. In normal adult lungs, pulmonary neuroendocrine cells (PNECs) are located through the length of the respiratory tract, extending from trachea to the terminal airways [1]. Diffuse idiopathic pulmonary neuroendocrine cell hyperplasia (DIPNECH), as the name implies, is a diffuse idiopathic form of neuroendocrine cell hyperplasia (NEC) [2]. A rare condition, it was first described by Aguayo et al. in 1992 in 6 non-smoking adults presenting with slowly progressive cough and breathlessness. These patients had diffuse NEC, multiple carcinoid tumorlets, and peribronchiolar fibrosis obliterating small airways [3]. Although still an orphan disease, the last two decades have witnessed an increasing recognition of this entity with attempts to better understand its pathophysiology as well as its relationship to more familiar illnesses originating from neuroendocrine cell lines.

T. Narula
Respiratory Critical Care and Sleep Medicine Associates, Baptist South, Baptist Medical Center, Jacksonville, FL, USA

C. Farver
Department of Pathology, Cleveland Clinic, Cleveland, OH, USA

A.C. Mehta (✉)
Pulmonary Medicine, Respiratory Institute, Cleveland Clinic, Cleveland, OH 44195, USA
e-mail: Mehtaa1@ccf.org

A.C. Mehta
Lerner College of Medicine, Buoncore Family Endowed Chair in Lung Transplantation, Respiratory Institute, Cleveland Clinic, Cleveland, OH, USA

© Springer International Publishing Switzerland 2016
A.C. Mehta et al. (eds.), *Diseases of the Central Airways*,
Respiratory Medicine, DOI 10.1007/978-3-319-29830-6_14

Epidemiology

To date, approximately 100 cases have been described in the literature and much remains to be learnt about DIPNECH. There is a gender bias with close to 90 % of sufferers being women. Although it can occur at any age, it is most commonly diagnosed in the fifth or sixth decades. As highlighted in the earliest descriptions from Aguayo, majority of the patients are non-smokers [4, 5]. Even though the clinical course is benign in most cases, a delay in diagnoses of months to years is not uncommon. With increasing awareness of this entity coupled with a much more liberal use of advanced cross-sectional imaging modalities of the chest, an increase in its incidence is anticipated.

Pathology and Etiopathogenesis

NECs reside along the length of the respiratory epithelium. These cells have the ability to synthesize, store, and secrete neuroamines and neuropeptides. Three manifestations of NEC proliferations have been described that occur in different clinical settings:

1. Reactive NEC that is typically a response to chronic hypoxia in the setting of pulmonary pathologies such as emphysema.
2. NEC proliferations associated with carcinoid tumors.
3. DIPNECH—a widespread NEC of the peripheral airways. Distinguishing it from other proliferations, the term DIPNECH is restricted to cases in which the hyperplasia is diffuse and primary in nature [6–8]. The challenges in diagnosis of DIPNECH can be appreciated from the multiplicity of presentations of the cases described in the literature. Cases with widespread diffuse lesions abound as do those that were subjected to a limited investigation of the lung in a radiographically affected region of interest [3, 9–11] (Figs. 14.1, 14.2, and 14.3).

Histopathological confirmation forms the cornerstone for diagnosis of DIPNECH [12]. The gold standard remains a surgical lung biopsy. This is frequently preceded by less invasive testing, typically bronchoscopy with biopsies and/or lavage in an effort to rule out infectious and more common diagnoses [13].

There is a suggestion that DIPNECH sits along a continuum of neuroendocrine cell abnormalities and possibly serves as a pre-neoplastic process for peripheral carcinoid tumors [14–16]. DIPNECH proliferations may proceed to breach the basement membrane and penetrate into the peribronchial soft tissue, forming small nodules. If less than 5 mm, the nodules are arbitrarily referred to as carcinoid tumorlets, and if greater than 5 mm, they are classified as carcinoids [17]. These proliferations can potentially become mechanically occlusive resulting in an

Fig. 14.1 Neuroendocrine
cell hyperplasia (*NE*) with
adjacent carcinoid tumorlet
(*T*) and carcinoid tumor (*C*).
(hematoxylin and eosin;
12/5×)

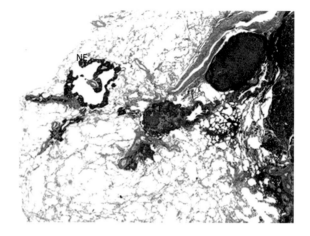

Fig. 14.2 Carcinoid tumorlet
with spindle cell morphology
impinging on airway
(hematoxylin and eosin; 40×)

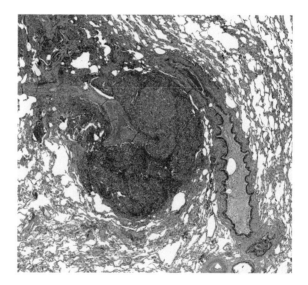

obstructive physiology. The World Health Organization recognizes the pre-invasive
nature of DIPNECH and its potential to form into carcinoid tumors [7]. Efforts are
being made to understand the sequence of events, including those at a genetic level,
and to explain the transformation of a relatively benign cell line of NEC to a
carcinoid tumor.

The other intriguing element is the tendency of patients to develop symptomatic
or asymptomatic constrictive bronchiolitis. Proliferating neuroendocrine cells are
believed to produce fibrogenic cytokines such as bombesin, gastrin-releasing
peptide, and other neuropeptides that can stimulate fibroblast proliferation with
subsequent airway fibrosis [8, 18].

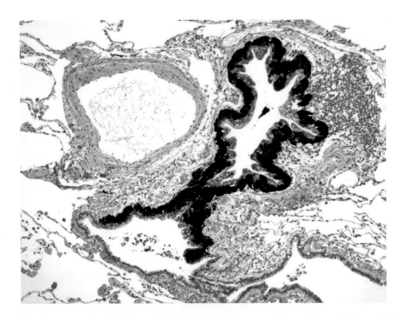

Fig. 14.3 Neuroendocrine cell hyperplasia undermining normal bronchial epithelium of airway highlighted with antibody staining to chromogranin (anti-chromogranin with methylene *blue* counterstain; 40×)

Clinical Features

Two distinct modes of clinical presentation are described—symptomatic and asymptomatic. Symptoms, when present, are typically non-specific with a protracted nonproductive cough and dyspnea. Many of the patients remain symptomatic for many years prior to diagnosis and are frequently misdiagnosed to have asthma or chronic bronchitis/bronchiolitis [11]. Descriptions of a relatively more acute presentation with less than a year of symptoms before the diagnosis of DIPNECH are noted in a minority of patients [13].

The second mode of presentation is an asymptomatic patient who is diagnosed to have DIPNECH on histopathology in the setting of resection of pulmonary nodule or nodules of unclear etiology. Frequently, DIPNECH is not considered in the differential diagnoses for these patients prior to resection [11].

Laboratory Investigations

Unfortunately, there is no diagnostic blood or serologic investigations to confirm or refute the diagnosis of DIPNECH. Expressions of neuroendocrine antigens as well as secretion of fibrogenic cytokines and neuropeptides though suggestive are not

diagnostic of DIPNECH. These can be seen in the whole spectrum of NEC proliferations ranging from the benign to the malignant variants. The usefulness of
serum biomarkers in DIPNECH is limited with only isolated case reports of elevated serum Chromogranin A and urinary 5-HIAA levels [19]. Studies investigating
the differential expression of key antigens involved in controlling cell kinetics
suggest early and fundamental differences between the 'reactive' process of PNEC
proliferation that occurs as part of the normal response to pulmonary injury as
against those that seen in the pre-neoplastic condition of DIPNECH. Expression of
p53, p16, and Ki67, proteins involved in cell proliferation and death, is seen more
consistently and earlier in proliferation in DIPNECH [4, 20]. Reports of multiorgan
endocrinopathies in patients with DIPNECH exist including those with coexistent
MEN1 syndrome and acromegaly [11, 21].

Imaging

Chest radiographs of patients with DIPNECH typically demonstrate multiple pulmonary micronodules [22]. These are better appreciated on high-resolution computed tomographic (HRCT) scan of the chest (Fig. 14.4a, b). Addition of expiratory
imaging, especially in those patients that have a suggestion of associated mosaic
attenuation, helps recognize air trapping, a radiological clue to constrictive bronchiolitis of the small airways. The micronodules can have a variable attenuation
ranging from ground glass to solid, and concerns for a metastatic malignancy are
frequent. Bronchiectasis, bronchial wall thickening, and atelectasis have also been
described. Although none of these abnormalities are pathognomonic, the association of small nodules with CT features of constrictive bronchiolitis is a clue to the
diagnosis of DIPNECH [11, 23, 24].

Pulmonary Function Testing

Physiologically, the disorder is most commonly associated with an obstructive
respiratory impairment due to progressive airways narrowing. However, lung
function tests may reveal a mixed obstructive/restrictive pattern or be normal in a
number of patients [4, 25]. Not all cases of DIPNECH or tumorlets that are
encountered pathologically are associated with clinical evidence of airflow
obstruction in the small airways. In a series of 25 consecutive patients undergoing
resection for peripheral carcinoid tumors, even though 76 % had histological evidence of NEC, only 32 % had airway changes of constrictive bronchiolitis, and two
of these patients had asymptomatic evidence of airflow obstruction. This series
suggests that only a minority of cases with NEC identified pathologically have
associated clinical evidence of airflow obstruction [10].

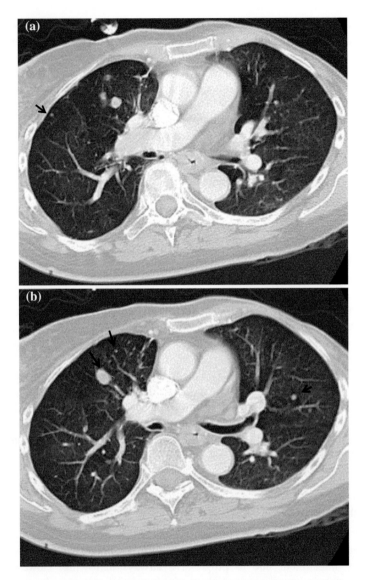

Fig. 14.4 a, b Contrast-enhanced computed tomography of the chest revealing multiple pulmonary nodules (*black arrows*) and interstitial infiltrates of DIPNEC

Bronchoscopy

In general, the large tissue sample size required for pathologically identifying tumorlets and neuroendocrine cell proliferation in airways renders transbronchial biopsies and lavage washings low yield for diagnosis of DIPNECH. However, in the appropriate setting, a presumptive diagnosis of DIPNECH-associated airway disease can be made in a small subset of patients based on bronchoscopically obtained pathological specimens so long as the clinical, functional, and radiological findings are compatible [13]. It is common place for interventional bronchoscopists to be invited to participate in care when lung nodules are detected, primarily with the intention of sampling. In cases with DIPNECH, these nodules are usually small and reliance on advanced diagnostic modalities such as navigational guidance and radial probe endobronchial ultrasound is frequently sought [26]. Our own anecdotal experience suggests that an awareness of this entity can prevent unnecessary bronchoscopic procedures, not just resulting in cost savings but also mitigating the risk of potential complications from the same.

Differential Diagnoses

Any etiology for constrictive (obliterative) bronchiolitis needs to be entertained in the differential diagnoses of DIPNECH. These range from connective tissue disorders, exposure to an inhaled toxins/mineral dusts, drug reactions, or diseases such as ulcerative colitis [27]. Patients with DIPNECH are frequently misdiagnosed to have asthma in light of their protracted course and symptomatic resemblance [11].

Prognosis and Treatment

Data on long-term treatment options and outcomes in patients diagnosed with DIPNECH are limited. Without any available guidelines, treatment strategies are based upon inferences drawn from case reports and small case series. Typically an indolent and non-progressive disorder, majority of patients with DIPNECH have excellent long-term survival [11, 28].

Treatment options have ranged from non-invasive strategies including a 'wait-and-watch' approach with close observation in minimally symptomatic stable patients to major interventions including lung transplantation in select cases with progressively worsening clinical course [28, 29].

Unsuccessful attempts at the use of cytotoxic agents in two patients with DIPNECH, one of whom ultimately died of progressive respiratory failure while receiving treatment with fluorouracil, were reported in the initial description of DIPNECH [3]. To date, there is no convincing evidence supporting the use of chemotherapeutic drugs in patients with DIPNECH. Current therapeutic options have focused on steroid-based therapies. A trial of inhaled or systemic corticosteroid therapy, coupled with bronchodilators, particularly in patients who demonstrate reversible airflow obstruction, is frequently advocated. Clinical improvement has been noted in some series with this approach. Reduction in the inflammatory response stimulated by the neuropeptide secretions from PNEC has been touted as the mechanistic rationale underlying this benefit [13, 30]. However, there is a paucity of defined predictors of a favorable response to steroids. Surgical excision of the dominant lesion, along with the use of somatostatin analogs has also been proposed with a suggestion of disease stabilization for symptomatic patients [4, 30].

Summary

Long considered a rare entity, DIPNECH is now being increasingly recognized as the use of computed tomography of the chest becomes rampant. Although the course is typically protracted and benign, severe cases with unfavorable outcomes are well reported. There remain major voids in our understanding of the pathogenesis as well as natural history of this illness translating into the absence of consistently effective management strategies. There exists a dire need for a database to systematically investigate the nuances that surround the uncommon clinical entity of DIPNECH.

References

1. Chong S, Lee KS, Chung MJ, Han J, Kwon OJ, Kim TS. Neuroendocrine tumors of the lung: clinical, pathologic, and imaging findings. Radiographics. 2006;26(1):41–57.
2. Benson RE, Rosado-de-Christenson ML, Martínez-Jiménez S, Kunin JR, Pettavel PP. Spectrum of pulmonary neuroendocrine proliferations and neoplasms. Radiographics 2013;33(6): 1631–49.
3. Aguayo SM, Miller YE, Waldron JA Jr, Bogin RM, Sunday ME, Staton GW Jr, Beam WR, King TE Jr. Brief report: idiopathic diffuse hyperplasia of pulmonary neuroendocrine cells and airways disease. N Engl J Med. 1992;327(18):1285–8.
4. Gorshtein A, Gross DJ, Barak D, Strenov Y, Refaeli Y, Shimon I, Grozinsky-Glasberg S. Diffuse idiopathic pulmonary neuroendocrine cell hyperplasia and the associated lung neuroendocrine tumors: clinical experience with a rare entity. Cancer. 2012;118(3):612–9.
5. Patel C, Tirukonda P, Bishop R, Mulatero C, Scarsbrook A. Diffuse idiopathic pulmonary neuroendocrine cell hyperplasia (DIPNECH) masquerading as metastatic carcinoma with multiple pulmonary deposits. Clin Imag. 2012;36(6):833–6.
6. Van Lommel A, Bollé T, Fannes W, Lauweryns JM. The pulmonary neuroendocrine system: the past decade. Arch Histol Cytol. 1999;62(1):1–16.
7. Gosney JR, Travis WD. Diffuse idiopathic neuroendocrine cell hyperplasia. In: Travis WD, Brambilla E, Müller-Hermelink HK, Harris CC, editors. Pathology and genetics: tumours of the lung, pleura, thymus and heart. Lyon: IARC; 2004. p. 76–7.
8. Oba H, Nishida K, Takeuchi S, Akiyama H, Muramatsu K, Kurosumi M, Kameya T. Diffuse idiopathic pulmonary neuroendocrine cell hyperplasia with a central and peripheral carcinoid and multiple tumorlets: a case report emphasizing the role of neuropeptide hormones and human gonadotropin-alpha. Endocr Pathol. 2013;24(4):220–8.
9. Adams H, Brack T, Kestenholz P, Vogt P, Steinert HC, Russi EW. Diffuse idiopathic neuroendocrine cell hyperplasia causing severe airway obstruction in a patient with a carcinoid tumor. Respir. 2006;73(5):690–3.

10. Miller RR, Müller NL. Neuroendocrine cell hyperplasia and obliterative bronchiolitis in patients with peripheral carcinoid tumors. Am J Surg Pathol. 1995;19(6):653–8.
11. Davies SJ, Gosney JR, Hansell DM, Wells AU, du Bois RM, Burke MM, Sheppard MN, Nicholson AG. Diffuse idiopathic pulmonary neuroendocrine cell hyperplasia: an under-recognised spectrum of disease. Thorax. 2007;62(3):248–52.
12. Dacic S. Pulmonary preneoplasia. Arch Pathol Lab Med. 2008;132(7):1073–8.
13. Nassar AA, Jaroszewski DE, Helmers RA, Colby TV, Patel BM, Mookadam F. Diffuse idiopathic pulmonary neuroendocrine cell hyperplasia: a systematic overview. Am J Respir Crit Care Med. 2011;184(1):8–16.
14. Gosney JR. Diffuse idiopathic pulmonary neuroendocrine cell hyperplasia as a precursor to pulmonary neuroendocrine tumors. Chest. 2004;125(5 Suppl):108S.
15. Lantuéjoul S, Salameire D, Salon C, Brambilla E. Pulmonary preneoplasia–sequential molecular carcinogenetic events. Histopathol. 2009;54(1):43–54.
16. Rizvi SM, Goodwill J, Lim E, Yap YK, Wells AU, Hansell DM, Davis P, Selim AG, Goldstraw P, Nicholson AG. The frequency of neuroendocrine cell hyperplasia in patients with pulmonary neuroendocrine tumours and non-neuroendocrine cell carcinomas. Histopathol. 2009;55(3):332–7.
17. Ruffini E, Bongiovanni M, Cavallo A, Filosso PL, Giobbe R, Mancuso M, Molinatti M, Oliaro A. The significance of associated pre-invasive lesions in patients resected for primary lung neoplasms. Eur J Cardiothorac Surg. 2004;26(1):165–72.
18. Kerr KM. Pulmonary preinvasive neoplasia. J Clin Pathol. 2001;54(4):257–71.
19. Seregni E, Ferrari L, Bajetta E, Martinetti A, Bombardieri E. Clinical significance of blood chromogranin a measurement in neuroendocrine tumours. Ann Oncol. 2001;12(Suppl 2): S69–72.
20. Gosney JR, Williams IJ, Dodson AR, Foster CS. Morphology and antigen expression profile of pulmonary neuroendocrine cells in reactive proliferations and diffuse idiopathic pulmonary neuroendocrine cell hyperplasia (DIPNECH). Histopathology. 2011;59(4):751–62.
21. Fessler MB, Cool CD, Miller YE, Schwarz MI, Brown KK. Idiopathic diffuse hyperplasia of pulmonary neuroendocrine cells in a patient with acromegaly. Respirology. 2004;9(2):274–7.
22. Koo CW, Baliff JP, Torigian DA, Litzky LA, Gefter WB, Akers SR. Spectrum of pulmonary neuroendocrine cell proliferation: diffuse idiopathic pulmonary neuroendocrine cell hyperplasia, tumorlet, and carcinoids. AJR Am J Roentgenol. 2010;195(3):661–8.
23. Lee JS, Brown KK, Cool C, Lynch DA. Diffuse pulmonary neuroendocrine cell hyperplasia: radiologic and clinical features. J Comput Assist Tomogr. 2002;26(2):180–4.
24. Darvishian F, Ginsberg MS, Klimstra DS, Brogi E. Carcinoid tumorlets simulate pulmonary metastases in women with breast cancer. Hum Pathol. 2006;37(7):839–44.
25. Ge Y, Eltorky MA, Ernst RD, Castro CY. Diffuse idiopathic pulmonary neuroendocrine cell hyperplasia. Ann Diagn Pathol. 2007;11(2):122–6.
26. Narula T, Machuzak MS, Mehta AC. Newer modalities in the work-up of peripheral pulmonary nodules. Clin Chest Med. 2013;34(3):395–415.
27. King MS, Eisenberg R, Newman JH, Tolle JJ, Harrell FE Jr, Nian H, Ninan M, Lambright ES, Sheller JR, Johnson JE, Miller RF. Constrictive bronchiolitis in soldiers returning from Iraq and Afghanistan. N Engl J Med. 2011;365(3):222–30.
28. Swigris J, Ghamande S, Rice T, Farver C. Diffuse idiopathic neuropathic cell hyperplasia. An interstitial lung disease with airway obstruction. J Bronch 2005;12:62–64.
29. Sheerin N, Harrison NK, Sheppard MN, Hansell DM, Yacoub M, Clark TJ. Obliterative bronchiolitis caused by multiple tumourlets and microcarcinoids successfully treated by single lung transplantation. Thorax. 1995;50(2):207–9.
30. Mitchell P, Kennedy M, Henry M. A case of DIPNECH and review of the current literature. Open J Respir Dis. 2013;3(2):68–72.

Chapter 15
Black Bronchoscopy

Pichapong Tunsupon and Atul C. Mehta

Introduction

The term black bronchoscopy has been used to describe the presence of black pigmentation in the airways during flexible bronchoscopy. This condition was first described in the literatures in association with occupational exposures in early 1940. However, Packham and Yeow used the term "black bronchoscopy" to describe endobronchial metastasis from a malignant melanoma in 2003 [1]. Since then, multiple case reports have been published describing the hyperpigmentation of the airway. It is a rare condition related to multiple etiologies such as congenital disease, inborn error metabolism, infections, environmental exposures, neoplasm, and iatrogenic causes. Although the majority of these conditions are benign, pulmonologists should be fully cognizant of the differential diagnosis of black bronchoscopy. In this chapter, we review the literature on causes of black discoloration of the airway, discuss the clinical presentation, and provide the guidelines for management.

P. Tunsupon (✉)
Department of Internal Medicine, Division of Pulmonary, Critical Care, and Sleep Medicine,
University of Buffalo, Buffalo, NY, USA
e-mail: ptunsupon@gmail.com

P. Tunsupon
120 Meyer Road, Apt. 519, Amherst, NY 14226, USA

A.C. Mehta
Pulmonary Medicine, Respiratory Institute, Cleveland Clinic, Cleveland, OH, USA
e-mail: Mehtaa1@ccf.org

A.C. Mehta
Lerner College of Medicine, Buoncore Family Endowed Chair in Lung Transplantation,
Respiratory Institute, Cleveland Clinic, Cleveland, OH, USA

© Springer International Publishing Switzerland 2016
A.C. Mehta et al. (eds.), *Diseases of the Central Airways*,
Respiratory Medicine, DOI 10.1007/978-3-319-29830-6_15

Fig. 15.1 Incidental finding
of endobronchial melanosis in
a patient undergoing
bronchoscopy for an unrelated
indication

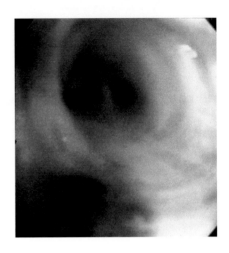

Congenital Disease

Melanosis

Tracheobronchial melanosis (TM) is an unusual finding in bronchoscopic examination. Previous case series have reported a prevalence of one in every 52 bronchoscopies performed and distributed equally between male and female gender [2].
TM is found incidentally during bronchoscopic examination for unrelated indications. The hyperpigmented areas can be isolated or present at multiple sites in the
secondary and tertiary carina without distortions of the airways or mucosal
abnormalities (Fig. 15.1) Although melanosis of the larynx and oropharyngeal
mucosa has been associated with occult malignancy, thus far no association has
been found between endobronchial melanosis and internal malignancy or smoking
[3]. Although TM is a benign condition, it is important for pulmonologists to
distinguish this condition from other causes of black bronchoscopy.

Inborn Error of Metabolism

Alkaptonuria (Ochronosis)

Alkaptonuria is a rare inborn error metabolism involving the catabolic pathway of
the amino acids phenylalanine and tyrosine. It is a disorder caused by mutation of
the *HGO* gene encoding a specific liver enzyme, homogentisate-1,2-dioxygenase
(HGD), which degrades homogentesic acid (HGA)—an intermediary metabolite in
the phenylalanine and tyrosine degradation pathway. Alkaptonuria is inherited in an
autosomal recessive pattern [4].

Fig. 15.2 Ochronosis. Note
black pigments involving
lower trachea. Courtesy of
Mohamad Bakry, MD,
Pulmonary and Critical Care
Medicine, New York
Methodist Hospital

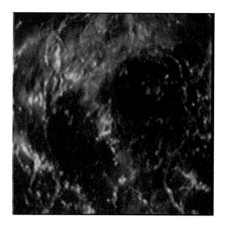

HGD deficiency results in elevated plasma HGA level, which polymerized to form a pigment and deposits throughout the body resulting in degenerative dark gray pigmentation of connective tissues and cartilages. This syndrome is also known as ochronosis. Signs and symptoms are primarily due to the accumulation of HGA in tissues. Affected patients are usually asymptomatic in childhood. The incidence and severity of ochronosis increases parallel to aging especially after the third decades of life. Ochronosis has wide spectrum of signs and symptoms depends on affecting organ systems.

Involvement of central airways with alkaptonuria was described in one case in 2005 [5]. Flexible bronchoscopy demonstrated hyperpigmented tracheal and main-stem bronchial mucosa extended distally to small bronchioles that could not be removed by saline irrigation or forceps extraction with the evidence of overlying dry black secretion (Fig. 15.2). Histologic features of tracheal mucosa and black secretion revealed acute bronchitis and necrotic debris, respectively. The diagnosis of alkaptonuria was confirmed by the quantitative measurement of plasma and urine HGA level by gas chromatographic-mass spectrophotometric assays [6]. Postmortem autopsy of another undiagnosed alkaptonuria revealed extensive grayish black discoloration of the epiglottis, laryngeal, and bronchial cartilages [7]. Histologic examination revealed extensive calcium pyrophosphate dehydrate (CPPD) deposition and generalized brownish yellow pigmentation of the matrix [7]. Multiple published case reports also demonstrate CPPD deposition with degenerative ochronotic arthritis involving synovial membrane and knee joints.

The optimal management of hyperpigmented airways related to alkaptonuria is not clearly elucidated. High-dose vitamin C and protein restriction are ineffective in reducing urinary HGA excretion. Nitisinone, a triketone herbicide that reversibly inhibits 4-hydroxyphenylpyruvate dioxygenase, an enzyme in the tyrosine catabolic pathway, decreases urinary HGA excretion by more than 80 % in an animal model and decreases HGA production in human with alkaptonuria in one short-term study. However, long-term efficacy and safety necessitate further evaluation [4].

(a)   (b)

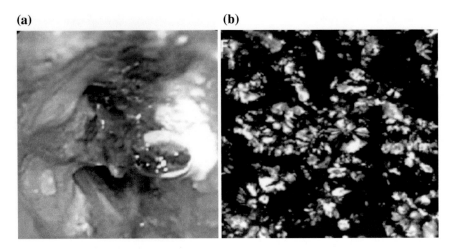

Fig. 15.3 **a** *Aspergillus niger* colonization involving right upper lobe bronchus in a lung transplant recipient. The white calcium oxalate particles are at the base. **b** Calcium oxalate crystals under the microscope. Reprinted from Singhal et al. [9] with the permission from Elsevier

Infection

Aspergillus Niger

Aspergillus species are commonly found in the environment. The most common route of exposure is accidental inoculation from the inhalation of aerosolized spores. The primary site of disease is the lung. There are several reports of black pigmentation in association with *Aspergillus niger* infection on bronchoscopic examination. One percent of all *Aspergillus* airway infections following lung transplantation are from the *A. niger* species [8]. It generally occurs in immuno-compromised population, in the nosocomial settings, patients with diagnosis of hypogammaglobulinemia and patients who are taking long-term itraconazole therapy. The fungus produces oxalic acid, which bind to airway calcium, which causes deposition of white mass of calcium oxalate in airway mucosa in addition to the black pigmentation due to *A. niger* [9] (Fig. 15.3). Management of endo-bronchial aspergillosis is discussed in Chap. 9.

Ochroconis Gallopava

Fungal infection caused by dematiaceous fungi (dark-pigmented fungi), such as mycetoma, chromoblastomycoses, and phaeohyphomycosis, characterizes by the presence of melanin or melanin-like pigmentation [10]. The incidence of this type of fungal infection has been increasing in solid-organ transplant recipients

Fig. 15.4 Black
pigmentation of *Ochroconis
gallopava* involving the left
upper lobe bronchus in an
immunocompetent patient.
Courtesy of Wes Shepherd,
MD, Interventional
Pulmonology, Virginia
Commonwealth University
Medical Center

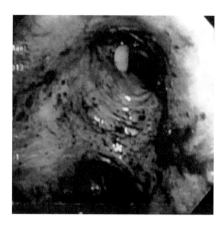

especially in the genus Ochroconis [10], which include species *gallopava, constrict,*
and *humicola.*

Ochroconis gallopava infection generally presents with the pulmonary or
extrapulmonary involvement especially of CNS and skin. Among solid-organ
transplant recipients, lung transplant recipients have the highest incidence of
O. gallopava infections [11]. Common pulmonary presentations include nodules
and non-resolving infiltrates with upper and middle lung predominance. Cough may
be present [12]. Involvements of airways could present with black pigmentation and
growth similar to *A. niger* (Fig. 15.4). Diagnosis is made by transbronchial biopsies
and fungal culture. Antifungal therapy anecdotally has been decided based on
sensitivities. Rarely, cases of *O. gallopava* have also been reported in the
non-solid-organ transplant population [13].

Healed Endobronchial Tuberculosis

Healed endobronchial *Mycobacterium tuberculosis* (MTB) infection often leaves
black pigmentation within the airways mucosa. Bronchoscopic examination reveals
multiple areas of dense fibrosis and the deposition of black pigment particle
(Fig. 15.5). Multiple calcified intrathoracic lymph nodes on computer tomography
of the chest raise suspicion for a prior infection with MTB [14]. The proposed
mechanism of dark pigmentation is intrabronchial microperforation of the lymph
nodes loaded with pigment-laden macrophages into the adjacent bronchial mucosa.
After years of healing and fibroblastic proliferation, airway stenosis may develop
[15]. The black pigments are assumed to be the residues of MTB organisms.
Anti-TB regimen can potentially resolve the atelectasis and bronchial narrowing,
but hyperpigmentation is considered irreversible [14].

Fig. 15.5 Healed
endobronchial
Mycobacterium tuberculosis
(MTB) involving the right
lower lobe bronchus

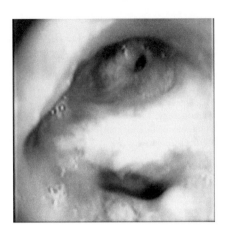

Environmental Causes

Anthracosis and Anthracofibrosis

Anthracosis is a condition in which inhaled carbon particles are deposited in the airways and the lung parenchyma. This condition is commonly found in cigarettes smokers and in individuals heavily exposed to atmospheric soot. The inhaled anthracotic particles are usually removed by mucociliary clearance, which is an important lung defensive mechanism. However, small amounts of carbon particles ingested by macrophages are retained within the bronchioles [16]. This, however, does not lead to inflammation or fibrosis.

Bronchial anthracofibrosis and anthracostenosis refer to luminal airway narrowing along with anthracotic (black) pigmentation overlying the bronchial mucosa without history of cigarette smoking [17–19] (Fig. 15.6). Anthracofibrosis is mainly reported in association with occupations such as coal mining, masonry, and in

Fig. 15.6 Severe narrowing
and black pigmentation of
anthracostenosis involving the
right lower lobe bronchus in
an elderly coal miner.
Reprinted from
Mireles-Cabodevila et al. [19]
with the permission from
Wolters Kluwer Health

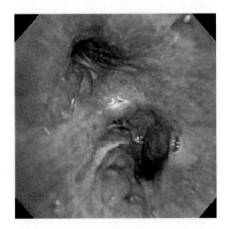

patients with chronic exposure to wood smoke [20–22]. Anthracofibrosis related to chronic biomass or wood-smoke exposure is typically found in non-smoking elderly women using biomass fuels for indoor cooking [20, 23].

The common presentation of anthracofibrosis is chronic cough, sputum, and airflow obstruction with a minimal response to bronchodilators therapy [23]. Other respiratory symptoms are dyspnea, wheezing, and rhonchi [18, 20, 23]. Characteristic findings of chest computerized tomography (CT) are thickening and narrowing of airways, leading to lobar atelectasis predominantly involving the right upper and middle lobes, surrounded by enlarged and/or calcified peribronchial, hilar, or mediastinal lymph nodes [15]. Microperforation of the airways by the enlarged lymph nodes during chronic healing process is believed to be the major cause of anthracofibrosis. A high proportion of crystalline silica and non-fibrous silicates (mica and kaolin particles) in hilar lymph nodes, lung tissues, and BAL fluid from mineralogical analyses by transmission electron microscopy is the gold standard for the diagnosis of anthrocofibrosis [22]. Several cases of bronchogenic carcinoma have been reported in association with anthracofibrosis [24]; particularly, poorly differentiated adenocarcinomas have been found to develop in severely anthracotic lungs [25]. This occurrence seems to be coincidental rather than a cause–effect relationship. Radiological diagnosis of this clinical entity is not sufficient and potentially misses the diagnosis of lung cancer. Thus, bronchoscopy is essential for diagnosis of unexplained localized central airway abnormality and atelectasis, especially if clinical history suggests a high probability for malignancy [22].

There is no definite guideline for management of anthracofibrosis. In a single case report, pharmacological treatment with corticosteroids and tamoxifen showed a partial resolution of bronchial narrowing [20]; however, the multiple patchy areas of black pigmentation remained unchanged [20]. Other alternative treatment options, such as antibiotics, bronchodilators, physiotherapy, and postural drainage, are of limited value [23].

Soot Inhalation (Smoke Inhalation)

The major causes of death in fire injury in the past decades include skin burns, systemic toxicity from carbon monoxide or nitric oxide poisoning, and wound sepsis. The recent data support that smoke inhalation injury is the most frequent causes of death in burn and fire injury [26]. The mortality rate from soot inhalation alone is approximately 10 %. A combination of smoke inhalation and skin burns increases the mortality rate to 30–90 % [27]. A targeted history and physical examination (e.g., facial burns, nostril edema) [28] are keys for diagnosis of smoke inhalation injury. Laryngeal edema following the smoke inhalation can rapidly progress to acute upper airway obstruction from thermal injury or chemical injury of the upper airways. Early intubation and mechanical ventilation is justified in this circumstance [29]. FB is a standard procedure for the diagnosis of smoke inhalation [30]. The characteristic bronchoscopic findings are multiple areas of large grayish

Fig. 15.7 Sooty inhalation:
thick layer of soot involving
the lower trachea. Reprinted
from Ribeiro et al. [32] with
the permission from Wolters
Kluwer Health

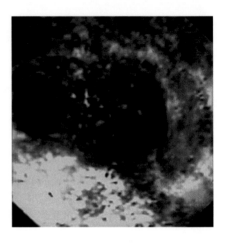

edematous plaques involving the mucosa of tracheobronchial tree. [31, 32] (Fig. 15.7). The smoke inhalation injury results in significant decrease in surfactant production [33] leading to atelectasis and pneumonia seen on chest radiographs. Histologic examination reveals disruption of the tracheobronchial mucosa with focal necrosis and the formation of a pseudomembrane composed of mucus, cell debris, fibrinous exudate, neutrophils, and bacteria [27].

An important concept in the management of smoke inhalation injury is secretion clearance by means of therapeutic coughing, chest physiotherapy, early ambulation, and airways suction. Pharmacological managements, such as bronchodilators, racemic epinephrine to induce vasoconstriction and reduction of mucosal edema [34], and mucolytic agents, also alleviate clearance of secretion. Flexible bronchoscopy is very effective for secretion and cell debris removal. Untreated airways can become completely obstructed, causing lobar atelectasis and post-obstructive pneumonia [33]. The combination of inhalation injury and pneumonia results in a 60 % increase in mortality from burns [27]. A retrospective study has revealed that patients with 30–59 % surface-area burn and pneumonia who underwent at least one bronchoscopy required shorter duration mechanical ventilation (21 vs. 28 days, $P < 0.0001$), ICU stay (35 vs. 39 days, $P < 0.04$), as well as overall hospital stay (45 vs. 49 days, $P < 0.009$). In addition, the mortality rate was reduced by 18 % in the bronchoscopy group [26]. A prospective study proposes a graded severity of soot inhalation according to the depth of mucosal injury. This classification is based on FB being performed within the first 24 h after the injury (Tables 15.1 and 15.2) [35]. FB helps predict outcomes and leads to the development of effective treatment guidelines. Deeper the mucosal damage on histology is associated with higher the rate of acute lung injury and mortality rate [35]. Thus, early bronchoscopy is strongly recommended for patients with an inhalation injury [35, 36].

Table 15.1 Classification of endobronchial burns according to the depth of mucosal damage

Group	Finding
G_0	Negative
G_b	Confirmed positive by biopsy
G_1	Mild mucosal edema and hyperemia, with or without carbon soot
G_2	Severe mucosal edema and reddening, with or without carbon soot
G_3	Ulcerations, necrosis, and absence of both cough reflex and bronchial secretions

G = group
Adapted from Chou et al. [35] with the permission from Springer Science + Business Media

Table 15.2 Correlation of acute lung injury (ALI) and mortality by group

	Number of patients	ALI (n, %)	Mortality (%)
G_0	53	2 (3.8)	0
G_b	6	0	0
G_1	49	2 (4)	2
G_2	46	15 (33)	15
G_3	13	10 (77)	62
Total	167	29	14

Adapted from Chou et al. [35] with the permission from Springer Science + Business Media

Argyria and Argyrosis

Argyria is a condition caused by chronic silver exposure results in an irreversible, bluish gray discoloration of the skin (argyria) and sclera (argyrosis) [37, 38]. Cases of occupational- and medication-related argyria have been reported since the early 1940s [39, 40]. The duration of exposure varies from months to years prior to the diagnosis [39, 40]. The routes of silver particles exposure via inhalation, ingestion, or a parenteral route have been reported [37, 41, 42]. The deposition of silver particles is commonly confined to one area (localized argyria) through prolonged direct contact or can be distributed throughout the organ systems (systemic argyria). Involvement of organs such as the trachea, skin, liver, kidneys, corneas, gingival, mucous membranes, nails, and spleen has been reported in literatures [43]. Argyria is proposed as a mechanism of detoxifying silver from the bloodstream by its excretion into the tissues in the form of a harmless silver–protein complex [44]. Sparse data are available on the possible toxic effects of silver deposition in organ tissues [37]. Patients who report high levels of silver exposure and present with plasma silver levels above the normal range can develop neuropathy [45]. Histologic examination reveals tiny dark-brown particles of silver deposited in the affected areas, especially the internal elastic lamina of small vessels [39]. This finding is visually distinguishable from the typical coarse deposition of black pigment seen in anthracosis [38, 43]. Chronic inhalation of silver vapors can lead to discoloration of bronchial mucosa and alveoli [39], which usually presents with

Fig. 15.8 Endobronchial
argyria. Well-demarcated area
of grayish black pigmentation
involving upper trachea in a
patient using a silver
tracheostomy tube over
30 years. Reprinted from
Schreiber et al. [43] with the
permission from Wolters
Kluwer Health

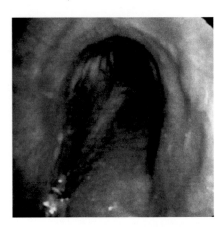

mild respiratory symptoms such as chronic cough, mild bronchitis, emphysematous change, and reduction in lung volumes. There have been no major clinical consequences reported thus far [46]. A single case report described an unusual bronchoscopic finding of a dark hyperpigmented area with a distinctive demarcation in a patient in prolonged contact with a silver tracheostomy tube (Fig. 15.8) [43]. Histologic examination revealed dark fine pigments underneath the epithelium, without the involvement of blood vessels [43].

Neoplasms

Endobronchial Melanoma

Several endobronchial neoplasms exhibit dark pigments. Primary melanoma of the lung is a rare tumor involving 0.01 % of all lung tumors [47]. Metastatic melanoma is the more common than the primary endobronchial melanoma. Metastatic melanoma usually presents months or years after the onset of the primary tumors. It is mandatory to look for primary tumor if melanoma of the lung is found on bronchoscopy. Kiryu et al. [48] classified the endobronchial melanomas into four different types: type 1, direct metastasis to the bronchus; type 2, bronchial invasion by a parenchymal metastatic lesion; type 3, bronchial invasion by mediastinal or hilar lymph node metastasis; and type 4, a peripheral lesion extending along the proximal bronchus.

Primary or metastatic melanoma is seen as a dark hyperpigment, sticky endobronchial lesion on FB examination [49] (Fig. 15.9) [50]. The differential diagnosis of endobronchial melanoma includes melanocytic carcinoid, schwannoma, and paraganglioma [47]. Histological examination is required to differentiate these tumors from endobronchial melanoma. Because primary melanoma of the lung is exceedingly rare, strict diagnostic criteria have been established: junctional changes

Fig. 15.9 Endobronchial
metastatic melanoma
producing total obstruction of
the left main-stem bronchus in
a patient with prior history of
melanoma. Reprinted from
Das et al. [50] with the
permission from Wolters
Kluwer Health

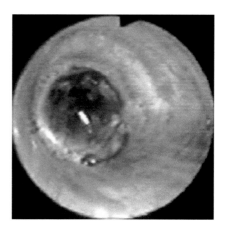

(e.g., dropping off or nesting of melanoma cells just beneath the bronchial epithelium), the invasion of the bronchial epithelium by melanoma cells in an area where the bronchial epithelium is not ulcerated, and absence of melanoma elsewhere in the body at the time of diagnosis [51]. The overall prognosis is poor for both primary and metastatic melanomas because the endobronchial lesions usually present at advanced stages of disease. Median survival after the diagnosis of metastatic disease is approximately 15 months [52]. Surgical resection followed by chemotherapy and immunotherapy has been reported in a few instances, but long-term prognosis is not well defined.

Teratomas

Teratoma composes of collections of tissue and organized structures derived from all three-cell layers, ectoderm, mesoderm, and endoderm. A mature teratoma may rupture and release its contents into airways, resulting in a recurrent cough, hemoptysis, and tricoptysis [53]. The term tricoptysis refers to the expectoration of hairs. Tricoptysis is seen in 15 % of the cases of intrapulmonary teratoma. Involved airways exhibit dark black areas due to the presence of hair. Even though the tumor is benign, there is risk of malignant transformation [54]. Histopathological examination is a gold standard for diagnosis of mature teratoma. Thus, surgical excision of the tumor is the treatment of choice.

Iatrogenic Causes

Charcoal Aspiration

Activated charcoal is used for the management of several drug intoxications. It binds directly to the toxic drug creating a passive diffusion gradient from the bloodstream, across the GI lumen (GI dialysis) [55] to prevent poisons from being absorbed into the systemic circulation. Patients with neurological deficits are at increased risk of activated charcoal aspiration into the lungs, especially if the airway is not adequately protected. Aspiration is reported in 1.7 % of patients who received activated charcoal alone and 2.3 % of those who also undergoes gastric emptying [56]. Simultaneous aspiration of gastric content and activated charcoal aspiration results in severe pulmonary complications. Acute complications of charcoal aspiration include airway obstruction, bronchospasm, hypoxemia, and aspiration pneumonia. Late complications include ARDS, bronchiolitis obliterans, bronchopleural fistula, and death [57]. Activated charcoal is thought to be an inert and nonabsorbable agent; however, it exerts a strong immunogenicity and provokes an inflammatory response in the lungs. Direct instillation of activated charcoal into the lungs of animal models results in increased microvasculature permeability and pulmonary edema. Interestingly, activated charcoal aspiration has been reported to present as a spiculated, PET-positive mass mimicking lung cancer [58].

Management is largely supportive with mechanical ventilation and inhaled bronchodilators. Aspirated charcoal should be removed from the endobronchial tree (Fig. 15.10) [55, 59], with bronchial washings as much as possible. Repeated bronchoscopies may be needed in some patients with severe aspiration. The key to prevention of charcoal aspiration is to provide adequate airway protection with endotracheal intubation, especially in patients with underlying neurological deficits [55].

Fig. 15.10 Activated charcoal aspiration in an obtunded patient. Reprinted from Rajamani and Allen [55] with the permission from Wolters Kluwer Health

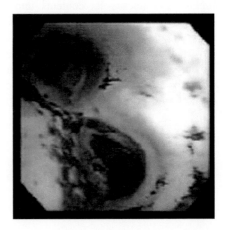

Fig. 15.11 *Black pigmentation* involving left lower lobe bronchus, in a patient on long-term high-dose amiodarone therapy. Reprinted from Lincoln et al. [63] with the permission from Wolters Kluwer Health

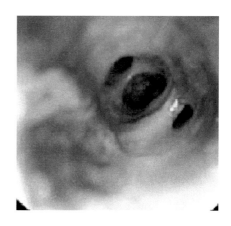

Amiodarone

Amiodarone is an antiarrhythmic agent used to control cardiac arrhythmias. Pulmonary complications develop in 5–15 % of patients on 500 mg or more daily and in 0.1–0.5 % of patients on doses up to 200 mg daily [60]. There are two possible mechanisms of pulmonary toxicity: (1) a direct toxic effect and (2) an immune-mediated hypersensitivity reaction [61]. Pulmonary complications that have been reported in the literatures include interstitial pneumonia, organizing pneumonia, ARDS, pulmonary nodules, alveolar hemorrhage, and pulmonary fibrosis [62]. In addition, airway hyperpigmentation is reported in one case [59, 63] possibly due to prolong exposure to high-dose amiodarone, which results in chronic accumulation in the submucosal tissue (Fig. 15.11) [59]. Bronchial hyperpigmentation is reversed by discontinuation of medication [59, 63].

Tricoptysis

Tricoptysis refers to the expectoration of hairs. In addition to benign tumor such as teratoma as discussed above, a case of iatrogenic tricoptysis has also been reported in the literature [64]. The patient presented with a gradual onset of shortness of breath, hoarseness, wheezing, and coughing of hair after he underwent reconstruction surgery for a benign laryngeal tumor, which used a mucosal flap. FB revealed an extensive meshwork of black hair filaments, below the epiglottis, partially covering the vocal cords [64]. Some hairs were covered by thick mucus. Most patients with a laryngeal tumor who undergo flap reconstruction require postoperative radiation to minimize ectopic hair growth. However, this patient had not received external beam radiation. Laser hair removal or fulguration techniques were necessary to remove hairs permanently from this location [64].

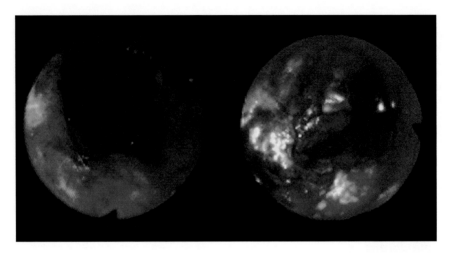

Fig. 15.12 Endobronchial ignition during laser photo-resection producing sloughing of the bronchial mucosa. Reprinted from Krawtz et al. [66] with the permission from American College of Chest Physicians

Endobronchial Ignition

Several cases of endobronchial ignition during thermal ablation have been reported in literatures. The incidence does not only occur during thermal ablation but also occur during laser, electrocautery, or argon plasma coagulation. Burned mucosa as a result of tracheal fire exhibits black debris, based on the degree of injury (Fig. 15.12) [65, 66]. The endobronchial ignition results in black discoloration of the airways. The black carbonaceous debris and the toxic vapors from a burn can produce chemical injury and chronic mucosal inflammation [67]. Severe endobronchial inflammation can also lead to the perforation of the airways creating a fistula tract with adjacent internal organs. Major factors contributing to the endobronchial ignition are types of endotracheal tube, type of bronchoscope and laser used, and high oxygen concentration (FiO2) [68].

Endobronchial ignition is an emergency condition regardless of the source of energy. Strategies have been proposed to minimize the incidence of endotracheal fire during laser photo-resection and argon plasma coagulation [66, 69–73]. The operating room personnel should be trained to properly manage the circumstances. A protocol when a flash fire is detected should be established. All anesthetic agents should be discontinued immediately and saline may be used to extinguish fire. The endotracheal tube should be removed. The patient should receive pure oxygen ventilation by mask prior to reintubation [67]. The tracheobronchial tree should be re-evaluated for the removal of any foreign particles. Surveillance FB should be performed daily to evaluate the extent of injury and detect early complications [67]. Steroids should be initiated with a gradual tapering as the patient's condition improves. Tracheal cultures should be obtained daily for the early detection of microbiology. Prophylactic antibiotics, such as penicillin and cephalosporin, should be initiated and later adjusted according to the result of cultures [67]. In severe laryngopharyngeal injury, tracheostomy is necessary to prevent airway obstruction. A high-humidity nebulizer will facilitate the clearing of secretions because burned airways with impaired mucociliary function are prone to form mucus plugs, resulting in post-obstructive pneumonia [67].

Iron Pill Aspiration

Iron pill aspiration (IPA) is a condition that frequently reported in the literatures. Iron supplements are available over the counter in different colors in the USA. Ferrous sulfate ($FeSO_4$) is the most common preparation involved in this condition; neither ferrous gluconate nor ferrous fumarate has been reported in the cases of aspiration. Once $FeSO_4$ dissolves in the lung secretions, the acidic property (pH < 3) of the $FeSO_4$ [74] leading to severe inflammation, acute mucosal damage, granuloma formation, fibrosis, or bronchial stenosis [75, 76]. A triad of history of IPA, intense airway inflammation, and histologic examination showing iron particles from bronchial biopsy in the absence of foreign body constitutes the syndrome of IPA [76]. Radiographic investigation could support the diagnosis despite the lack of classic triad of IPA. CT scan of the chest demonstrating circumferential thickening of the bronchus intermedius in the context of IPA has been reported [77]. PET-CT scans showing evidence of airway inflammation and necrosis due to iron deposition have also been reported [78].

Bronchoscopic examination in majority of IPA cases reveals greenish dark-brown necrotic material overlying bronchial mucosa. Although the $FeSO_4$ pill rapidly disintegrates in the airway and may not be visually detected during bronchoscopic examination, an endobronchial biopsy specimen may show iron particles' deposition even after a year of aspiration [76]. Bronchial washing may reveal reactive epithelial cells and histiocytes with both intracellular and extracellular, refractile, crystalline material positive for Prussian blue iron stain [78].

Measure to prevent IPA is to avoid oral iron pills supplement in patients with swallowing disorders. An alternative route of supplementation is parenteral administration. Bronchial stenosis resulting from IPA can be managed by bronchoscopic intervention. Failure to diagnose IPA in patients with previously compromised lung function can lead to lethal consequences [76, 79].

Minocycline-induced Endobronchial Tree Hyperpigmentation

Minocycline is a broad-spectrum tetracycline antibiotic. Most common indications for minocycline administration are for treatment of skin acne, chronic infection from gram-positive, gram-negative, and atypical microorganism [80].

Minocycline-induced abnormal pigmentation is a common side effect after exposure to the medicine. An accumulation of dark blue minocycline-degraded product in various tissues is a potential source of abnormal pigmentation [81]. The cumulative dose and duration of minocycline-exposure-induced hyperpigmentation is not clearly defined. There are numerous case reports of minocycline-induced hyperpigmentation in systemic organs such as dermatology (skin, nail), ophthalmology (sclera and conjunctivae), oral cavity (teeth, mucous membrane, gingiva, hard palate, and alveolar bone), bone and cartilage, and internal organ tissue such as thyroid, aortic and mitral valves, atherosclerotic plaques, and breast milk [80]. In addition, Asakura et al. [82] reported the first case of minocycline-induced tracheal ring hyperpigmentation, which partially resolved in 6 months after the medication was discontinued. Pulmonologist who perform bronchoscopy should rise suspicious of minocycline side effect if encounter areas of dark blue discoloration of the

Table 15.3 Diagnostic approach to black bronchoscopy

Etiology	Differential diagnoses	Diagnostic method
Congenital	Melanosis	By excluding other conditions
Inborn error metabolism	Alkaptonuria (ochronosis)	Measurement of urine and plasma HGA levels
Infection	*Aspergillus niger* *Ochroconis gallopava*	Endobronchial biopsy and culture Transbronchial biopsy and culture
	Healed TB	Prior history of TB infection and pigment location at lymph node stations
Environmental exposures	Anthracosis and anthracofibrosis	By history, endobronchial biopsy and microscopic examination under polarized light
	Sooty inhalation	History of exposure to fire
	Argyria	By history and endobronchial biopsy
Neoplasm	Primary malignant melanoma	Endobronchial biopsy
	Metastatic malignant melanoma	Endobronchial biopsy
	Melanotic carcinoid tumor	Endobronchial biopsy
	Melanotic schwannoma	Endobronchial biopsy
	Melanotic paraganglioma	Endobronchial biopsy
	Teratoma (tricoptysis)	Chest CT scan
Iatrogenic	Charcoal aspiration	History of charcoal use
	Amiodarone	History of amiodarone use and resolution after discontinuation of the drug
	Tricoptysis	History of prior airway reconstruction surgery
	Endobronchial ignition	History of thermal ablation
	Iron pill aspiration	History and endobronchial biopsy

HGA Homogentisic acid

endobronchial tree particularly at the cartilaginous part of the trachea. It is a benign condition, and a detailed history and review of medication list is an important key leading to final diagnosis without unnecessary investigation.

Conclusions

This chapter provides a comprehensive review of differential diagnoses, diagnostic studies, and optimal management guidelines for airway hyperpigmentation. Despite most of the etiologies are benign, pulmonologist should also be cognizant of malignant etiologies. The majority of the cases can be diagnosed by clinical history of exposure, endobronchial biopsies, and tissue cultures. However, specific diagnostic tests may be required to guide the diagnosis in particular cases (Table 15.3). Overall, it is very important for pulmonologist to recognize the entities of these airway abnormalities for proper diagnosis and management.

References

1. Packham S, Jaiswal P, Kuo K, Goldsack N. Black bronchoscopy. Respir Int Rev Thorac Dis. 2003;70(2):206.
2. Pagliaccio L, Mehta AC. Endobronchial melanosis: occurrence and possible significance. Chest. 1989;96:222S.
3. Babin RW, Ceilley RI, DeSanto LW. Oral hyperpigmentation and occult malignancy—report of a case. J Otolaryngol. 1978;7(5):389–94.
4. Phornphutkul C, Introne WJ, Perry MB, et al. Natural history of alkaptonuria. N Engl J Med. 2002;347(26):2111–21.
5. Parambil JG, Daniels CE, Zehr KJ, Utz JP. Alkaptonuria diagnosed by flexible bronchoscopy. Chest. 2005;128(5):3678–80.
6. Lustberg TJ, Schulman JD, Seegmiller JE. The preparation and identification of various adducts of oxidized homogentisic acid and the development of a new sensitive colorimetric assay for homogentisic acid. Clin Chim Acta Int J Clin Chem. 1971;35(2):325–33.
7. McClure J, Smith PS, Gramp AA. Calcium pyrophosphate dihydrate (CPPD) deposition in ochronotic arthropathy. J Clin Pathol. 1983;36(8):894–902.
8. Karnak D, Avery RK, Gildea TR, Sahoo D, Mehta AC. Endobronchial fungal disease: an under-recognized entity. Respir Int Rev Thorac Dis. 2007;74(1):88–104.
9. Singhal P, Usuda K, Mehta AC. Post-lung transplantation Aspergillus niger infection. J Heart Lung Transplant Official Publ Int Soc Heart Transplant. 2005;24(9):1446–7.
10. Singh N, Chang FY, Gayowski T, Marino IR. Infections due to dematiaceous fungi in organ transplant recipients: case report and review. Clin Infect Dis Official Publ Infect Dis Soc Am. 1997;24(3):369–74.
11. Qureshi ZA, Kwak EJ, Nguyen MH, Silveira FP. Ochroconis gallopava: a dematiaceous mold causing infections in transplant recipients. Clin Transplant. 2012;26(1):E17–23.
12. Shoham S, Pic-Aluas L, Taylor J, et al. Transplant-associated Ochroconis gallopava infections. Transplant Infect Dis Official J Transplant Soc. 2008;10(6):442–8.

13. Odell JA, Alvarez S, Cvitkovich DG, Cortese DA, McComb BL. Multiple lung abscesses due to Ochroconis gallopavum, a dematiaceous fungus, in a nonimmunocompromised wood pulp worker. Chest. 2000;118(5):1503–5.

14. Long R, Wong E, Barrie J. Bronchial anthracofibrosis and tuberculosis: CT features before and after treatment. AJR. Am J Roentgenol. 2005;184(3 Suppl):S33–36.

15. Kim HY, Im JG, Goo JM, et al. Bronchial anthracofibrosis (inflammatory bronchial stenosis with anthracotic pigmentation): CT findings. AJR. Am J Roentgenol. 2000;174(2):523–527.

16. Reginato AJ, Schumacher HR, Martinez VA. Ochronotic arthropathy with calcium pyrophosphate crystal deposition. A light and electron microscopic study. Arthritis Rheum. 1973;16(6):705–14.

17. Chua AP, Mehta AC. New disease—new terminology. Chest. 2010;137(2):503–504 (author reply 504–505).

18. Chung MP, Lee KS, Han J, et al. Bronchial stenosis due to anthracofibrosis. Chest. 1998;113 (2):344–50.

19. Mireles-Cabodevila EKD, Shah S, Mehta AC. Anthracostenosis. J Bronchology. 2006;13 (3):153–5.

20. Boonsarngsuk V, Suwatanapongched T, Rochanawutanon M. Bronchial anthracostenosis with mediastinal fibrosis associated with long-term wood-smoke exposure. Respirology (Carlton, Vic.). 2009;14(7):1060–63.

21. Dumortier P, De Vuyst P, Yernault JC. Comparative analysis of inhaled particles contained in human bronchoalveolar lavage fluids, lung parenchyma and lymph nodes. Environ Health Perspect. 1994;102(Suppl 5):257–9.

22. Naccache JM, Monnet I, Nunes H, et al. Anthracofibrosis attributed to mixed mineral dust exposure: report of three cases. Thorax. 2008;63(7):655–7.

23. Amoli K. Bronchopulmonary disease in Iranian housewives chronically exposed to indoor smoke. Eur Respir J. 1998;11(3):659–63.

24. Liao QH. [A clinicopathological study of 16 autopsy cases of anthracosilicosis with lung cancer]. *Zhonghua lao dong wei sheng zhi ye bing za zhi = Zhonghua laodong weisheng zhiyebing zazhi.* Chin J Ind Hygiene Occup Dis. 2005;23(5):340–342.

25. Wang D, Minami Y, Shu Y, et al. The implication of background anthracosis in the development and progression of pulmonary adenocarcinoma. Cancer Sci. 2003;94(8):707–11.

26. Carr JA, Phillips BD, Bowling WM. The utility of bronchoscopy after inhalation injury complicated by pneumonia in burn patients: results from the National Burn Repository. J Burn Care Res Official Publ Am Burn Assoc. 2009;30(6):967–974.

27. Mlcak RP, Suman OE, Herndon DN. Respiratory management of inhalation injury. Burns J Int Soc Burn Injuries. 2007;33(1):2–13.

28. Moylan JA, Chan CK. Inhalation injury—an increasing problem. Ann Surg. 1978; 188(1):34–7.

29. Haponik EF, Meyers DA, Munster AM, et al. Acute upper airway injury in burn patients. Serial changes of flow-volume curves and nasopharyngoscopy. Am Rev Respir Dis. 1987;135 (2):360–6.

30. Wanner A, Cutchavaree A. Early recognition of upper airway obstruction following smoke inhalation. Am Rev Respir Dis. 1973;108(6):1421–3.

31. Diaz JV, Koff J, Gotway MB, Nishimura S, Balmes JR. Case report: a case of wood-smoke-related pulmonary disease. Environ Health Perspect. 2006;114(5):759–62.

32. Ribeiro C, Guimaraes M, Antunes A, et al. "The black bronchoscopy": a case of airway soot deposition. J Bronchology Intervent Pulmonol. 2013;20(3):271–3.

33. Arakawa A, Fukamizu H, Hashizume I, et al. Macroscopic and histological findings in the healing process of inhalation injury. Burns J Int Soc Burn Injuries. 2007;33(7):855–9.

34. Herndon DN. Inhalation injury. In: Total burn care. 2nd ed. Philadelphia, PA: Elsevier; 2002, p. 242–53.

35. Chou SH, Lin SD, Chuang HY, Cheng YJ, Kao EL, Huang MF. Fiber-optic bronchoscopic classification of inhalation injury: prediction of acute lung injury. Surg Endosc. 2004;18 (9):1377–9.

36. Masanes MJ, Legendre C, Lioret N, Saizy R, Lebeau B. Using bronchoscopy and biopsy to diagnose early inhalation injury. Macroscopic Histologic Find. Chest. 1995;107(5):1365–1369.
37. Drake PL, Hazelwood KJ. Exposure-related health effects of silver and silver compounds: a review. Ann Occup Hygiene. 2005;49(7):575–85.
38. Greene RM, Su WP. Argyria. Am Fam Physician. 1987;36(6):151–4.
39. Barrie HJ, Harding HE. Argyro-siderosis of the lungs in silver finishers. Br J Ind Med. 1947;4 (4):225–9.
40. Hill WR, Pillsbury PD. Argyria. The pharmacology of silver. Baltimore, MD: Williams & Wilkins; 1939.
41. Bowden LP, Royer MC, Hallman JR, Lewin-Smith M, Lupton GP. Rapid onset of argyria induced by a silver-containing dietary supplement. J Cutan Pathol. 2011;38(10):832–5.
42. Brooks SM. Lung disorders resulting from the inhalation of metals. Clin Chest Med. 1981;2 (2):235–54.
43. Schreiber JSC, Hege S, Knolle J. Localized argyria of the proximal trachea. J Bronchology. 2005;12(4):234–5.
44. Venugopal BLT, eds. Metal toxicity in mammals, vol. 2: chemical toxicology of metals and metalloids. NewYork, NY: Academic Press; 1978. P. 32–36.
45. Williams N, Gardner I. Absence of symptoms in silver refiners with raised blood silver levels. Occup Med (Oxford, England). 1995;45(4):205–208.
46. Perrone S, Clonfero E, Gori G, Simonato L. 4 cases of occupational argyrosis. La Medicina del lavoro. 1977;68(3):178–86.
47. Dountsis A, Zisis C, Karagianni E, Dahabreh J. Primary malignant melanoma of the lung: a case report. World J Surg Oncol. 2003;1(1):26.
48. Kiryu T, Hoshi H, Matsui E, et al. Endotracheal/endobronchial metastases: clinicopathologic study with special reference to developmental modes. Chest. 2001;119(3):768–75.
49. Abul Y, ERYÜKSEL E, Çelikel C, Tosuner Z, Yazici Z, Karakurt S. Endobronchial metastasis of malignant melanoma presenting with dyspnea: case report and review of literature. Turkiye Klinikleri J Med Sci. 2011;31(2):468–470.
50. Das R, Dasgupta A, Tewari S, Mehta AC. Malignant melanoma of the bronchus. J Bronchology. 1998;5(1):59–60.
51. Reddy VS, Mykytenko J, Giltman LI, Mansour KA. Primary malignant melanoma of the lung: review of literature and report of a case. Am Surg. 2007;73(3):287–9.
52. Teo YK, Kor AC. "Black bronchoscopy"—a case of endobronchial metastases from melanoma. J Bronchology Intervent Pulmonol. 2010;17(2):146–8.
53. Ustun MO, Demircan A, Paksoy N, Ozkaynak C, Tuzuner S. A case of intrapulmonary teratoma presenting with hair expectoration. Thorac Cardiovasc Surg. 1996;44(5):271–3.
54. Rawat J, Saini S, Raghuvanshi S, Sindhwani G, Kesarwani V. Intrapulmonary teratoma presenting with tricoptysis: a case report and review of the literature. Indian J Chest Dis Allied Sci. 2011;53(4):237–9.
55. Rajamani S, Allen P. Accidental charcoal aspiration. J Bronchology. 2004;11(2):130–131.
56. Bond GR. The role of activated charcoal and gastric emptying in gastrointestinal decontamination: a state-of-the-art review. Ann Emerg Med. 2002;39(3):273–86.
57. Justiniani FR, Hippalgaonkar R, Martinez LO. Charcoal-containing empyema complicating treatment for overdose. Chest. 1985;87(3):404–5.
58. Seder DB, Christman RA, Quinn MO, Knauft ME. A 45-year-old man with a lung mass and history of charcoal aspiration. Respir Care. 2006;51(11):1251–4.
59. Kupeli E, Khemasuwan D, Lee P, Mehta AC. "Pills" and the air passages. Chest. 2013;144 (2):651–60.
60. Ott MC, Khoor A, Leventhal JP, Paterick TE, Burger CD. Pulmonary toxicity in patients receiving low-dose amiodarone. Chest. 2003;123(2):646–51.
61. Martin WJ 2nd. Mechanisms of amiodarone pulmonary toxicity. Clin Chest Med. 1990;11 (1):131–8.
62. Brinker A, Johnston M. Acute pulmonary injury in association with amiodarone. Chest. 2004;125(4):1591–2.

63. Lincoln MJ, Zanders TB, Morris MJ. Bronchial pigmentation as a manifestation of amiodarone pulmonary toxicity. J Bronchology. 2007;14(4):275–277.
64. Bakry MB, Arshad S, Haq S, et al. Hairy hoarseness [abstract]. Chest. 2004;126(4_Meeting Abstracts):943S–a–944S.
65. Hasegawa YTS, Okudera K, et al. Intratracheal fire ignited by a gallium-arsenide-aluminum diode laser during treatment of airway obstruction with lung cancer. J Bronchology. 2003;10 (3):198–200.
66. Krawtz S, Mehta AC, Wiedemann HP, DeBoer G, Schoepf KD, Tomaszewski MZ. Nd-YAG laser-induced endobronchial burn. Management and long-term follow-up. Chest. 1989;95 (4):916–18.
67. Schramm VL Jr, Mattox DE, Stool SE. Acute management of laser-ignited intratracheal explosion. Laryngoscope. 1981;91(9 Pt 1):1417–26.
68. Kumar SDZH, Myers JR. Carbon dioxide laser-induced endotracheal fire: a case report and review of the literature. J Bronchology. 1998;5(3):216–9.
69. Mathur PN. Chapter 15. In: Wang KPMA, Turner JF, editors. Flexible bronchoscopy. 3rd ed. Hoboken, NJ: Wiley-Blackwell Science Publisher; 2012. p. 201–11.
70. Reichle GFL, Kullman H-J, Prenzel R, Macha H-N, Farin G. Argon plasma coagulation in bronchology: a new method alternative or complementary? J Bronchology. 2000;7(2):109–17.
71. Sosis MB, Dillon FX. A comparison of CO_2 laser ignition of the Xomed, plastic, and rubber endotracheal tubes. Anesth Analg. 1993;76(2):391–3.
72. Takanashi S, Hasegawa Y, Ito A, Sato M, Kaji K, Okumura K. Airflow through the auxiliary line of the laser fiber prevents ignition of intra-airway fire during endoscopic laser surgery. Lasers Surg Med. 2002;31(3):211–5.
73. Rampil IJ. Anesthesia for laser surgery. In: Miller DR, editors. Anesthesia. 5th ed. Philadelphia, PA: Churchill Livingstone; 2000:2199–12.
74. Carlborg B, Densert O. Esophageal lesions caused by orally administered drugs. An experimental study in the cat. Eur Surg Res. Europaische chirurgische Forschung. Recherches chirurgicales europeennes. 1980;12(4):270–282.
75. Jimenez Rodriguez BM, de Jesus SC, Merinas Lopez CM, Gonzalez de Vega San Roman JM, Romero Ortiz AD. Bronchial stenosis after iron pill aspiration. J Bronchology Intervent Pulmonol. 2013;20(1):96–97.
76. Lee P, Culver DA, Farver C, Mehta AC. Syndrome of iron pill aspiration. Chest. 2002;121 (4):1355–7.
77. Grosu HB, Jimenez CA, Eapen GA, Ost D, Moran C, Morice RC. The iron lady. Am J Respir Crit Care Med. 2012;186(5):460.
78. Cimino-Mathews A, Illei PB. Cytologic and histologic findings of iron pill-induced injury of the lower respiratory tract. Diagn Cytopathol. 2013;41(10):901–3.
79. Eliashar R, Eliachar I, Esclamado R, Gramlich T, Strome M. Can topical mitomycin prevent laryngotracheal stenosis? Laryngoscope. 1999;109(10):1594–600.
80. Eisen D, Hakim MD. Minocycline-induced pigmentation. Incidence, prevention and management. Drug Saf. 1998;18(6):431–40.
81. Hendrix JD Jr, Greer KE. Cutaneous hyperpigmentation caused by systemic drugs. Int J Dermatol. 1992;31(7):458–66.
82. Asakura T, Nukaga S, Namkoong H, et al. Blue-black trachea as a result of minocycline-induced hyperpigmentation. Am J Respir Crit Care Med. 2015 Oct 1. [Epub ahead of print].

Chapter 16
Airway Complications After Lung Transplantation

Jose F. Santacruz, Satish Kalanjeri and Michael S. Machuzak

Introduction

Airway complications (AC) have had a significant impact on the morbidity and mortality in lung transplantation since the first human lung transplant in 1963. Early incidence of complications were exceedingly high at 60–80 %, but improvement in many facets led complication rates to drop significantly into the 10–15 % range with a related mortality rate of 2–3 % [1–6].

AC have a variety of presentations and while their treatments are often institution dependent, they are all individualized to the type of AC (stenosis, dehiscence, etc.), timing, location, and severity. While most early reports of AC dealt primarily with the anastomosis, we now are aware of complications distal to the suture line, such as the "vanishing bronchus syndrome" [7].

AC can be grouped anatomically (anastomotic or distal to the anastomosis), descriptively (stricture, granulation tissue, infection, necrosis, dehiscence, and fistula formation), temporally (early or late) or by etiology (ischemic, infectious, iatrogenic, or idiopathic). In addition to the associated mortality, patients with AC experience increased morbidity, most notably in of quality of life. The number of procedures, repeated office visits, hospitalizations, and associated costs can all significantly affect one's satisfaction with lung transplant and in some cases minimize or completely negate benefits from this complicated undertaking.

J.F. Santacruz (✉)
Bronchoscopy and Interventional Pulmonology, Houston Methodist Lung Center,
6560 Fannin, Suite 1632, Houston, TX 77030, USA
e-mail: jfsantacruz@houstonmethodist.org

S. Kalanjeri
Section of Pulmonary, Critical Care and Sleep Medicine, Louisiana State University
Health Sciences Center, Shreveport, LA, USA

M.S. Machuzak
Respiratory Institute, Cleveland Clinic, Cleveland, OH, USA

© Springer International Publishing Switzerland 2016
A.C. Mehta et al. (eds.), *Diseases of the Central Airways*,
Respiratory Medicine, DOI 10.1007/978-3-319-29830-6_16

The goals of this chapter include a brief description of the history of AC, transplant-specific anatomy, surgical techniques of lung transplantation, classification of AC, etiologies, management, and potential future directions for prevention and treatment.

Historical Background

James Hardy performed the first human lung transplantation at the University of Mississippi in 1963. The patient had lung cancer and died 18 days after the transplant due to renal failure [8].

The first successful lung transplant occurred at the University of Toronto in 1983. Prior to it, multiple attempts were performed around the world without success; many of those cases had deficient healing of the bronchial anastomosis [8].

In the early days of lung transplantation, AC were a significant source of morbidity and mortality, making AC the "Achilles heel" of lung transplantation short-term survival [1–3, 8, 9].

With improved surgical techniques, new immunosuppressant regimens, and overall better medical management, survival has significantly improved over the years [1–10].

Anatomy

Lung transplantation patients have a unique situation compared to other solid organ recipients. Human lungs contain dual blood supplies, a pulmonary and separate bronchial circulation. The bronchial circulation provides the blood supply to the major airways and supporting structures of the lungs, and this is not re-established in standard lung transplantation. Previous anatomic studies have defined fairly consistent origins of the bronchial arteries. These vessels arise either as branches of the aorta or intercostal arteries and travel through the hila where small arteries enter into the muscular layer of the airway and eventual terminate in a plexus within the bronchial mucosa. This submucosal plexus gives rise to a collateral circulation between the pulmonary and the bronchial vessels. The bronchial circulation provides primary blood supply to both proximal mainstem bronchi, although the pulmonary circulation can contribute through retrograde collaterals. While the pulmonary circulation is re-established during the transplantation procedure, bronchial circulation is not. This feature places bronchial viability and anastomotic healing completely dependent upon retrograde blood flow from the pulmonary to bronchial circulation. As a result, there is potential for perioperative ischemia jeopardizing the anastomosis and distal airways. The main carina and both proximal mainstem bronchi are supplied via the coronary collateral system arising from atrial branches of the left and right coronary arteries. This may explain why the proximal airways seem to suffer less ischemic injury.

Incidence and Prevalence

There is a wide range in the reported incidence of anastomotic complications in the lung transplant population. Reports of complication rates range from 1.6–33 % over the past several decades, though numbers around 15 % seem to be the expert consensus. The incidence of AC in heart–lung transplant recipients is low [2, 11, 12]. Many theories exist for the rationale of why AC rates have declined from the 60–80 % range. These include advances in graft preservation, donor and recipient selection, progress in perioperative management, and immunosuppression as well as improvements in surgical techniques. Most recently, Shoffer et al. [13] and Dutau et al. [14] reported institutional rates of AC of 13 and 14.5 %, respectively, again on a par with recent observations [1–6, 10, 11, 15–18]. There is controversy regarding the incidence of AC in transplantation using donation after cardiac death, but in our experience it is similar to that reported for lung from brain-dead donors [19, 20].

This is clearly a complex issue with much interplay, but one of the most likely reasons for this wide range may be the lack of a standardized classification system. What has been classified as a complication at one institution may not have been listed as one in another. We will discuss AC classifications later in this chapter.

Risk Factors

Several proposed risk factors to the development of AC have been identified. These can be subdivided into donor/recipient factors, surgical techniques, infections, medications or immunosuppression, and miscellaneous [21].

Historically, AC have been mainly attributed to ischemia of the donor bronchus during the immediate post-transplant period [1, 22, 23].

Donor and Recipient Risk Factors

Several risk factors may be attributed to the donor. Van De Wauwer et al. [9]; identified the duration of donor's mechanical ventilation (50–70 h) prior to organ recovery and a greater height mismatch (likely related to a larger bronchial diameter) with a taller donor being more likely to lead to an AC. In such cases, the surgical technique of minimizing the length of the anastomosis as well as telescoping may be the best solution [10].

Other risk factors thought to be involved include ischemia of the donor bronchus (particularly in the immediate postoperative period), the length of the donor bronchus, the type of surgical anastomosis, infections, size difference between the donor and the recipient bronchi, type of immunosuppressive regimen used, pulmonary fungal infections, and the need for a postoperative tracheostomy [2, 16, 24–28].

Surgical

Which anastomotic technique is best is a matter of debate and controversy [10, 29]. Many techniques and variations including telescoping, end-to-end, wrapping vascular pedicles, and bronchial artery revascularization (BAR) have been tried and studied, though opinions vary on which is best, no consensus is present. The initial experience of end-to-end anastomoses was poor but fortunately these outcomes prompted changes and led to a variety of techniques [2, 22].

After initial disappointing results, the practice of wrapping the anastomosis became more popular, first with omentum, later pericardial, peribronchial, or intercostal tissue [2, 4, 26, 27, 29]. However, the added technical complexity of the wrap in addition to lack of randomized controlled trials showing benefit has decreased enthusiasm for this technique and it is rarely used today [30].

The technique of telescoping the anastomosis has also been tried to address complications, particularly dehiscence [2, 18, 23, 31]. Although it initially gained support, this technique has been largely abandoned as it has demonstrated increased complication rates, as high as 48 % [16]. The major issue limiting the usefulness of the telescoping technique was increased stenosis but increased concern for infection has also been cited. These complications are likely related to this technique starting with a narrowed airway by virtue of the telescoping and possibly trapping bacteria between the airway walls [10, 16].

Presently, the end-to-end bronchial anastomosis without a wrap, performed, as close to the secondary carina as possible, is the preferred technique at most centers [10, 32]. Performing the anastomosis close to the secondary carina is desirable, as donor bronchus length has been shown to be crucial. Excessive length of this donor bronchus increases the likelihood for ischemia as all flow in the post-transplant period is via collaterals and inversely proportional to length [2, 9, 22].

Though it may seem logical that a longer ischemic time will increase the incidence of AC, this has not necessarily proven true. This has been best supported in bilateral sequential lung transplantation [4, 10, 18, 23]. Despite the longer ischemic time, the second anastomosis of a bilateral sequential transplant is not more prone to AC [26].

Regardless of the approach, the bronchial anastomosis remains ischemic in the postoperative period possibly leading to AC. BAR has been presented as an approach to avoid this and will be discussed later [10, 18, 27, 29–33].

Infections

Infections in both the preoperative and the postoperative periods have long been postulated to be a factor predisposing to AC. The rationale of increased inflammation and decreased healing certainly has merit [11, 22].

In some patients, a high inoculum of pathogenic organisms may be present immediately after transplantation and often the anastomosis is sutured on a contaminated field, not infrequently with multidrug-resistant bacteria [10, 34, 35].

Combining this with the evidence supporting bacterial and fungal airway colonization increasing patient risk for infections in suppurative lung disease may add support [34, 35]; however, the actual role of infection leading to dehiscence, stricture, granulation tissue, and malacia is not firmly established.

Medications/Immunosuppression

Considerable improvements in lung transplant survival have been achieved; however, other solid organ transplants demonstrate superior survival. While AC may play a role in this regard, other factors contribute as well. Despite lung transplant patients being maintained at higher levels of immunosuppression, both acute and chronic rejection rates remain higher than most solid organ transplants. Chronic rejection manifests as bronchiolitis obliterans syndrome (BOS) and occurs earlier with more severity compared to other solid organ transplants [36].

Immunosuppression is critical for the survival of an allograft; however, this may predispose the airways to complications due to increased susceptibility to infection and reduced healing. The use of corticosteroids in the preoperative period was once considered a contraindication due to concern for anastomotic healing [25, 37]. Later studies showed not only adverse effect and possibly less granulation tissue formation but also improved survival in the face of corticosteroids [2, 12, 26, 37, 38].

Typical post-transplant immunosuppressive regimens are three-tiered and consist of a calcineurin inhibitor (typically tacrolimus), an anti-lymphocyte (mycophenolate mofetil or azathioprine), and corticosteroid. Sirolimus (rapamycin, Rapamune) should specifically be discussed as it has been shown to play a role in airway healing. Sirolimus is a novel macrolide first developed as an antifungal agent, later found to have potent immunosuppressive and anti-proliferative properties. First used in renal and later in lung transplants since the major complication associated with calcineurin inhibitors is renal toxicity, this is much less common with sirolimus. Sirolimus has been shown to significantly increase the rate of catastrophic AC in de novo recipients. In particular, unacceptably high rate of anastomotic dehiscence was found in the early transplant period. The current recommendation is to avoid sirolimus for at least 90 days of post-transplantation [25, 28, 39].

Miscellaneous

Multiple other risk factors have been described as potential etiologic features for AC. These include primary graft dysfunction, acute cellular rejection, positive pressure mechanical ventilation, positive end-expiratory pressure (PEEP), organ preservation technique, recipient/donor sex or age, body mass index, acute kidney injury, among others [1, 9, 10, 21, 22, 40–42].

Primary graft dysfunction, a type of reperfusion injury may compromise pulmonary flow and increase the length of mechanical ventilation and the degree of PEEP required. Positive pressure ventilation and PEEP have the potential to increase the bronchial wall and the anastomosis stress, with the potential of inhibiting collateralization and graft perfusion especially when high inflation pressures are needed [1, 10]. Even though studies have described, more AC with prolonged mechanical ventilation controversy exits [29].

Classification of Airway Complications

AC are quite diverse and vary in presentation, severity, complexity, and timing. Bronchial stenosis is identified as the most common complication but others should be included in the discussion such as granulation tissue, malacia, infection, dehiscence, and fistula. Anastomotic complications, particularly early in the history of lung transplantation, played a major role in high morbidity and mortality with the procedure. Management of such problems can be complex and is best handled as a multidisciplinary team approach. Over the past decade, novel techniques have played a major role in the management of these complications. Balloon bronchoplasty, laser photoresection, electrocautery, high-dose rate brachytherapy, cryotherapy, and stent placement among others have been described. While there is little doubt these endoscopic techniques have played an important role, they certainly are not the only advancements in transplant medicine as enhancements in medical management such as understanding graft dysfunction, immunologic reactions, and antimicrobial prophylaxis as well as postoperative care have paved the way to improved outcomes [1, 6, 18, 22, 23, 43, 44].

As previously mentioned, there is a wide range in the reported incidence of AC. One explanation may be the lack of a universal classification system. There have been several attempts at a classification system; however, none has been unanimously accepted [2, 45, 46].

We have previously described the basic classification of AC [1]. The classification described the six types of AC with a brief description of the bronchoscopic, radiological, and clinical observations (Table 16.1).

Recently, Dutau et al. [14] published a proposed grading system for central AC following lung transplantation and this is known as the MDS classification. The first parameter is the macroscopic aspect (M), the next d is the diameter (D), and a third describes the appearance of the sutures (S) (Table 16.2).

Table 16.1 Classification of airway complications

1. Stenosis	**Anastomotic bronchial stenosis**	
		– Stenosis <50 % of bronchial diameter
		– Stenosis >50 % of bronchial diameter
	Segmental non-anastomotic bronchial stenosis	
		– Stenosis <50 % of bronchial diameter
		– Stenosis >50 % of bronchial diameter
		– Vanishing Bronchus Intermedius Syndrome (VBIS)
2. Necrosis and Dehiscence	Grade I	No slough or necrosis reported. Anastomosis healing well
	Grade II	Any necrotic mucosal slough reported, but no bronchial wall necrosis
	Grade III	Bronchial wall necrosis within 2 cm of anastomosis
	Grade IV	Extensive bronchial wall necrosis extending >2 cm from anastomosis
3. Exophytic granulation tissue	Exophytic granulation tissue	
		– Granulation tissue with <50 % diameter narrowing
		– Granulation tissue with >50 % diameter narrowing
4. Malacia	– Diffuse tracheobronchial malacia	
		– Anastomotic malacia (1 cm proximal or distal)
5. Fistulae	– Bronchopleural fistula	
		– Bronchomediastinal fistula
		– Bronchovascular fistula
6. Infections	– Anastomotic infections	
		– Non-anastomotic infections (tracheitis, bronchitis, etc.)

Reprinted with the permission from American Thoracic Society. Copyright © 2015 American Thoracic Society: Santacruz and Mehta [1]. The Annals of the American Thoracic Society is an official journal of the American Thoracic Society

In the MDS classification system, the M designation is divided into 4 subgroups. M0 or the healed scar aspect is considered by most to represent the normal response of healing. M1 (cartilaginous protrusion) is most commonly present in the cases of size mismatch from the donor to recipient bronchi. This is typically associated with a telescoping anastomosis, though there may be no abnormal healing and the lumen is narrowed simply due to the diameter of the donor bronchus. M2 (granulomatous component) is related to exuberant inflammation at the anastomotic site. The M3 lesion describes ulceration, ischemia, and necrosis.

The D classifications are divided into 4 subgroups classifying the diameter. The D parameter is separated by the amount of reduction with D0 including a normal to fixed reduction up to 33 %; D1 including malacia greater than 50 %; D2 a stenosis from 33 to 66 %; and D3 any stenosis >66 %.

Table 16.2 The MDS
endoscopic standardized
grading system for
macroscopic central airway
complications following lung
transplantation

M (macroscopic aspect)
• M0: scar tissue
• M1: protruding cartilage
• M2: inflammation/granulomas
• M3: ischemia/necrosis
Extent of abnormalities in regard to the anastomosis: a. Abnormalities localized to the anastomosis b. Abnormalities extending from the anastomosis to the bronchus intermedius or to the extremity of the left main bronchus, without lobar involvement c. Abnormalities extending from the anastomosis to lobar or segmental bronchi d. Abnormalities affecting the lobar and/or segmental bronchi, without anastomotic involvement
D (diameter)
• D0: normal to a fixed reduction <33 %
• D1: expiratory reduction (malacia) >50 %
• D2: fixed reduction from 33 to 66 %
• D3: fixed reduction >66 %
Extent of abnormalities in regard to the anastomosis: a. Abnormalities localized to the anastomosis b. Abnormalities extending from the anastomosis to the truncus intermedius or to the extremity of the left main bronchus, without lobar involvement c. Abnormalities extending from the anastomosis to lobar or segmental bronchi d. Abnormalities affecting the lobar and/or segmental bronchi, without anastomotic involvement
S (sutures)
• S0: absence of dehiscence
• S1: limited dehiscence (<25 % of circumference)
• S2: extensive dehiscence (from 25 to 50 %)
• S3: very extensive dehiscence (>50 %)
Localization: e: anteriorly; f: other localizations

Reprinted from Dutau et al. [14] with the permission from Oxford University Press

The S designation was developed to include dehiscence ranging from S0 or absence of dehiscence to limited dehiscence of <25 %; S2 categorizing dehiscence from 25 to 50 %; and S3 extensive dehiscence >50 %.

It is the hope of these authors that we can universally agree on a nomenclature and classification system that will be universally accepted. This may be the first step to scientifically approach this morbid complication. Until we are able to consistently report an issue such as AC, we cannot fully understand its incidence, prevalence, morbidity, and mortality, and develop consistent techniques for treatment and possibly prevention.

Fig. 16.1 Necrosis and
stenosis of the distal right
bronchus intermedius (*RBI*)
and right middle lobe
bronchus (*RML*). Severe
necrosis extending into the
subsegmental level of the
right middle lobe

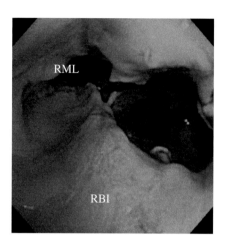

Bronchial Stenosis

Bronchial stenosis is the most common complication with published reports between 1.6 and 32 % [11, 16, 47, 48].

Extensive necrosis and dehiscence will predispose to the formation of strictures (Fig. 16.1). Infectious etiologies may play a role as well and Aspergillus has been identified as one potential causative agent. As discussed, the surgical technique may predispose an airway to stenosis with a 7 % incidence seen in a telescoping anastomotic technique [4, 16]. Recently, an association between the early rejection and the incidence of strictures was described [49].

Another important distinction when discussing bronchial stenosis is the location. The most commonly discussed bronchial stenosis involves a stricture at the anastomotic line (Fig. 16.2a, b). However, recent publications have highlighted another troubling finding of stenosis distal to the anastomotic line. This non-anastomotic stenosis can be quite troubling as the strictures can extend segmentally and even sub-segmentally. This incidence is lower, though with the caveat that in many publications this type of stricture was not specifically labeled separately, so the reported rates of 2.5–3 % may be inaccurate [3, 48, 50].

This can be severe enough to cause the loss of a segmental or larger airway, as in the case of the vanishing bronchus intermedius syndrome (VBIS). The bronchus intermedius may be particularly susceptible likely due to the fact that it is already a narrower airway (Fig. 16.3). This symptomatic narrowing occurs in approximately 2 % of the airways. The most devastating form can lead to a complete atresia. VBIS can be seen as early as 6 months and adversely affects survival with a mean survival of 25 months after initial diagnosis [7, 50].

The underlying etiology of bronchial stenosis is poorly understood but may be related to increased airway inflammation and a mononuclear infiltration.

Fig. 16.2 **a** Right mainstem
bronchus stricture. Note the
suture embedded with the
scar/stricture. **b** This image
demonstrates the same airway
after dilation and placement
of a modified silicone stent

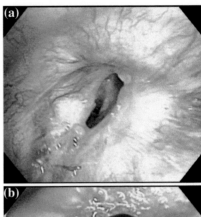

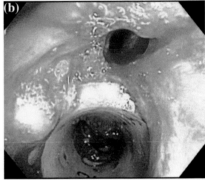

Fig. 16.3 Stenosis distal to
anastomosis: Right bronchus
intermedius

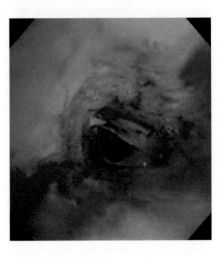

This coupled with ischemic injury can lead to changes in the underlying cartilage, epithelium, and re-formation of airway vessels [3, 12]. Stenosis is typically seen 2- to 9-month post-transplant [3, 26, 47, 51].

Bronchial strictures may present asymptomatically and be diagnosed on routine post-transplant bronchoscopic surveillance, as early stenosis may have minimal clinical signs or symptoms. More frequently, it manifests as increasing dyspnea, cough, post-obstructive pneumonia, radiographic abnormalities, or dropping flow rate on spirometry [6].

The pulmonary function tests may show in spirometry a decrease in the forced and peak expiratory flow. Also, a spirometry failure to improve the first few months post-transplant may be seen [2]. Abnormal flow-volume loop patterns have been described [52, 53].

Flexible bronchoscopy is the gold standard for diagnosis. Computed tomography (CT) of the chest is also useful in the diagnosis and for intervention planning. Axial, helical, and multi-planar reconstruction CT chest-imaging techniques have been described to have an accuracy of more than 90 % in the diagnosis of bronchial stenosis [54, 55].

Multiple individual techniques have been described though a multimodality approach is most common. Successful techniques are in continuous evolution but the armamentarium typically includes a multi-tiered approach with dilation, ablation, and stent placement in ascending order dependent upon the severity. Dilation can be accomplished by many means with an endoscopic balloon, rigid scope, or a bougie. Ablation modalities are also numerous with cryotherapy, electrocautery, laser, argon plasma coagulation (APC), brachytherapy, or even photodynamic therapy (PDT) being described. Stenting should be left as a last resort, though beneficial in many ways, not without potentially serious complications [2, 6, 11, 56–59].

Dilation is usually the first therapeutic procedure performed and can be accomplished safely in multiple ways, as we will discuss. Balloon bronchoplasty is the most common and has been shown to be an excellent palliative technique improving spirometry and relieving symptoms immediately in 50 and 94 % of patients, respectively [47]. While more than one procedure is typical, balloon bronchoplasty may be the only procedure required in 26 % of cases [56].

No single method has proven superiority, but personal experiences have shown several potential advantages with the inflatable balloon. These balloons come in a variety of sizes allowing for incremental and customized dilations. Balloon dilation can also be done quickly and safely, often under conscious sedation without the need for fluoroscopy [56, 58]. The procedural aspects have been well described previously and vary from device to device and so are beyond the scope of this chapter [47, 60]. Balloon bronchoplasty is a simple and quick task to change a balloon size rather than upsizing rigid bronchoscopes for dilation, though more costly.

The rigid bronchoscopic technique has advantages other than cost, as it allows for direct visualization during dilation, tissue debulking, and tamponade while simultaneously ventilating one or both lungs. An inflated balloon will completely occlude the airway it is dilating, preventing ventilation and can be an issue when dealing with a single-lung transplant or a tracheal lesion (less commonly). An additional benefit of the rigid bronchoscope includes ease of stent placement, particularly if a silicone stent is being placed. While rigid dilation is effective, care must be taken to avoid injury, endobronchial, or otherwise, and should only be done by an experienced operator [61, 62].

Strictures can assume many shapes, some are focal and web-like, and others dense and long. The type of stricture encountered will dictate the intervention. A focal web-like stricture may be best handled with a mucosal sparing technique such as endobronchial electrosurgery or laser, followed by dilation [63].

Adjunctive techniques such as submucosal steroid injection or Mitomycin-C have also been described. In a technique adapted from published articles describing endoscopic treatment for tuberculosis strictures, small volumes of dexamethasone or a similar steroid are injected submucosally at the area of the stricture [64]. While no controlled trial evidence exists for this technique, it has been described in lung transplant patients as well [63].

In a similar fashion, borrowing an idea from ear, nose, and throat (ENT) literature endobronchial Mitomycin-C has also been described [65].

Stenting may be required in the cases of recurrent stenosis, although in this immune-compromised population, placement of any foreign body must be carefully considered. Historically, self-expanding metallic stents (SEMS) have been described more commonly in transplant patients. Published use of SEMS in anastomotic and post-anastomotic stenosis can provide almost immediate relief in 80–94 % of individuals, as well as "long-term" maintenance of patency in 45 % of patients [47, 66].

Despite the reported success in these patients, numerous complications have been described. This is not uncommon in any non-malignant condition, particularly in a complex group of immune-compromised patients. The types and rates of complications vary and include infections (16–33 %), granulation tissue formation (12–36 %), and stent migration (5 %) [6, 66]. This not an all-inclusive list as bacterial colonization, halitosis, and fatigue-related stent fracture are also well described. The halitosis may be related to bacterial colonization and bio-film formation within the stent. Colonization is seen in up to 78 % of patients [6, 66, 67]. While not all colonization is significant or needs to be treated, emerging data in stented patients may suggest that stents increase respiratory infections. While these data come from patients with malignant airway disease, care must be taken in those immunosuppressed to the level of transplant patients [68].

One must also keep in mind that once a SEMS is deployed the next thought should be on removal. The longer a SEMS is in place the more difficult it may be to remove and the removal process can be quite complicated [69–71]. Fernandez-Bussy et al. [72] used completely covered SEMS to successfully treat transplant-related AC, and described the potential removal in experienced hands.

Stent-related complication rates as high as 54 % are reported in transplant patients. These echoes concern for stent placement in any benign disease [73–75].

Although many experts feel silicone stents are the preferred types of stents in benign diseases, particularly transplant airways, SEMS may have some advantages. Their ease of deployment, especially without a rigid bronchoscope, favorable external to internal diameter ratio, and superior flexibility allowing the stent to conform to the abnormalities associated with anastomoses can make them particularly useful [76].

An approach that may negate at least some of the above issues such as removal of stent is the use of a biodegradable stent. Although use of biodegradable stents needs to be evaluated further, its feasibility and relative safety was demonstrated in a case series of 6 patients who received customized biodegradable stents made of polydioxanone, the material that absorbable sutures used in airway anastomosis in lung transplantation. In this series [77], all patients had immediate relief of symptoms after stent placement, with stent absorption in 4–6 months time. Median time for re-stenting was about 5 months (Range: 2–15 months). One patient died of pulmonary embolism a year after the biodegradable stent placement. The 5 survivors despite requiring at least one re-stenting remained clinically well over the 4-year follow-up period, with a median intervention-free period of 24 months (Range: 7–44 months.) There were no instances of bleeding, perforation, or stent displacement. Although this method appears to be attractive and feasible, larger studies are needed to validate benefit and safety.

Given many concerns associated with SEMS, particularly in benign airway disease, silicone stents are gaining popularity (Fig. 16.2b). Many features of silicone stents make them ideal for lung transplant AC including lower rates of granulation tissue, ability to be modified, and the ease of removal. The ability to customize these stents cannot be overestimated, as the exact length can be cut; customized holes fashioned to allow ventilation and mucus clearance from airways that would otherwise be compromised from a fully covered SEMS [46, 76, 78]. Stenting of the bronchus intermedius may be challenging due the probable occlusion of the right upper lobe, in such case a customized silicone stent or a modified Montgomery T-tube has been used [79]. Sundset et al. [80] reported the successful use of silicone stents for stenotic AC, and that after removal, the airways remained patent and had an improved spirometry value for as long as 24 months. In our experience, this can be a very useful tool.

Silicone stents are not without complication including increased rates of migration and mucus plugging, reinforcing that the decision to place any kind of stent must be carefully evaluated [24].

Hybrid stents exist as well and have been described in transplant patients. The self-expanding silicone stent, Polyflex (Boston Scientific; Boston, MA), is one example. Our experience with this was reported. We found this stent suboptimal with a 100 % migration rate and have since abandoned its use in our practice [75].

Regardless of the type of stent used, there can be complications and one must be cognizant of this fact. No stent is perfect and multiple authors have previously published the advantage and disadvantages [74, 75, 81]. Presently, our practice is to reserve the use of any stent only after other techniques have been exhausted, particularly in patients with recalcitrant symptomatic bronchial strictures in whom repeated balloon dilations have failed.

Dutau et al. retrospectively evaluated the clinical efficacy and safety of silicone stents in lung transplant patients. They described the insertion of 17 silicone stents in 117 patients over a range of 5–360 days to palliate 23 airways. Symptomatic improvement was seen in all, with an increase in mean forced expiratory volume in 1 s (FEV1) of 672 ± 496 ml. The stent-related complication rate was 0.13/patient per month, with obstructive granulomas [10], mucus plugging [7], and migration [7] being the most common. Stents were successfully removed in 16/23 airways and the stented patients had a similar survival to those without AC [82].

An area of interest related to the significance of AC, specifically stenosis; Castleberry et al., looked at risk factors and outcomes of bronchial stricture as it may be associated with acute rejection. A total of 9,335 patients were analyzed with a stricture incidence of 11.5 %. They found that early rejection was associated with a significantly greater incidence of strictures. Also associated with increased incidence of stricture were male gender, restrictive lung disease, and pretransplant requirement of hospitalization. Those with a stricture had a lower postoperative peak percent predicted FEV1, shorter unadjusted survival, and an increased risk of death after adjusting for potential confounders [49].

In a single-center retrospective review, Shofer et al. evaluated lung transplant patients with central airway stenosis (CAS) with the objective of determining its association with chronic rejection or worse survival. Also, risk factors associated with CAS were identified. In this review, 467 patients were evaluated with 60 (13 %) developing CAS. Of the patients with CAS, 22 (37 %) had resolution with bronchoplasty alone and 32 % required stent. This retrospective review determined that CAS requiring intervention was not a risk factor for developing BOS or worse survival, though a significant complication. Pulmonary fungal infections and the need for postoperative tracheostomy were identified as risk factors for the development of CAS based on their time-dependent multivariable model [13].

The multimodality approaches discussed have been shown to be effective, safe, and reproducible over time, but are not infallible. When endoscopic techniques fail, a surgical approach can be considered. Bronchial anastomoses reconstruction, sleeve resections, bronchoplasty, lobectomy, pneumonectomy, and even re-transplantation have all been described. As one can imagine, this comes at a cost of considerable morbidity and mortality.

Necrosis and Dehiscence

Whether isolated at the anastomotic line or extending from it, some necrosis is seen almost universally after transplant. Since this finding is so common, it is often not referred to as a complication, but rather part of the normal healing process. Necrotic changes are typically seen early in the healing process characteristically between weeks 1 and 5. The necrotic area is often circumferential, originating at the anastomosis and can extend into lobar or even segmental bronchi (Fig. 16.4a, b). This finding peaks early on and resolves quickly in most cases as the airway will either heal or progress to frank dehiscence. Bronchial necrosis and subsequent dehiscence can thus be viewed as a continuum from the normal to the catastrophic [10, 83] (Fig. 16.5).

Fig. 16.4 a Mild necrosis at
the left mainstem bronchial
anastomosis. **b** Right
mainstem and Bronchus
Intermedius showing severe
necrosis

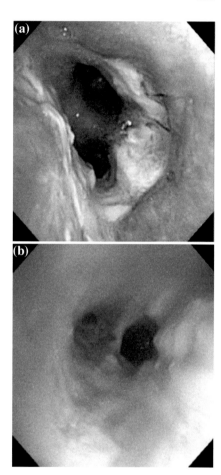

While necrosis is commonplace, dehiscence is seen much less often with commonly reported incidences between 1 and 10 % [84], though a single report describes this finding in as many as 24 % of airways, again likely owing to the variance in reporting [16].

Though much is still not known of the inciting events leading to necrosis and dehiscence, it is likely that ischemia and infection play major roles in the most severe cases. Significant morbidity and mortality can be attributed to a frankly dehiscing airway. This devastating complication may still arise despite the most meticulous surgical techniques and uneventful postoperative course. A key to preventing the disastrous event may be early diagnosis and this is best realized by always considering the diagnosis.

This is particularly important in any lung transplant patient with a prolonged air leak, pneumothorax, or pneumomediastinum. Overt dehiscence is a diagnostic challenge as many of the signs or symptoms of dehiscence are commonly seen in the post-transplant period due to other more common complications. A chest

Fig. 16.5 a This is an
example of minimal focal
breakdown; this is likely to
heal without intervention.
b This image shows a
complete dehiscence which
will require either stenting or
a repeat operation

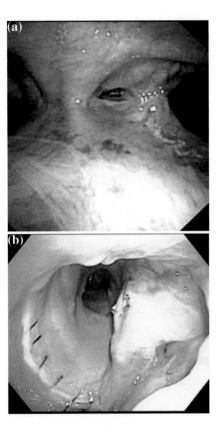

roentgenogram is crude but may intimate dehiscence by a pneumothorax or pneumomediastinum, while a chest CT has higher sensitivity and specificity [85].

A CT scan may show dehiscence as evidenced by peribronchial air. Although this is not uncommon immediately after a transplant, additional factors may alert one to a dehiscence. In addition to a prolonged air leak, extensive amounts of peribronchial air in conjunction with bronchial wall abnormalities, dissection into the mediastinum, or fascial planes should increase a clinician's concern [86–88].

The gold standard for diagnosis is bronchoscopy, as radiographic studies cannot reliably image the mucosa. In the setting of severe necrosis, it may be difficult to see the actual site of dehiscence; however, there are a number of clues seen endoscopically. Significant necrosis and loose sutures can be evidenced that the anastomosis is at risk, presently dehiscing or already dehisced. Ultimately the management of dehiscence will vary based on its severity. The most severe cases may require an open surgical repair, flap bronchoplasty, or even re-transplantation, though quite risky with less than ideal results [23].

No intervention, except close observation is typically required for grades I and II bronchial dehiscence though antibiotic regimens, including inhaled delivery methods may be practical. Fortunately, grades III and IV bronchial dehiscence are not common, approximately 1.6 % in our experience, as they can have devastating complications. Most patients with grade III or IV dehiscence eventually develop infection and this is the usual source of mortality. The severity of the dehiscence and its clinical impact will dictate the management. Both bronchoscopic and surgical techniques exist for the treatment, though more invasive approaches are fraught with a high morbidity and mortality. Surgical options for repair include re-anastomosis, a flap bronchoplasty, or in severe cases a re-transplantation [23].

Bronchoscopic techniques described include cyanoacrylate glue, growth factors, and autologous platelet-derived factors. Although some reports have been successful, the general impression in these techniques is lacking [89].

Utilizing the temporary placement of non-covered SEMS, our institution has described a novel bronchoscopic approach for grades III and IV dehiscence. This technique utilizes the propensity to cause granulation tissue, a well-known complication of SEMS as an advantage. Once airway patency is optimized with gently dilation and/or debulking, a non-covered SEMS is deployed in the airway covering the dehiscence and closely followed. Healing may be appreciated in as little as one week with a removal/replacement occurring once epithelialization/granulation tissue develops, typically within a few weeks. Several cycles of this technique have demonstrated healing of the bronchial wall. In our experience 37.5 days was the mean time to removal [83].

Incumbent in this technique is expertise not only in placing but also (and possibly more importantly) in the removal of the SEMS. Improper stent placement or manipulation can easily extend the airway injury as can an over-aggressive removal, so great care must be taken. Complications such as stenosis and malacia are more frequently encountered even if the dehiscence is successfully closed. Continue close surveillance is recommended.

Exophytic Granulation Tissue

In about 7–24 % of lung transplant patients, benign hyperplastic endoluminal granulation tissue may cause significant airway obstruction [90]. Typically occurs at the anastomotic site few months after transplantation [57].

The etiology of the formation of the hyperplastic tissue may be related to ischemia and inflammation with a subsequent remodeling process [57, 91]. Similar to keloid reactions, exaggerated immune response may be present. Anastomotic infections, especially Aspergillus, may intensify its formation [22]. Also, therapeutic interventions, such as airway stenting, promote the formation of granulation tissue [83, 91]. After stent placement, the estimated incidence of granulation tissue formation is about 12–36 % [66, 92]. The incidence of granulation tissue formation related to airway stents has been described to be less in post-transplant patients, theoretically related to the immunosuppressant medications used [93].

Depending upon the degree of airway obstruction, excessive granulation tissue formation may present with progressive dyspnea, cough, hypoxia, hemoptysis, decreased secretions clearance, or post-obstructive pneumonia [1, 57]. Decreasing spirometry values may be seen. Chest CT may show the obstructive granulation tissue at the bronchi that is typically confirmed by direct visualization of the airway.

Its management requires a multidisciplinary approach, and often multiple procedures are needed due to its tendency to recur. Debridement is the management of choice. Based on the amount of granulation tissue, the degree of obstruction, and the location, several techniques for debridement may be used including forceps (flexible or rigid), cryotherapy, APC, electrocautery, or laser [1, 12, 92, 94, 95].

Cryotherapy, APC, and laser techniques have been described elsewhere and are beyond the scope of this chapter. Cryotherapy advantages are the safety profile, the cryo-sensitivity of granulation tissue, its excellent hemostasis, and the ability of using high oxygen concentrations. Cryotherapy causes cell lysis due to cellular crystallization. Although historically described its use as a delayed effect, cryoablation of endobronchial tissue with cryo-recanalization an immediate result may be employed [96]. Furthermore, cryotherapy may be used around granulation tissue in silicone stents without the risk of ignition. APC, electrocautery, and Nd:YAG laser have also been described successfully for granulation tissue management after lung transplantation.

Despite the above methods, recurrence is common and difficult to treat. Retrospectives studies have shown the use of high-dose-rate endobronchial brachytherapy (HDR-EB) for recalcitrant cases. By using Iridium-192, a high dose of conformal dose of ionizing radiation is used to treat excessive granulation tissue at the anastomosis and related to endobronchial stents, while minimizing radiation exposure to the surrounding structures [57, 91]. Serious and fatal complications, such as massive hemoptysis, have been described with HDR-EB, and extreme caution must be used when considering this approach [76].

Approaches to prevent the formation of granulation tissue have been used. Specifically, topical Mitomycin-C may be applied to reduce the proliferation of granulation tissue due to its ability to inhibit the proliferation of fibroblast [97, 98]. The antineoplastic agent is applied at the airway after granulation tissue debridement by any of the above-mentioned methods to reduce its recurrence [98, 99]. A dose from 0.5 to 1 mg/mL may be used via pledget and swabbed to the area for few minutes [76]. Randomized trials are lacking, however, given its safety profile and potential advantages; is frequently used.

Tracheobronchomalacia

Tracheomalacia or bronchomalacia has been defined as a luminal narrowing of 50 % or more on expiration [61]. The diameter reduction may be related to the loss of cartilaginous support or due to excessive dynamic airway collapse. It may be seen after lung transplantation diffusely, at the anastomotic site or associated with bronchial stenosis. Pathological airway cartilage changes have been described, but its pathophysiology is poorly understood. The cartilage may be damaged by peri-transplant ischemia or infections.

Signs and symptoms include cough, dyspnea, recurrent infections, wheezing, and the inability to clear secretions. A common "barking" cough has been described. Reductions in the FEV1, forced expiratory flow at 25–75 %, and a low peak expiratory flow rate may be encountered. The flow-volume loops may show a variable obstruction, more marked during expiration. Bronchoscopic airway examination is the gold standard for diagnosis; however, a dynamic CT of the chest may suggest the process [51, 61, 74].

Tracheobronchomalacia management is a therapeutic dilemma. The intervention will depend on the severity of its presentation. Most of the recommendations are extrapolated from non-transplant-related malacia. Medical management includes pulmonary hygiene, mucolytics, and noninvasive positive pressure ventilation (NIPPV) [1, 100]. In cases with severe functional impairment and symptomatology despite medical interventions, airway stenting may be used. The stent will allow restoring and maintaining airway patency, improving secretion clearance and infection improvement. Small studies have shown that stent placement for transplant-related bronchomalacia improves spirometry values [56]. Silicone stents are preferred, and once deployed, close surveillance is needed. Rarely, after all other alternatives have been exhausted, a SEMS may be used, taking into consideration the concerns about metallic stents and benign diseases [76] (Fig. 16.6).

Fistulas

Airway fistulas after lung transplantation are uncommon, but a very challenging complication to treat. Fistulas can develop between the airway and the pleura, mediastinum, aorta, pulmonary arteries, and the left atrium 1 [101–106]. Fortunately, this complication is quite rare.

A bronchopleural fistula is rarely seen and it is probably related to bronchial ischemia. It is associated with high morbidity and mortality and typically occurs early in the postoperative period. It may present as dyspnea, hypotension, sepsis, and pneumothorax including tension, subcutaneous emphysema, or persistent air leaks. It is usually encountered in the setting of dehiscence. Initial management includes infection control with antibiotics and thoracostomy drainage. Endoscopic closure of the fistula may attempt, as the initial choice and usually, the success depends on the size and location. Endoscopic techniques include cyanoacrylate glue, fibrinogen plus thrombin, or bronchial stents. Also, intrabronchial one-way valves may be an option. Surgical options include flaps, open drainage, or thoracoplasty [1, 76, 100].

A bronchomediastinal fistula with or without dehiscence has a high mortality rate due to sepsis [2]. The presentation may be as bacteremia, sepsis, mediastinitis,

Fig. 16.6 a Demonstrates
malacia of the left mainstem
bronchus (*LMSB*). **b** Shows a
modified silicone stent in the
LMSB of the same patient

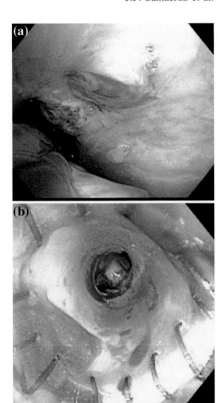

mediastinal abscess, or cavitation. The fistula usually develops anastomosis site, but
may occur at any place in the airway.

Bronchovascular fistulas are very rare and associated with high mortality.
A minor premonitory hemoptysis episode may be seen, followed by a fatal bleed.
A fistula should be suspected in the cases of infectious complications (Aspergillus)
combined with moderate hemoptysis [1, 76, 107]. In addition to hemoptysis, air
embolism and sepsis have been described [100, 108]. Its management literature is
limited to the case reports of pneumonectomy and bilobectomy.

Anastomotic Infections

In lung transplantation, the susceptibility to infections is determined by various
factors, including the degree of immunosuppression, use of steroids, airway anatomy, ischemic complications, sutures misfortunes, impaired mucociliary function,
altered phagocytosis in alveolar macrophages, interrupted lymphatic drainage,
direct communication of the lungs with the atmosphere, and the lack of

tracheobronchial cough reflex due to organ denervation [109, 110]. Furthermore, the allograft is exposed not only to the external environment, but also to the flora of the native and donor's airways [111]. Also, many patients even in the pretransplant period are already colonized with multidrug-resistant organisms.

Overall infections are common after lung transplantation. An incidence of 34–59 % has been described and is significantly higher when compared to other solid organ transplants [112]. Bacterial and fungal infections are most frequently seen in the first month after transplant, while viral infections are more common in the second and third postoperative months [112]. Bacterial pneumonia is the most common infection in lung transplant recipients. About 75 % of lung transplant patients will developed a bacterial infection within 3 months after transplantation [110].

Endobronchial infections are common as well, and usually opportunistic infections are involved. The infection may involve the entire airway, such as bronchitis or tracheitis, or involve the anastomosis area. Pseudomonas and Staphylococcus are the most frequently acquired bacterial infections [1, 113]. Saprophytic fungal organisms are also quite common. Aspergillus is the most frequently involved. Other reported fungal organisms include Cladosporium, Candida, Zygomycetes (mucormycosis), and Scedosporium species.

Aspergillus colonizes about 20 % of lung transplant patients in the immediate postoperative period. Clinically, Aspergillus infection post-transplant may present as invasive pulmonary aspergillosis, colonization, or tracheobronchitis, and precise diagnosis of these syndromes can be very difficult [114]. Locally invasive or disseminated Aspergillus infection accounts for 2–33 % of infections following lung transplantation and have a high reported mortality. Airway colonization with Aspergillus fumigatus in the first 6-month post-transplant has a 11-fold increase risk to develop invasive disease [110]. Aspergillus also is associated with an ulcerative tracheobronchitis that can lead to anastomotic dehiscence [110]. Anastomotic complications are more common in patients with Aspergillus infection [114, 115].

Anastomotic infections represent an airway complication and may predispose to all the other AC as well. The mechanisms are not well understood, but infection may lead to dehiscence, fistula formation, stenosis, and granulation tissue formation and if it invades directly the bronchial wall to airway collapse and malacia.

Diagnosis of anastomotic infections is usually done at bronchoscopy. The infections tend to be relatively asymptomatic, although some patients may complain of fever, cough, secretions, wheezing, and/or hemoptysis. At bronchoscopic exam airway erythema, ulceration and pseudo-membranes may be seen. Positive cultures are vital, to identify the organism and tailor treatment, especially in fungal etiologies.

Treatment includes bronchoscopic debridement of devitalized tissue and antibiotic therapy. With regard to fungal infections, given the potential consequences of Aspergillus colonization or infection, prevention is a key. In the first 6-month post-transplant, most programs routinely use antifungal prophylaxis. Voriconazole, itraconazole, and inhaled amphotericin-B formulas are the most commonly used chemotherapy agents [114, 115]. Stent placement in the presence of infection is not recommended, despite reports of such use in aspergillus infection-related AC [116].

Management Summary

Management of AC is complicated. Many modalities are available and which is optimal may not be clear, as no randomized trials exist to direct the clinician. The optimal management is a multidisciplinary approach performed by individuals experienced in not only the techniques discussed but also the nuances of a post-transplant patient.

Bronchial Artery Revascularization

As previously discussed, routine lung transplantation does not restore the bronchial artery supply posing a unique problem in this population. An attempt to improve this process was developed and studied. Allowing the anastomosis of bronchial arteries and preservation of blood flow to the airways showed early promising results. BAR has been described as a successful alternative in small series [117–120]. In the largest series of BAR to date, a single institution demonstrated improved survival over sequential bilateral lung transplantation [121, 122].

The BAR procedure has been described in detail in the referenced articles; however, a brief summary has merit in this review. During BAR, the donor lungs are procured en bloc via sternotomy, including both the esophagus and the descending aorta, thus securing inclusion of the retroesophageal right intercostobronchial artery. One internal thoracic artery is harvested. When double-lung transplantation is performed, cardiopulmonary bypass (CPB) is utilized with a tracheal anastomosis. For the en bloc transplants, BAR anastomoses are performed first, followed by the trachea, pulmonary trunk, and left atrium. The internal thoracic artery is then anastomosed to at least 1 bronchial artery ostia in the donor descending aorta. Single-lung transplantation is not performed on CPB and the bronchial anastomosis occurs at the secondary carina, as in non-BAR transplants and is the final anastomosis after giving 10,000 IU of heparin and pulmonary artery reperfusion [117, 118, 123–128].

This technique was recently re-addressed at our institution. The vascular re-anastomosis was successful in 26 of 27 patients. This pilot showed that this technique was feasible, associated with less airway ischemia, and required no airway interventions. A higher risk of bleeding was found, but safety was comparable between BAR and non-BAR patients. Additional findings that may show future relevance included less early rejection, fewer infections, and delay of BOS. While these findings are encouraging, a multicenter study will be needed to firmly establish these benefits [129].

Future Directions

Biodegradable stent placement is an attractive strategy, and in theory addresses issues with SEMS such as timing of removal, risk involved with removal of metallic stents, migration, stent fracture, inability to customize metallic stents, and infection [77, 130]. Feasibility of such a study has been demonstrated in a case series of 6 patients as described above [77]. The indications for the use of biodegradable stents included non-anastomotic necrosis, grade III–IV malacia, and anastomotic stenosis. Although larger studies are needed to confirm safety and efficacy, and determine infection rates, this approach, at least in theory, may be particularly useful in anastomotic stenosis and dehiscence.

Paclitaxel-coated balloon (PCB) dilation of non-anastomotic airway stenosis has been recently described [131]. In this proof of concept cohort study, 12 patients with non-anastomotic airway stenosis underwent PCB bronchoplasty following recurrence of stenosis after standard measure such as balloon dilation, APC, and stent placement. 8/12 (75 %) patients remained intervention-free at 90-day follow-up. 2 patients required repeat PCB dilation and both remained intervention-free at 90-day follow-up. 5/10 (50 %) of the lesions remained intervention-free at 180-day follow-up. One patient developed pneumothorax requiring hospitalization for 4 days. One patient died of unrelated sepsis 70 days after PCB. This study demonstrates the feasibility of the concept already success-fully used in coronary angioplasty and may well gain popularity provided further studies validate the above findings.

A seemingly far-fetched strategy in post-lung-transplant AC, yet a potentially exciting approach is tissue-engineered airway transplantation [132]. This may be potentially useful in large airway fistulas that need definitive repair of the airway defect. Although the first successful tissue-engineered tracheal transplant was performed for tracheomalacia (non-lung transplant patient), the approach may well be an option for transplant-related AC. Recently, 5-year follow-up data for this patient were published, addressing questions about long-term feasibility and safety [133]. A human decellularized matrix of a trachea (obtained from a deceased human donor) was bioengineered with chemotactic and angiogenic properties. The matrix was then implanted into the recipient after in vitro differentiation of epithelial cells and chondrocytes derived from mesenchymal stem cells. Post-lung-transplant air-way defects may be treated in the future with this approach, and one important reason for this is because this patient did not need immunosuppression after about 4 months. The patient developed subglottic stenosis at the anastomosis site requiring balloon dilations and multiple episodes of stent placement. Although now subjected to regular bronchoscopies, the patient's quality of life remains intact. If this technique is to be extrapolated to be used in the management of post-lung-transplant AC, then the potential benefit of placing a tissue graft over fistulas may have to be traded for airway stenosis. However, at this point, the role of stem cell-derived graft in post-lung-transplant AC is purely speculative.

Conclusion

Lung transplant anatomy and the techniques associated with it pose a unique problem in transplantation. Many etiologies may be responsible for causing AC and similarly many techniques are available to deal with these. AC can have a significant impact on the quality of life of the patient post-transplantation. Frequent visits to specialists, interventions, and recurrence of symptoms can be quite frustrating and although bronchoscopic interventions may significantly improve the patient's symptoms and FEV1, these repeated visits and procedures could be troubling, time-consuming, and costly. Many patients who undergo a transplant do so understanding that their survival may not be significantly extended but rather they will have an improved quality of life. The symptoms associated with AC as well as the need for frequent procedures undoubtedly have a detrimental effect on this proposed benefit. The impact on survival may not be obvious. The overall 5-year survival after lung transplantation is approximately 50 %. The early mortality rates are equivalent for patients treated for anastomotic AC and those without complications. There appears to be an increase in late risk beginning at approximately 18 months. In patients who undergo no treatment for their AC, there is a higher early mortality, but their late risk is equivalent to patients who have no AC. Lung transplant patients are varied and complex and so are their complications; this is particularly true relating to AC. Multiple presentations of AC are described and as such a myriad of management strategies may be employed. Different techniques are used due to the differences in the types of complications but many yield a successful outcome. Improvements in many areas such as surgical techniques, peri-procedural and ICU management, immunosuppression, endoscopic treatments, donor, and recipient selection may lead to optimal outcomes. Currently, there are no blinded, randomized control trials demonstrating a superior algorithm of management of AC. The management of each individual complication requires an individualized multidisciplinary approach by a team with considerable expertise and experience. Future studies in this heterogeneous population will hopefully lead to optimal treatment in this complex patient group.

References

1. Santacruz JF, Mehta AC. Airway complications and management after lung transplantation: ischemia, dehiscence, and stenosis. Proc Am Thorac Soc. 2009;6(1):79–93.
2. Shennib H, Massard G. Airway complications in lung transplantation. Ann Thorac Surg. 1994;57(2):506–11.
3. Hasegawa T, Iacono AT, Orons PD, Yousem SA. Segmental nonanastomotic bronchial stenosis after lung transplantation. Ann Thorac Surg. 2000;69(4):1020–4.
4. Schmid RA, Boehler A, Speich R, Frey HR, Russi EW, Weder W. Bronchial anastomotic complications following lung transplantation: still a major cause of morbidity? Eur Respir J. 1997;10(12):2872–5.

5. Wildevuur CR, Benfield JR. A review of 23 human lung transplantations by 20 surgeons. Ann Thorac Surg. 1970;9(6):489–515.
6. Kapoor BS, May B, Panu N, Kowalik K, Hunter DW. Endobronchial stent placement for the management of airway complications after lung transplantation. J Vasc Interv Radiol JVIR. 2007;18(5):629–32.
7. Shah SS, Karnak D, Minai O, Budev MM, Mason D, Murthy S, et al. Symptomatic narrowing or atresia of bronchus intermedius following lung transplantation vanishing bronchus intermedius syndrome (vbis). CHEST J. 2006;130(4_MeetingAbstracts):236S-a-236S (October 1).
8. Samano MN, Minamoto H, Junqueira JJ, et al. Bronchial complications following lung transplantation. Transpl Proc. 2009;41(3):921–6.
9. Van De Wauwer C, Van Raemdonck D, Verleden GM, et al. Risk factors for airway complications within the first year after lung transplantation. Eur J Cardio-thorac Surg Off J Eur Assoc Cardio-Thorac Surg. 2007;31(4):703–10.
10. Murthy SC, Blackstone EH, Gildea TR et al. Impact of anastomotic airway complications after lung transplantation. Ann Thorac Surg. 2007;84(2):401–9, 409.e1-4.
11. Herrera JM, McNeil KD, Higgins RS et al. Airway complications after lung transplantation: treatment and long-term outcome. Ann Thorac Surg. 2001;71(3):989–93 (discussion 993-4).
12. Kaditis AG, Gondor M, Nixon PA, et al. Airway complications following pediatric lung and heart-lung transplantation. Am J Respir Crit Care Med. 2000;162(1):301–9.
13. Shofer SL, Wahidi MM, Davis WA, et al. Significance of and risk factors for the development of central airway stenosis after lung transplantation. Am J Transplant Off J Am Soc Transplant Am Soc Transplant Surg. 2013;13(2):383–9.
14. Dutau H, Vandemoortele T, Laroumagne S, et al. A new endoscopic standardized grading system for macroscopic central airway complications following lung transplantation: the MDS classification. Eur J Cardio-thorac Surg Off J Eur Assoc Cardio-Thorac Surg. 2014;45 (2):e33–8.
15. Meyers BF, de la Morena M, Sweet SC, et al. Primary graft dysfunction and other selected complications of lung transplantation: a single-center experience of 983 patients. J Thorac Cardiovasc Surg. 2005;129(6):1421–9.
16. Garfein ES, McGregor CC, Galantowicz ME, Schulman LL. Deleterious effects of telescoped bronchial anastomosis in single and bilateral lung transplantation. Ann Transplant Q Polish Transplant Soc. 2000;5(1):5–11.
17. Schroder C, Scholl F, Daon E, et al. A modified bronchial anastomosis technique for lung transplantation. Ann Thorac Surg. 2003;75(6):1697–704.
18. Alvarez A, Algar J, Santos F, et al. Airway complications after lung transplantation: a review of 151 anastomoses. Eur J Cardio-thorac Surg Off J Eur Assoc Cardio-Thorac Surg. 2001;19 (4):381–7.
19. Mason DP, Brown CR, Murthy SC et al. Growing single-center experience with lung transplantation using donation after cardiac death. Ann Thorac Surg. 2012;94(2):406–11 (discussion 411-2).
20. De Oliveira NC, Osaki S, Maloney JD, et al. Lung transplantation with donation after cardiac death donors: long-term follow-up in a single center. J Thorac Cardiovasc Surg. 2010;139 (5):1306–15.
21. Ruttmann E, Ulmer H, Marchese M, et al. Evaluation of factors damaging the bronchial wall in lung transplantation. J Heart Lung Transplant Off Publ Int Soc Heart Transplant. 2005;24 (3):275–81.
22. Mulligan MS. Endoscopic management of airway complications after lung transplantation. Chest Surg Clin N Am. 2001;11(4):907–15.
23. Kshettry VR, Kroshus TJ, Hertz MI, Hunter DW, Shumway SJ, Bolman RM 3rd. Early and late airway complications after lung transplantation: incidence and management. Ann Thorac Surg. 1997;63(6):1576–83.
24. Murthy SC, Gildea TR, Machuzak MS. Anastomotic airway complications after lung transplantation. Curr Opin Organ Transplan. 2010;15(5):582–7.

25. Schafers HJ, Wagner TO, Demertzis S, et al. Preoperative corticosteroids. A contraindication to lung transplantation? Chest. 1992;102(5):1522–5.

26. Colquhoun IW, Gascoigne AD, Au J, Corris PA, Hilton CJ, Dark JH. Airway complications after pulmonary transplantation. Ann Thorac Surg. 1994;57(1):141–5.

27. Schafers HJ, Haverich A, Wagner TO, Wahlers T, Alken A and Borst HG. Decreased incidence of bronchial complications following lung transplantation. Eur J Cardio-thorac Surg Off J Eur Assoc Cardio-Thorac Surg. 1992;6(4):174–8 (discussion 179).

28. Groetzner J, Kur F, Spelsberg F, et al. Airway anastomosis complications in de novo lung transplantation with sirolimus-based immunosuppression. J Heart Lung Transplant Off Publ Int Soc Heart Transplant. 2004;23(5):632–8.

29. Date H, Trulock EP, Arcidi JM, Sundaresan S, Cooper JD and Patterson GA. Improved airway healing after lung transplantation. An analysis of 348 bronchial anastomoses. J Thorac Cardiovasc Surg. 1995;110(5):1424–32 (discussion 1432-3).

30. Khaghani A, Tadjkarimi S, al-Kattan K et al. Wrapping the anastomosis with omentum or an internal mammary artery pedicle does not improve bronchial healing after single lung transplantation: results of a randomized clinical trial. J Heart Lung Transplant Off Publ Int Soc Heart Transplant. 1994;13(5):767–773.

31. Griffith BP, Magee MJ, Gonzalez IF et al. Anastomotic pitfalls in lung transplantation. J Thorac Cardiovasc Surg. 1994;107(3):743–53; discussion 753-4.

32. Garfein ES, Ginsberg ME, Gorenstein L, McGregor CC, Schulman LL. Superiority of end-to-end versus telescoped bronchial anastomosis in single lung transplantation for pulmonary emphysema. J Thorac Cardiovasc Surg. 2001;121(1):149–54.

33. Choong CK, Sweet SC, Zoole JB, et al. Bronchial airway anastomotic complications after pediatric lung transplantation: incidence, cause, management, and outcome. J Thorac Cardiovasc Surg. 2006;131(1):198–203.

34. Davis RD Jr, Pasque MK. Pulmonary transplantation. Ann Surg. 1995;221(1):14–28.

35. de Pablo A, Lopez S, Ussetti P, et al. Lung transplant therapy for suppurative diseases. Arch Bronconeumol. 2005;41(5):255–9.

36. Bloom RD, Goldberg LR, Wang AY, Faust TW and Kotloff RM. An overview of solid organ transplantation. Clinics in chest medicine. 2005;26(4):529–43, v.

37. Park SJ, Nguyen DQ, Savik K, Hertz MI and Bolman RM, 3rd. Pre-transplant corticosteroid use and outcome in lung transplantation. J Heart Lung Transplant Off Publ Int Soc Heart Transplant. 2001;20(3):304–309.

38. McAnally KJ, Valentine VG, LaPlace SG, McFadden PM, Seoane L, Taylor DE. Effect of pre-transplantation prednisone on survival after lung transplantation. J Heart Lung Transplant Off Publ Int Soc Heart Transplant. 2006;25(1):67–74.

39. King-Biggs MB, Dunitz JM, Park SJ, Kay Savik S, Hertz MI. Airway anastomotic dehiscence associated with use of sirolimus immediately after lung transplantation. Transplantation. 2003;75(9):1437–43.

40. Yokomise H, Cardoso PF, Kato H, et al. The effect of pulmonary arterial flow and positive end-expiratory pressure on retrograde bronchial mucosal blood flow. J Thorac Cardiovasc Surg. 1991;101(2):201–8.

41. Porhownik NR. Airway complications post lung transplantation. Curr Opin Pulm Med. 2013;19(2):174–80.

42. Eberlein M, Arnaoutakis GJ, Yarmus L, et al. The effect of lung size mismatch on complications and resource utilization after bilateral lung transplantation. J Heart Lung Transplant Off Publ Int Soc Heart Transplant. 2012;31(5):492–500.

43. Lonchyna VA, Arcidi JM,Jr, Garrity ER,Jr et al. Refractory post-transplant airway strictures: successful management with wire stents. Eur J Cardio-thorac Surg Off J Eur Assoc Cardio-Thorac Surg. 1999;15(6):842–9; discussion 849-50.

44. Christie JD, Carby M, Bag R, et al. Report of the ISHLT Working Group on Primary Lung Graft Dysfunction part II: definition. A consensus statement of the International Society for Heart and Lung Transplantation. J Heart Lung Transplant Off Publ Int Soc Heart Transplant. 2005;24(10):1454–9.

45. Couraud L, Nashef SA, Nicolini P, Jougon J. Classification of airway anastomotic healing. Eur J Cardio-thorac Surg Off J Eur Assoc Cardio-Thorac Surg. 1992;6(9):496–7.
46. Thistlethwaite PA, Yung G, Kemp A, et al. Airway stenoses after lung transplantation: incidence, management, and outcome. J Thorac Cardiovasc Surg. 2008;136(6):1569–75.
47. De Gracia J, Culebras M, Alvarez A, et al. Bronchoscopic balloon dilatation in the management of bronchial stenosis following lung transplantation. Respir Med. 2007;101 (1):27–33.
48. Marulli G, Loy M, Rizzardi G, et al. Surgical treatment of posttransplant bronchial stenoses: case reports. Transpl Proc. 2007;39(6):1973–5.
49. Castleberry AW, Worni M, Kuchibhatla M et al. A comparative analysis of bronchial stricture after lung transplantation in recipients with and without early acute rejection. Ann Thorac Surg. 2013;96(3):1008–17 (discussion 1017-8).
50. Souilamas R, Wermert D, Guillemain R, et al. Uncommon combined treatment of nonanastomotic bronchial stenosis after lung transplantation. J Bronchol Interv Pulmonol. 2008;15(1):54.
51. Krishnam MS, Suh RD, Tomasian A et al. Postoperative complications of lung transplantation: radiologic findings along a time continuum. Radiogr Rev Publ Radiol Soc North Am Inc. 2007;27(4):957–974.
52. Neagos GR, Martinez FJ, Deeb GM, Wahl RL, Orringer MB and Lynch JP, 3rd. Diagnosis of unilateral mainstem bronchial obstruction following single-lung transplantation with routine spirometry. Chest. 1993;103(4):1255–1258.
53. Anzueto A, Levine SM, Tillis WP, Calhoon JH, Bryan CL. Use of the flow-volume loop in the diagnosis of bronchial stenosis after single lung transplantation. Chest. 1994;105(3):934–6.
54. Garg K, Zamora MR, Tuder R. Armstrong JD,2nd and Lynch DA. Lung transplantation: indications, donor and recipient selection, and imaging of complications. Radiogr Rev Publ Radiol Soc North Am Inc. 1996;16(2):355–67.
55. Quint LE, Whyte RI, Kazerooni EA, et al. Stenosis of the central airways: evaluation by using helical CT with multiplanar reconstructions. Radiology. 1995;194(3):871–7.
56. Chhajed PN, Malouf MA, Tamm M, Spratt P, Glanville AR. Interventional bronchoscopy for the management of airway complications following lung transplantation. Chest. 2001;120 (6):1894–9.
57. Tendulkar RD, Fleming PA, Reddy CA, Gildea TR, Machuzak M, Mehta AC. High-dose-rate endobronchial brachytherapy for recurrent airway obstruction from hyperplastic granulation tissue. Int J Radiat Oncol Biol Phys. 2008;70(3):701–6.
58. Mayse ML, Greenheck J, Friedman M, Kovitz KL. Successful bronchoscopic balloon dilation of nonmalignant tracheobronchial obstruction without fluoroscopy. Chest. 2004;126 (2):634–7.
59. Mathur PN, Wolf KM, Busk MF, Briete WM, Datzman M. Fiberoptic bronchoscopic cryotherapy in the management of tracheobronchial obstruction. Chest. 1996;110(3):718–23.
60. McArdle J, Gildea T, Mehta A. Balloon bronchoplasty: Its indications, benefits, and complications. J Bronchol Interv Pulmonol. 2005;12(2):123–7.
61. Simoff M, Sterman D and Ernst A. Thoracic endoscopy. advances in interventional pulmonology. Malden: Wiley-Blackwell; 2006:376.
62. Dutau H, Vandemoortele T, Breen DP. Rigid bronchoscopy. Clin Chest Med. 2013;34 (3):427–35.
63. Tremblay A, Coulter T and Mehta A. Modification of a mucosal-sparing technique using electrocautery and balloon dilatation in the endoscopic management of web-like benign airway stenosis. J Bronchol Interv Pulmonol 2003;10(4):268–271.
64. Verhaeghe W, Noppen M, Meysman M, Monsieur I, Vincken W. Rapid healing of endobronchial tuberculosis by local endoscopic injection of corticosteroids. Monaldi archives for chest disease=Archivio Monaldi per le malattie del torace / Fondazione clinica del lavoro, IRCCS [and] Istituto di clinica tisiologica e malattie apparato respiratorio, Universita di Napoli, Secondo ateneo. 1996;51(5):391–393.

65. Cosano-Povedano J, Muñoz-Cabrera L, Jurado-Gámez B, Fernández-Marín M, Cobos-Ceballos M, Cosano-Povedano A. Topical mitomycin C for recurrent bronchial stenosis after lung transplantation: a report of 2 cases. J Bronchol Interv Pulmonol. 2008;15 (4):281–3.

66. Saad CP, Ghamande SA, Minai OA, et al. The role of self-expandable metallic stents for the treatment of airway complications after lung transplantation. Transplantation. 2003;75 (9):1532–8.

67. Bolliger CT, Sutedja TG, Strausz J, Freitag L. Therapeutic bronchoscopy with immediate effect: laser, electrocautery, argon plasma coagulation and stents. Eur Respir J. 2006;27 (6):1258–71.

68. Grosu HB, Eapen GA, Morice RC, et al. Stents are associated with increased risk of respiratory infections in patients undergoing airway interventions for malignant airways disease. Chest. 2013;144(2):441–9.

69. Doyle DJ, Abdelmalak B, Machuzak M, Gildea TR. Anesthesia and airway management for removing pulmonary self-expanding metallic stents. J Clin Anesth. 2009;21(7):529–32.

70. Murthy SC, Gildea TR, Mehta AC. Removal of self-expandable metallic stents: is it possible? Semin Respir Crit Care Med. 2004;25(4):381–5.

71. Lunn W, Feller-Kopman D, Wahidi M, Ashiku S, Thurer R, Ernst A. Endoscopic removal of metallic airway stents. Chest. 2005;127(6):2106–12.

72. Fernandez-Bussy S, Akindipe O, Kulkarni V, Swafford W, Baz M, Jantz MA. Clinical experience with a new removable tracheobronchial stent in the management of airway complications after lung transplantation. J Heart Lung Transplant Off Publ Int Soc Heart Transplant. 2009;28(7):683–8.

73. Madden BP, Loke TK, Sheth AC. Do expandable metallic airway stents have a role in the management of patients with benign tracheobronchial disease? Ann Thorac Surg. 2006;82 (1):274–8.

74. Murgu SD, Colt HG. Complications of silicone stent insertion in patients with expiratory central airway collapse. Ann Thorac Surg. 2007;84(6):1870–7.

75. Gildea TR, Murthy SC, Sahoo D, Mason DP, Mehta AC. Performance of a self-expanding silicone stent in palliation of benign airway conditions. Chest. 2006;130(5):1419–23.

76. Machuzak M. Principles and practice of interventional pulmonology. In: Ernst A, Herth F, editors. Management of posttrasnplant disorders. Springer: New York; 2013. p. 463.

77. Lischke R, Pozniak J, Vondrys D, Elliott MJ. Novel biodegradable stents in the treatment of bronchial stenosis after lung transplantation. Eur J Cardio-thorac Surg Off J Eur Assoc Cardio-Thorac Surg. 2011;40(3):619–24.

78. Alraiyes AH, Machuzak MS, Gildea TR. Intussusception technique of intrabronchial silicone stents: description of technique and a case report. J Bronchol Interv Pulmonol. 2013;20 (4):342–4.

79. Lari SM, Gonin F and Colchen A. The management of bronchus intermedius complications after lung transplantation: a retrospective study. J Cardiothorac Surg. 2012;7:8–8090-7-8.

80. Sundset A, Lund MB, Hansen G, Bjortuft O, Kongerud J, Geiran OR. Airway complications after lung transplantation: long-term outcome of silicone stenting. Respir Int Rev Thorac Dis. 2012;83(3):245–52.

81. Wang K, Mehta A, Turner J. Flexible bronchoscopy. 2nd ed. Malden: Blackwell Publishing; 2004.

82. Dutau H, Cavailles A, Sakr L, et al. A retrospective study of silicone stent placement for management of anastomotic airway complications in lung transplant recipients: short- and long-term outcomes. J Heart Lung Transplant Off Publ Int Soc Heart Transplant. 2010;29 (6):658–64.

83. Mughal MM, Gildea TR, Murthy S, Pettersson G, DeCamp M, Mehta AC. Short-term deployment of self-expanding metallic stents facilitates healing of bronchial dehiscence. Am J Respir Crit Care Med. 2005;172(6):768–71.

84. Usuda K, Gildea T, Pandya C, Mehta A. Bronchial dehiscence. J Bronchol Interv Pulmonol. 2005;12(3):164–5.

85. Herman SJ, Weisbrod GL, Weisbrod L, Patterson GA, Maurer JR. Chest radiographic findings after bilateral lung transplantation. AJR Am J Roentgenol. 1989;153(6):1181–5.
86. Semenkovich JW, Glazer HS, Anderson DC, Arcidi JM Jr, Cooper JD, Patterson GA. Bronchial dehiscence in lung transplantation: CT evaluation. Radiology. 1995;194(1):205–8.
87. O'Donovan PB. Imaging of complications of lung transplantation. Radiogr Rev Publ Radiol Soc North Am, Inc. 1993;13(4):787–796.
88. Schlueter FJ, Semenkovich JW, Glazer HS, Arcidi JM Jr, Trulock EP, Patterson GA. Bronchial dehiscence after lung transplantation: correlation of CT findings with clinical outcome. Radiology. 1996;199(3):849–54.
89. Maloney JD, Weigel TL, Love RB. Endoscopic repair of bronchial dehiscence after lung transplantation. Ann Thorac Surg. 2001;72(6):2109–11.
90. Meyer A, Warszawski-Baumann A, Baumann R et al. HDR brachytherapy: an option for preventing nonmalignant obstruction in patients after lung transplantation. Strahlentherapie und Onkologie: Organ der Deutschen Rontgengesellschaft … 2012;188(12):1085–1090.
91. Kennedy AS, Sonett JR, Orens JB, King K. High dose rate brachytherapy to prevent recurrent benign hyperplasia in lung transplant bronchi: theoretical and clinical considerations. J Heart Lung Transplant Off Publ Int Soc Heart Transplant. 2000;19(2):155–9.
92. Madden BP, Kumar P, Sayer R, Murday A. Successful resection of obstructing airway granulation tissue following lung transplantation using endobronchial laser (Nd:YAG) therapy. Eur J Cardio-thorac Surg Off J Eur Assoc Cardio-Thorac Surg. 1997;12(3):480–5.
93. Redmond J, Diamond J, Dunn J, Cohen GS, Soliman AM. Rigid bronchoscopic management of complications related to endobronchial stents after lung transplantation. Ann Otol Rhinol Laryngol. 2013;122(3):183–9.
94. Maiwand MO, Zehr KJ, Dyke CM, et al. The role of cryotherapy for airway complications after lung and heart-lung transplantation. Eur J Cardio-thorac Surg Off J Eur Assoc Cardio-Thorac Surg. 1997;12(4):549–54.
95. Keller CA, Hinerman R, Singh A, Alvarez F. The use of endoscopic argon plasma coagulation in airway complications after solid organ transplantation. Chest. 2001;119(6):1968–75.
96. Yilmaz A, Aktas Z, Alici IO, Caglar A, Sazak H, Ulus F. Cryorecanalization: keys to success. Surg Endosc. 2012;26(10):2969–74.
97. Ubell ML, Ettema SL, Toohill RJ, Simpson CB, Merati AL. Mitomycin-c application in airway stenosis surgery: analysis of safety and costs. Otolaryngol Head Neck Surg Off J Am Acad Otolaryngol Head Neck Surg. 2006;134(3):403–6.
98. Erard AC, Monnier P, Spiliopoulos A, Nicod L. Mitomycin C for control of recurrent bronchial stenosis: a case report. Chest. 2001;120(6):2103–5.
99. Penafiel A, Lee P, Hsu A, Eng P. Topical mitomycin-C for obstructing endobronchial granuloma. Ann Thorac Surg. 2006;82(3):e22–3.
100. Puchalski J, Lee HJ, Sterman DH. Airway complications following lung transplantation. Clin Chest Med. 2011;32(2):357–66.
101. Chang CC, Hsu HH, Kuo SW, Lee YC. Bronchoscopic gluing for post-lung-transplant bronchopleural fistula. Eur J Cardio-thorac Surg Off J Eur Assoc Cardio-Thorac Surg. 2007;31(2):328–30.
102. Mora G, de Pablo A, Garcia-Gallo CL, et al. Is endoscopic treatment of bronchopleural fistula useful? Arch Bronconeumol. 2006;42(8):394–8.
103. Hoff SJ, Johnson JE, Frist WH. Aortobronchial fistula after unilateral lung transplantation. Ann Thorac Surg. 1993;56(6):1402–3.
104. Karmy-Jones R, Vallieres E, Culver B, Raghu G, Wood DE. Bronchial-atrial fistula after lung transplant resulting in fatal air embolism. Ann Thorac Surg. 1999;67(2):550–1.
105. Rea F, Marulli G, Loy M, et al. Salvage right pneumonectomy in a patient with bronchial-pulmonary artery fistula after bilateral sequential lung transplantation. J Heart Lung Transplant Off Publ Int Soc Heart Transplant. 2006;25(11):1383–6.

106. Guth S, Mayer E, Fischer B, Lill J, Weiler N, Oelert H. Bilobectomy for massive hemoptysis after bilateral lung transplantation. J Thorac Cardiovasc Surg. 2001;121(6):1194–5.
107. Verleden GM, Vos R, van Raemdonck D, Vanaudenaerde B. Pulmonary infection defense after lung transplantation: does airway ischemia play a role? Curr Opin Org Transplant. 2010;15(5):568–71.
108. Knight J, Elwing JM, Milstone A. Bronchovascular fistula formation: a rare airway complication after lung transplantation. J Heart Lung Transplant Off Publ Int Soc Heart Transplant. 2008;27(10):1179–85.
109. Parada MT, Alba A, Sepulveda C. Early and late infections in lung transplantation patients. Transpl Proc. 2010;42(1):333–5.
110. Ahuja J, Kanne JP. Thoracic infections in immunocompromised patients. Radiol Clin North Am. 2014;52(1):121–36.
111. Nunley DR, Gal AA, Vega JD, Perlino C, Smith P, Lawrence EC. Saprophytic fungal infections and complications involving the bronchial anastomosis following human lung transplantation. Chest. 2002;122(4):1185–91.
112. Diez Martinez P, Pakkal M, Prenovault J et al. Postoperative imaging after lung transplantation. Clin Imaging. 2013;37(4):617–623.
113. Shteinberg M, Raviv Y, Bishara J, et al. The impact of fluoroquinolone resistance of Gram-negative bacteria in respiratory secretions on the outcome of lung transplant (non-cystic fibrosis) recipients. Clin Transplant. 2012;26(6):884–90.
114. Felton TW, Roberts SA, Isalska B, et al. Isolation of Aspergillus species from the airway of lung transplant recipients is associated with excess mortality. J Infect. 2012;65(4):350–6.
115. Weder W, Inci I, Korom S et al. Airway complications after lung transplantation: risk factors, prevention and outcome. Eur J Cardio-thorac Surg Off J Eur Assoc Cardio-Thorac Surg. 2009;35(2):293–8 (discussion 298).
116. Xie BX, Zhu YM, Chen C, et al. Outcome of TiNi stent treatments in symptomatic central airway stenoses caused by Aspergillus fumigatus infections after lung transplantation. Transpl Proc. 2013;45(6):2366–70.
117. Couraud L, Baudet E, Martigne C, et al. Bronchial revascularization in double-lung transplantation: a series of 8 patients. Bordeaux Lung and Heart-Lung Transplant Group. Ann Thorac Surg. 1992;53(1):88–94.
118. Couraud L, Baudet E, Nashef SA, et al. Lung transplantation with bronchial revascularisation. Surgical anatomy, operative technique and early results. Eur J Cardio-thorac Surg Off J Eur Assoc Cardio-Thorac Surg. 1992;6(9):490–5.
119. Daly RC, McGregor CG. Routine immediate direct bronchial artery revascularization for single-lung transplantation. Ann Thorac Surg. 1994;57(6):1446–52.
120. Pettersson G, Arendrup H, Mortensen SA, et al. Early experience of double-lung transplantation with bronchial artery revascularization using mammary artery. Eur J Cardio-thorac Surg Off J Eur Assoc Cardio-Thorac Surg. 1994;8(10):520–4.
121. Pettersson G, Norgaard MA, Arendrup H, et al. Direct bronchial artery revascularization and en bloc double lung transplantation–surgical techniques and early outcome. J Heart Lung Transplant Off Publ Int Soc Heart Transplant. 1997;16(3):320–33.
122. Burton CM, Milman N, Carlsen J, et al. The Copenhagen National Lung Transplant Group: survival after single lung, double lung, and heart-lung transplantation. J Heart Lung Transplant Off Publ Int Soc Heart Transplant. 2005;24(11):1834–43.
123. Schreinemakers HH, Weder W, Miyoshi S et al. Direct revascularization of bronchial arteries for lung transplantation: an anatomical study. Ann Thorac Surg 1990;49(1):44–53; discussion 53-4.
124. Laks H, Louie HW, Haas GS, et al. New technique of vascularization of the trachea and bronchus for lung transplantation. J Heart Lung Transplant Off Publ Int Soc Heart Transplant. 1991;10(2):280–7.
125. Dubrez J, Clerc F, Drouillard J, Couraud L. Anatomical bases for bronchial arterial revascularization in double lung transplantation. Ann Chir. 1992;46(2):97–104.

126. Svendsen U, Arendrup H, Norgaard M, et al. Double lung transplantation with bronchial artery revascularization using mammary artery. Transpl Proc. 1995;27(6):3485.
127. Norgaard MA, Olsen PS, Svendsen UG, Pettersson G. Revascularization of the bronchial arteries in lung transplantation: an overview. Ann Thorac Surg. 1996;62(4):1215–21.
128. Pettersson G, Norgaard A, Andersen et al. Lung transplantation, 1999. In: Hetzer R, editor. Lung and heart-lung transplantation with direct bronchial artery revascularization. Darmstadt, Germany: Darmstadt; 2003. p. 51–69.
129. Pettersson GB, Karam K, Thuita L et al. Comparative study of bronchial artery revascularization in lung transplantation. J Thorac Cardiovasc Surg 2013;146(4):894–900.e3.
130. Fuehner T, Suhling H, Greer M, et al. Biodegradable stents after lung transplantation. Transplant Int Off J Eur Soc Org Transplant. 2013;26(7):e58–60.
131. Greer M, Fuehner T, Warnecke G, et al. Paclitaxel-coated balloons in refractory nonanastomostic airway stenosis following lung transplantation. Am J Transplant Off J Am Soc Transplant Am Soc Transplant Surg. 2014;14(10):2400–5.
132. Macchiarini P, Jungebluth P, Go T, et al. Clinical transplantation of a tissue-engineered airway. Lancet. 2008;372(9655):2023–30.
133. Gonfiotti A, Jaus MO, Barale D, et al. The first tissue-engineered airway transplantation: 5-year follow-up results. Lancet. 2014;383(9913):238–44.

Chapter 17
Chronic Cough: An Overview for the Bronchoscopist

Umur Hatipoğlu and Claudio F. Milstein

Chronic Cough: Definition and Etiology

Chronic cough is one of the most common reasons for primary care physician visits and referrals to pulmonologists [1]. Chronic cough, defined as lasting more than 8 weeks, may have diverse and frequently multifactorial etiology (Table 17.1) with significant effect on quality of life. Various pulmonary parenchymal and airway diseases (e.g., interstitial lung disease and bronchiectasis) which present with abnormal chest imaging also have cough as one of the presenting symptoms. In this chapter, we focus on relatively uncommon etiologies of chronic cough related to airway disease which occur in the setting of a normal or near-normal chest X-ray. As such, these conditions are well within the practice realm of the bronchoscopist.

It has been suggested that a systematic approach to chronic cough employing an anatomic diagnostic protocol which includes empirical therapy has an extremely high diagnostic and therapeutic yield [2, 3]. Accordingly, upper airway cough syndrome (postnasal drip), asthma, and reflux disease account for over 80 % of the disorders that lead to chronic cough. In clinical practice, targeted diagnostic evaluation and empirical therapy, without any particular sequence, are used in conjunction with the management of these patients. An optimal cost-effective approach to the management of chronic cough has not been agreed upon. Moreover, recent data from a specialized cough center indicate a different distribution of etiologies for chronic cough, emphasizing the importance of referral bias when considering diagnostic possibilities [4].

U. Hatipoğlu (✉)
Respiratory Institute, Cleveland Clinic, 9500 Euclid Avenue, A-90, Cleveland,
OH 44195, USA
e-mail: hatipou@ccf.org

C.F. Milstein
Head and Neck Institute, Cleveland Clinic, 9500 Euclid Avenue, A-90, Cleveland,
OH 44195, USA

© Springer International Publishing Switzerland 2016   357
A.C. Mehta et al. (eds.), *Diseases of the Central Airways*,
Respiratory Medicine, DOI 10.1007/978-3-319-29830-6_17

Table 17.1 Uncommon reasons for chronic cough

Airway-related cough
Upper airway cough syndrome
Laryngopharyngeal reflux
Cough due to swallowing disorders
Vocal cord dysfunction
Laryngeal sensory neuropathy
Obstructive sleep apnea
Cough hypersensitivity syndrome
Inflammatory airway disease
Cough variant asthma
Non-asthmatic eosinophilic bronchitis
Systemic disorders
Connective tissue disorders (Sjogren syndrome)
Inflammatory bowel disease
Vasculitis (granulomatosis with polyangiitis, giant cell arteritis)

The use of invasive testing in the diagnosis of chronic cough is controversial as well. In general, fiberoptic bronchoscopy has low clinical yield in patients with chronic cough [5]. However, clinical judgment is always necessary to determine whether invasive testing should be utilized. For instance, fiberoptic bronchoscopic examination may be indicated to investigate persistent change in the character of cough after antibiotic treatment in a smoker, to exclude endobronchial malignancy.

Physiology of Cough: Cough Reflex Arc, Cough Receptors

Cough is a protective physiologic reflex which facilitates the removal of foreign objects and debris from the airway. In order for an effective cough, an intact respiratory neuromuscular unit and optimal interaction between gas and mucus layers have to be present. Afferent nerve endings are most concentrated in the epithelia of the upper and lower respiratory tracts, but they are also located in the external auditory meatus, tympanic membrane, esophagus, stomach, pericardium, and diaphragm. The afferent limb of the arc is the vagus nerve and its many branches include tracheobronchial, superior laryngeal, Arnold's nerve, pharyngeal, pleural, and gastric branches. The vagal afferent nerve types involved in the transmission of the impulse are rapidly adapting receptor (RAR), slowly adapting receptor (SAR) which most likely modify the cough reflex by processing mechanical stimuli (lung inflation, pulmonary edema), and C-fibers which respond primarily to chemical changes (pH, carbon dioxide, capsaicin and bradykinin) [6]. Activated C-fibers are also capable of inducing neuropeptide release without the activation of reflex arc and thus may play a role in neurogenic inflammation [7]. The vagal afferent impulse reaches the cough center which is located diffusely in the medulla oblongata. The efferent limb of the cough reflex starts from the cough center and the ventral respiratory group, a column of neurons located ventrolaterally in the medulla. The efferent impulse is conducted by the phrenic nerve and the spinal motor nerves to the inspiratory and expiratory muscles and by the recurrent laryngeal nerve to the larynx and bronchial tree.

The cough reflex is characterized by the generation of high intrathoracic pressures against a closed glottis, followed by forceful expulsion of air and secretions on glottic opening. High-velocity stream of air tears mucus off the airway walls and expel droplets into the air. Mucus clearance is facilitated by the greater depth of mucus but reduced by increasing mucus viscosity and elasticity [8].

Airway-Related Cough

Chronic cough due to primary airway disorders is relatively rare. Most of these conditions have been discussed elsewhere in the text. Table 17.2 provides a list of these.

Upper Airway Cough Syndrome

Upper airway cough syndrome, formerly known as postnasal drip syndrome, remains a poorly defined clinical definition that is largely defined by patient's symptomatology without specific signs. It is a common cause of chronic cough. Typical patient presents with a sensation of mucus in the oropharynx and persistent need for frequent throat clearing. The condition may be caused by various upper airway inflammatory syndromes that span the spectrum of rhinosinusitis. The

Table 17.2 Chronic cough due to primary airway disorders	
	Airway foreign bodies
	Airway stenosis
	Amyloidosis of the airway
	Broncholithiasis
	Endobronchial tumors (carcinoid, adenoid cystic carcinoma, and mucoid epidermoid carcinoma)
	Endobronchial sarcoidosis
	Extrinsic compression
	Relapsing polychondritis
	Tracheobronchomalacia
	Tracheobronchomegaly
	Tracheobronchopathia osteochondroplastica

etiology may be bacterial, fungal, allergic, vasogenic (vasomotor rhinitis), or medication related (rhinitis medicamentosa). Unfortunately, there are no specific findings that would alert the bronchoscopist to the diagnosis of upper airway cough syndrome [9]. Oropharyngeal mucus and cobblestone changes may be present but are nonspecific. The diagnosis is generally one of exclusion and confirmed with favorable response to antihistamines and decongestants.

Cough and Reflux

Gastroesophageal reflux disease (GERD) is generally considered among the most common etiologies of chronic cough. Numerous studies have proposed a correlation between reflux and cough, and it is common clinical practice to initiate a trial of proton pump inhibitors (PPI) in patients that present with chronic cough. Irritation of the laryngeal mucosa is a common otolaryngological finding in patients suspected of suffering from GERD or laryngopharyngeal reflux (LPR). It is well known that GERD/LPR can cause ear, nose, and throat symptoms, secondary to tissue irritation. Most signs of laryngeal irritation have been traditionally attributed to LPR. However, many signs of laryngeal irritation, such as the presence of an interarytenoid bar, pseudosulcus, erythema of the medial wall of the arytenoids, and pharyngeal wall cobblestoning, showed a substantial overlap with normal subjects with no LPR, suggesting a lack of diagnostic specificity [10, 11]. The signs that were found to be more sensitive and specific to LPR include posterior commissure erosion or erythema (Fig. 17.1), vocal fold erythema, edema, and lesions (Figs. 17.2 and 17.3).

Treatment of GERD may result in marked improvement or complete resolution of symptoms in some patients with chronic cough. On the other hand, many patients with documented reflux do not have cough. Moreover, the response to reflux treatment in the management of chronic cough is highly variable [12]. The

Fig. 17.1 Posterior commissure erosion and erythema

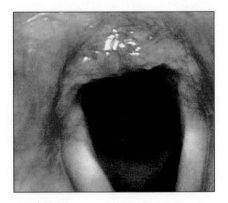

Fig. 17.2 Bilateral vocal fold posterior granulomas. Larger on the left side

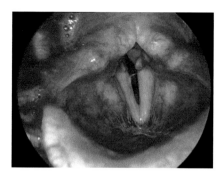

Fig. 17.3 Vocal fold erythema and bilateral nodular swelling on the middle third

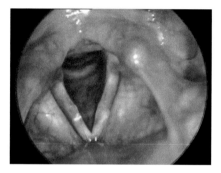

pathophysiology of reflux as it relates to cough remains elusive. Three main mechanisms have been proposed as possible initiators of cough related to acid exposure [13].

(A) Reflux in the esophagus provokes coughing via an esophago-bronchial reflex that stimulates vagal afferents from the airway and esophagus.
(B) Reflux into the larynx and pharynx may cause chronic laryngeal inflammation, increasing sensitivity of nerve terminals and stimulating cough receptors.
(C) Reflux enters the airway by means of micro-aspiration, leading to chronic inflammation and stimulating airway cough receptors.

There are multiple known triggers for chronic cough including sensitivity to perfumes, chemicals, environmental irritants, changes in temperature, or laryngeal activities that directly stimulate vocal fold mucosa such as talking and laughing. In line with the more recent view on laryngeal neuronal hypersensitivity, GERD-LPR itself is probably not a direct cause of cough, but one additional trigger that stimulates an already hyper-reactive laryngeal—pharyngeal—or upper airway mucosa.

The current recommendations for the management of LPR in patients with signs of laryngeal irritation and chronic cough include initial empiric therapy with twice-daily PPI for two to four months [14]. If the cough responds to therapy, tapering to once-daily therapy and eventually to non-drug treatment such as behavioral and dietary guidelines is advisable.

Swallowing and Cough

An important function of the larynx is to protect the airways, and deficits in the motor or sensory status of the larynx and pharynx, and esophagus can lead aspiration of food, liquids, or secretions into the airways. As alluded to earlier, cough reflex is a brainstem-mediated protective mechanism that helps expectorate material before it enters the airway. Cough that occurs during or immediately after meals may be a sign of swallowing difficulty or dysphagia. The most common symptoms of oropharyngeal dysphagia include (a) aspiration, or entry of food into the airway below the level of the true vocal folds, (b) entry of material into the larynx at some level down to but not below the true vocal folds, (c) residue or food that is left behind in the mouth or pharynx after the swallow, and d) regurgitation of food from the esophagus into the pharynx and nasal cavity. Cough is an important diagnostic sign that can help detect patients at high risk for pneumonia, malnutrition, or dehydration.

Coughing to prevent penetration or aspiration is part of a normal sensory mechanism. It is important to remember that if there is sensory deficit, patients may be "silent aspirators," where material goes past the true vocal folds into the airway without a proper cough response. Reports show that up to 60 % of in-patients in large hospitals or clinics may aspirate in the absence of a protective cough mechanism. High-risk populations include individuals with Parkinson's disease, amyotrophic lateral sclerosis, dementia, head and neck cancer, vocal fold paralysis or paresis, stroke, and brain injury.

When patients complain about coughing or choking around mealtimes, they should be referred to an ear, nose, and throat specialist with expertise in swallowing disorders to evaluate the etiology of the cough. It is important to differentiate patients who cough around mealtimes due to acid reflux exposure, or due to a hypersensitive larynx, from those with dysphagia who are at risk for aspiration.

Esophageal adenocarcinoma (EAC) represents one of the most rapidly rising malignancies in the USA. The diagnosis of EAC is usually made in the later stages of the disease, and most patients diagnosed with EAC have incurable disease at the time of detection. The majority of these patients are unaware of the presence of Barrett's esophagus prior to cancer diagnosis and many do not report typical symptoms of GERD. Several studies have shown that LPR symptoms, in particular chronic refractory cough, may be a predictor for EAC. Moreover, chronic cough has been suggested to be a better predictor of the presence of cancer and Barrett's esophagus than typical gastroesophageal reflux symptoms such as heartburn. Therefore, endoscopic screening for Barrett's esophagus and EAC should be considered for patients with refractory chronic cough of unknown etiology [15].

Aberrant Laryngeal Sensitivity and Reactivity

The term Irritable Larynx Syndrome (ILS) was introduced by Morrison and Rammage in 1999, and described as a condition in which a person experiences laryngeal muscle spasms, triggered by a sensory stimulus [16]. The laryngeal muscle spasm can cause episodes of coughing without apparent cause, a sense of a lump in the throat (globus sensation), laryngospasm, hoarseness, and paradoxical vocal fold motion.

ILS was initially thought to be related to altered brain stem control of laryngeal sensory-motor processes. However, in a 2010 update, the authors proposed that ILS is a central sensitivity syndrome where laryngeal and paralaryngeal muscles overreact to normal sensory stimuli [17]. They reported that out of 195 patients with ILS, more than half presented with one or two comorbidities related to central nervous system dysfunction such as irritable bowel syndrome, fibromyalgia, chronic fatigue syndrome, and migraines, concluding that ILS is secondary to central nervous system hypersensitivity.

Laryngeal hypersensitivity is a challenging condition since its constellation of symptoms can defy easy diagnosis and lead to under-recognition or misdiagnosis. Many subspecialties may be the entry point for patients who present with episodes of severe shortness of breath, chronic refractory cough, a prominent sensation of chest and throat constriction, dramatic stridor and hypersensitivity to fumes and strong smells. These can include pulmonary, allergy, otolaryngology, speech-language pathology, gastroenterology, and neurology. Adding to the challenge is the fact that the multidisciplinary involvement has resulted in a lack of unifying terminology. The following terms, all referring to similar conditions, have been used in recent literature: Chronic Refractory Cough, Post-Viral Vagal Neuropathy, Sensory Neuropathic Cough, Cough Hypersensitivity Syndrome, Laryngeal Sensory Neuropathy, Irritable Larynx Syndrome, Airway Hyper-responsiveness, and Cough Reflex Hypersensitivity.

A growing body of literature supports the idea that the aberrant laryngeal activity in these conditions is caused by peripheral sensory and motor neuropathies. All involve sensory dysfunction. There appears to be a complex interaction between peripheral nervous system and central nervous system processes with the evidence of both having excitatory and inhibitory influences.

Recently, Mazzone and colleagues have demonstrated that evoked cough is not only a brainstem-mediated reflex response to irritation of the airways, but it requires active facilitation by cortical regions and is further regulated by distinct higher order inhibitory processes [18]. Recent investigations indicate that there is an inverse relationship between the mechanical and the chemical responses of the airway mucosa to stimuli [19], suggesting that there is hyposensitivity to mechanical stimulation and hypersensitivity to chemical stimulation of the laryngeal airway mucosa.

The mounting evidence that central system sensitization is a relevant mechanism in refractory chronic cough, has led to the use of neuroleptic and psychotropic medications in the treatment of chronic cough and associated conditions. Clinical evidence along with a small cohort of studies recommends the use of the following for treatment of refractory chronic cough that has been non-responsive to more traditional treatment options: (a) Gabapentin, an antiepileptic also used to treat neuropathic pain [20]; (b) Tricyclic antidepressants, also used in chronic pain and fibromyalgia [21, 22]; (c) Selective serotonin re-uptake inhibitors, and combined serotonin and norepinephrine re-uptake inhibitors [23]; and (d) Baclofen, a centrally acting spasmolytic drug [24, 25].

Behavioral therapy is another effective management intervention for chronic cough that persists despite an adequate trial of medical treatments. This therapeutic intervention is conducted by a speech-language pathologist with expertise in treatment of cough. Therapy addresses lifestyle modifications, avoidance of sensory stimuli with treatment of LPR and minimizing exposure to triggers, and voice and breathing exercises in order to reprogram the habituated (laryngeal) motor response [26].

Chronic cough and laryngeal hypersensitivity are challenging and difficult to manage conditions because the constellation of symptoms can defy easy diagnosis. The impact that these can have on daily life is substantial. Some patients experience relentless symptoms that can persist for years, even decades, and frequent hospitalizations are not uncommon. Significant disability is seen in some cases, with noticeable impact on quality of life. Chronic cough is currently considered truly a multidisciplinary disease. The degree of cooperation between pulmonary, allergy, ENT, and speech pathology subspecialties is becoming more common in major healthcare facilities, and it can become a part of community practice as well. A "chronic cough clinic" offers the promise of many benefits:

- Improve the timing of diagnosis.
- Lower healthcare costs by [1] avoiding duplication of tests and [2] reducing the number of patient visits.
- Streamline management recommendations.
- Shorten the time necessary to achieve successful treatment.
- Improve outcomes.
- Improve patient satisfaction.

Professionals in subspecialties that commonly see these patients should make an effort to work with their colleagues and develop their own alliances that ultimately result in better patient care.

Obstructive Sleep Apnea

Obstructive sleep apnea is a clinical syndrome that results from an exaggerated propensity of upper airway collapse during sleep which occurs due to a complex interaction between anatomical (narrow, long, collapsible airway) and ventilatory control-related factors.

In a series of carefully documented cases, Birring et al. found obstructive sleep apnea to be the sole reason for chronic cough [27]. These patients experienced diagnostic delays of up to 3 years. The magnitude of the chronic cough symptom overshadowed their obstructive sleep apnea symptoms. Remarkably, within days of starting nasal CPAP, patients experienced significant and objectively documented reduction in their cough.

Chan and colleagues studied 55 patients with obstructive sleep apnea syndrome and no history of lung disease, recent upper respiratory tract infection, or use of ACE inhibitor [28]. 18 of these patients (33 %) had cough and 37 (67 %) did not. The patients with obstructive sleep apnea and cough were more likely to report symptoms of nocturnal heartburn and rhinitis. Presence or severity of cough had no relationship to the respiratory disturbance index.

The pathophysiological relationship between obstructive sleep apnea and cough is open to speculation. However, the two established causes for cough, upper airway inflammation and reflux disease, may explain the association. Repetitive collapse and opening of the airway has been shown to be associated with upper airway inflammation [29–31]. Furthermore, reversal of upper airway and systemic inflammation has been demonstrated after the use of nasal CPAP in patients with obstructive sleep apnea [32]. Obstructive sleep apnea also predisposes to gastroesophageal reflux as a consequence of marked swings in transdiaphragmatic pressure (suction effect) [33].

Patients with obstructive sleep apnea may pose specific challenges to the bronchoscopist. In a series of lung transplant recipients, patients with obstructive sleep apnea had significantly higher rates of procedural hypoxemia due to upper airway collapse [34]. When performing bronchoscopy for the investigation of chronic cough, presence of redundant upper airway, intraprocedural snoring, and hypoxemia may provide clues to the bronchoscopist for the diagnosis of obstructive sleep apnea. In those patients with known obstructive sleep apnea, performing the procedure in the presence of a nasopharyngeal tube [34], or while the patient receives noninvasive positive pressure ventilation [35], can alleviate upper airway obstruction and hypoxemia.

Cough Hypersensitivity Syndrome

In 2005, investigators at the Royal Brompton Hospital cough clinic reported their experience with 100 consecutive patients who were referred to this tertiary care center [4]. These patients were investigated and managed according to the anatomical protocol which involves systematic investigation and empirical treatment of the 3 common conditions which cause cough, i.e., asthma, upper airway cough syndrome, and GERD. The authors determined that the 3 conditions only account for 45 % of the patients. In additional 13 %, miscellaneous etiologies including post-viral cough, ACE inhibitor cough, COPD, bronchiectasis, Bordetella pertussis infection, and yellow nail syndrome were suggested. The remaining 42 % had no diagnosis after exhaustive work-up. These patients were said to have "chronic idiopathic cough" (CIC). Compared to patients with known etiology, patients with CIC had longer duration of the symptom, higher cough sensitivity as measured by capsaicin challenge, a higher incidence of precedent upper respiratory tract infection, and symptoms of sensitive cough reflex (such as coughing while talking, laughing, or eating crumbly foods). Chronic cough hypersensitivity syndrome was suggested as a more descriptive label for the condition since the entity represented a constellation of symptoms and signs associated with objective cough hypersensitivity, not explained by any specific medical condition [36]. It is important to note that cough hypersensitivity does not equate bronchial hyperreactivity.

Diagnosis of chronic cough hypersensitivity syndrome is one of exclusion; however, typical clinical characteristics, i.e., presence of allotussia and hypertussia, long duration, and precedent respiratory infection are helpful to the clinician. Treatment of the condition remains a challenge. Success has been reported with neuroactive agents such as gabapentin [20] and amitriptyline [22, 37]. As alluded to earlier, the relationship of chronic cough hypersensitivity syndrome and other similar entities such as aberrant laryngeal sensitivity remains a topic of discussion and research.

Inflammatory Airway Disease

Eosinophilic Inflammation of the Airway

Chronic cough can be a consequence of a continuum of inflammatory airway disorders associated with eosinophilic infiltration. These encompass the relatively common classic and cough variant asthma and less common and less-known entities of non-asthmatic eosinophilic bronchitis and atopic cough. Since cough is an accompanying and not main symptom of classical asthma, we will focus our discussion to cough variant asthma, non-asthmatic eosinophilic bronchitis, and atopic cough.

In essence, classical asthma is characterized by intermittent reversible airflow obstruction (bronchial hyperreactivity) and eosinophilic airway inflammation. Symptoms are dominated by the consequence of airflow obstruction, i.e., wheezing and shortness of breath. Eosinophilic inflammation is seen in the smooth muscle layer as well as airway epithelium. Cough variant asthma presents with the sole symptom of cough. There is evidence of bronchial hyperreactivity on challenge testing. Non-asthmatic eosinophilic bronchitis also presents with cough, but there is no evidence of bronchial hyperreactivity on objective testing. Here, eosinophilic inflammation is limited to airway epithelium. Atopic cough is a controversial entity described in Japan, where cough variant asthma is extremely prevalent. The

Table 17.3 Eosinophilic airway diseases

Clinical characteristic	Cough variant asthma	NAEB[a]	Atopic cough
Atopy	+	±	+
Cough reflex	±	+	+
Bronchial hyperreactivity	+	−	−
Response to antihistamines	−	?	+
Sputum eosinophilia	+	+	+
Mast cell infiltration in smooth muscle	+	−	?

[a]*NAEB* Non-asthmatic eosinophilic bronchitis
Based on data from Brightling [60]

hallmark of atopic cough is response to antihistaminic medications and presence of eosinophilic airway inflammation. Clinical nuances of these disorders are summarized in Table 17.3.

Cough Variant Asthma

Cough variant asthma is a subtype of asthma characterized by cough as the only presenting symptom [38]. It is one of the most common etiologies for chronic cough [1] accounting up to 30-40 % of cases. Atopy and seasonal variation are almost as common as classical asthma albeit lesser in magnitude [39]. Pulmonary function testing is essentially within normal limits. Sine a qua non is the presence of airway hyperreactivity on pulmonary function testing. Cough hypersensitivity as determined by capsaicin challenge is also present and improves after a 2-week course of leukotriene antagonists [40]. Cough variant asthma characteristically responds well to bronchodilators; however, inhaled corticosteroids are frequently necessary for the treatment of persistent cough [41]. Cough variant asthma can progress to classical asthma up to 40 % of the time [42].

Non-asthmatic Eosinophilic Bronchitis

Eosinophilic bronchitis is a pathological entity shared by various clinical conditions. In addition to asthma, rhinitis, COPD, and healthy individuals, patients with GERD may have evidence of eosinophilic bronchitis on pathology. Non-asthmatic eosinophilic bronchitis (eosinophilic bronchitis without asthma) as a cause of chronic cough was first described by Gibson et al. [43]. Patients with the condition presented with sputum eosinophilia (>3 %), normal spirometry without airway hyper-responsiveness, and an excellent response to corticosteroids [44]. Nevertheless, frank asthma (9 %) or fixed airflow obstruction (16 %) can develop over time [45].

Systemic Disorders that Affect the Airways

Connective Tissue Disease

Although cough can occur with various connective tissue disease (scleroderma, lupus, rheumatoid arthritis), this is mostly in the setting of parenchymal pulmonary involvement. In the case of Sjogren's syndrome however, cough can occur with airway involvement without significant abnormality in the lung tissue.

Sjogren Syndrome

Sjogren syndrome is a systemic inflammatory disorder that chiefly affects the exocrine glands. Diagnosis of Sjogren (primary) syndrome is made by using subjective and objective data for xerostomia and keratoconjunctivitis sicca and one of the criteria for autoimmunity (inflammatory infiltrates detected in minor saliva glands, and/or presence of Ro/La autoantibodies). Positive Schirmer's test, sialometry, ultrasound, or MRI of the saliva glands may be considered as confirmatory tests.

Sjogren syndrome is associated with multiple interstitial lung diseases such as nonspecific interstitial pneumonia, organizing pneumonia, lymphocytic interstitial pneumonia, follicular bronchiolitis, and granulomatous lung disease [46]. All of these entities may also be associated with chronic cough.

Chronic cough can also occur in primary Sjogren syndrome, however, without the presence of any interstitial lung disease. In a study by Bellido-Casado [47], 72 % of patients had respiratory symptoms such as cough and dyspnea without any radiological abnormalities. Interestingly, cough was more prevalent among patients with normal sputum inflammatory cell count in this study. In contrast, bronchodilator response or methacholine challenge test positivity was more prevalent among those with abnormal sputum (lymphocytosis). Cough in the absence of airway inflammation suggests that extrapulmonary etiologies for cough may be prevalent among patients with Sjogren syndrome, e.g., reflux disease. Indeed, three quarters of the patients with Sjogren syndrome may report dysphagia and presence of reflux disease has also been demonstrated [48]. Notably, methacholine challenge testing can be positive in up to 60 % of patients with Sjogren syndrome [49].

Inflammatory Bowel Disease

Inflammatory bowel diseases, i.e., Crohn's disease and ulcerative colitis, are associated with a myriad of pulmonary manifestations. Common embryological origin from the primitive foregut, similar luminal structure, and presence of submucosal lymphoid tissue in both tracts has been proposed as explanation for the pathophysiological link [50]. Lung parenchyma may be involved with pulmonary nodules, organizing pneumonia, nonspecific interstitial pneumonia, and granulomatous inflammation similar to sarcoidosis. The bronchoscopist may encounter large airway involvement manifesting as bronchiectasis, chronic bronchitis, or sometimes life-threatening purulent tracheobronchitis [51]. Severe inflammation in the major airways can lead to inflammatory pseudotumors and frank stenosis of the airway. Inflammatory bowel disease-related airway inflammation responds well to corticosteroids administered systemically or via inhaled therapy. The bronchoscopist should exclude concurrent infection, particularly non-tuberculous Mycobacterium species in these patients [52].

Vasculitis

Vasculitides comprise a group of disorders characterized by immune-mediated inflammation and destruction of blood vessels. Among these, granulomatosis with polyangiitis (GPA) formerly known as Wegener's granulomatosis and giant cell arteritis (GCA) are the most commonly associated with airway symptoms. GPA involves the central airways commonly and is associated with subglottic and tracheobronchial stenosis. Cough and hemoptysis are common. This disorder has been covered in detail, elsewhere in this text.

Giant cell arteritis is a vasculitic disorder of large- and medium-sized blood vessels characterized by the onset of disease after the age of 50, high sedimentation rate, headache, and vasculitis found on temporal artery biopsy [53]. Respiratory involvement is rare and may take the form of pleural effusion [54], mild interstitial lung disease [55], and in situ pulmonary artery thrombosis [56]. However, a puzzling clinical presentation is with a dry, nagging cough. In fact, dry cough is the most common respiratory manifestation of GCA [57]. It can also be the presenting symptom in approximately 8 % of the patients [57, 58]. Bronchoscopic examination may reveal nonspecific bronchitis [59]. Therefore, the bronchoscopist should be alert to the unusual presentation of this potentially morbid but treatable condition in the elderly patient who presents with a nagging, dry cough and an unexplained inflammatory disease.

References

1. Irwin RS. Introduction to the diagnosis and management of cough: ACCP evidence-based clinical practice guidelines. Chest. 2006;129(1 Suppl):25S–7S.
2. Irwin RS, Corrao WM, Pratter MR. Chronic persistent cough in the adult: the spectrum and frequency of causes and successful outcome of specific therapy. Am Rev Respir Dis. 1981;123 (4 Pt 1):413–7.
3. Smyrnios NA, Irwin RS, Curley FJ, French CL. From a prospective study of chronic cough: diagnostic and therapeutic aspects in older adults. Arch Intern Med. 1998;158(11):1222–8.
4. Haque RA, Usmani OS, Barnes PJ. Chronic idiopathic cough: a discrete clinical entity? Chest. 2005;127(5):1710–3.

5. Barnes TW, Afessa B, Swanson KL, Lim KG. The clinical utility of flexible bronchoscopy in the evaluation of chronic cough. Chest. 2004;126(1):268–72.
6. Canning BJ. Anatomy and neurophysiology of the cough reflex: ACCP evidence-based clinical practice guidelines. Chest. 2006;129(1 Suppl):33S–47S.
7. Barnes PJ. Neurogenic inflammation in the airways. Respir Physiol. 2001;125(1–2):145–54.
8. McCool FD. Global physiology and pathophysiology of cough: ACCP evidence-based clinical practice guidelines. Chest. 2006;129(1 Suppl):48S–53S.
9. Pratter MR. Chronic upper airway cough syndrome secondary to rhinosinus diseases (previously referred to as postnasal drip syndrome): ACCP evidence-based clinical practice guidelines. Chest. 2006;129(1 Suppl):63S–71S.
10. Hicks DM, Ours TM, Abelson TI, Vaezi MF, Richter JE. The prevalence of hypopharynx findings associated with gastroesophageal reflux in normal volunteers. J Voice. 2002;16 (4):564–79.
11. Milstein CF, Charbel S, Hicks DM, Abelson TI, Richter JE, Vaezi MF. Prevalence of laryngeal irritation signs associated with reflux in asymptomatic volunteers: impact of endoscopic technique (rigid vs. flexible laryngoscope). Laryngoscope. 2005;115(12):2256–61.
12. Smith JA, Abdulqawi R, Houghton LA. GERD-related cough: pathophysiology and diagnostic approach. Curr Gastroenterol Rep. 2011;13(3):247–56.
13. Kahrilas PJ, Smith JA, Dicpinigaitis PV. A causal relationship between cough and gastroesophageal reflux disease (GERD) has been established: A Pro/Con debate. Lung. 2014;192(1):39–46.
14. Barry DW, Vaezi MF. Laryngopharyngeal reflux: More questions than answers. Cleve Clin J Med. 2010;77(5):327–34.
15. Reavis KM, Morris CD, Gopal DV, Hunter JG, Jobe BA. Laryngopharyngeal reflux symptoms better predict the presence of esophageal adenocarcinoma than typical gastroesophageal reflux symptoms. Ann Surg 2004;239(6):849–56 (discussion 856-8).
16. Morrison M, Rammage L, Emami AJ. The irritable larynx syndrome. J Voice. 1999;13 (3):447–55.
17. Morrison M, Rammage L. Revue Cannadienne d'orthophonie et d'audiologie. 2010;34–4.
18. Mazzone SB, Cole LJ, Ando A, Egan GF, Farrell MJ. Investigation of the neural control of cough and cough suppression in humans using functional brain imaging. J Neurosci. 2011;31 (8):2948–58.
19. Phua SY, McGarvey L, Ngu M, Ing A. The differential effect of gastroesophageal reflux disease on mechanostimulation and chemostimulation of the laryngopharynx. Chest. 2010;138 (5):1180–5.
20. Ryan NM, Birring SS, Gibson PG. Gabapentin for refractory chronic cough: a randomised, double-blind, placebo-controlled trial. Lancet. 2012;380(9853):1583–9.
21. Bastian RW, Vaidya AM, Delsupehe KG. Sensory neuropathic cough: a common and treatable cause of chronic cough. Otolaryngol Head Neck Surg. 2006;135(1):17–21.
22. Jeyakumar A, Brickman TM, Haben M. Effectiveness of amitriptyline versus cough suppressants in the treatment of chronic cough resulting from postviral vagal neuropathy. Laryngoscope. 2006;116(12):2108–12.
23. Zylicz Z, Krajnik M. What has dry cough in common with pruritus? Treatment of dry cough with paroxetine. J Pain Symptom Manage. 2004;27(2):180–4.
24. Xu X, Chen Q, Liang S, Lu H, Qiu Z. Successful resolution of refractory chronic cough induced by gastroesophageal reflux with treatment of baclofen. Cough 2012;8(1):8. doi:10. 1186/1745-9974-8-8.
25. Dicpinigaitis PV, Dobkin JB, Rauf K, Aldrich TK. Inhibition of capsaicin-induced cough by the gamma-aminobutyric acid agonist baclofen. J Clin Pharmacol. 1998;38(4):364–7.
26. Ryan NM, Vertigan AE, Bone S, Gibson PG. Cough reflex sensitivity improves with speech language pathology management of refractory chronic cough. Cough. 2010;28(6):5.
27. Birring SS, Ing AJ, Chan K, Cossa G, Matos S, Morgan MD, et al. Obstructive sleep apnoea: a cause of chronic cough. Cough. 2007;2(3):7.

28. Chan KK, Ing AJ, Laks L, Cossa G, Rogers P, Birring SS. Chronic cough in patients with sleep-disordered breathing. Eur Respir J. 2010;35(2):368–72.
29. Sekosan M, Zakkar M, Wenig BL, Olopade CO, Rubinstein I. Inflammation in the uvula mucosa of patients with obstructive sleep apnea. Laryngoscope. 1996;106(8):1018–20.
30. Paulsen FP, Steven P, Tsokos M, Jungmann K, Muller A, Verse T, et al. Upper airway epithelial structural changes in obstructive sleep-disordered breathing. Am J Respir Crit Care Med. 2002;166(4):501–9.
31. Hatipoglu U, Rubinstein I. Inflammation and obstructive sleep apnea syndrome: how many ways do I look at thee? Chest. 2004;126(1):1–2.
32. Karamanli H, Ozol D, Ugur KS, Yildirim Z, Armutcu F, Bozkurt B, et al. Influence of CPAP treatment on airway and systemic inflammation in OSAS patients. Sleep Breath. 2012.
33. Demeter P, Pap A. The relationship between gastroesophageal reflux disease and obstructive sleep apnea. J Gastroenterol. 2004;39(9):815–20.
34. Chhajed PN, Aboyoun C, Malouf MA, Hopkins PM, Plit M, Grunstein RR, et al. Management of acute hypoxemia during flexible bronchoscopy with insertion of a nasopharyngeal tube in lung transplant recipients. Chest. 2002;121(4):1350–4.
35. Murgu SD, Pecson J, Colt HG. Bronchoscopy during noninvasive ventilation: indications and technique. Respir Care. 2010;55(5):595–600.
36. Chung KF. Chronic 'cough hypersensitivity syndrome': a more precise label for chronic cough. Pulm Pharmacol Ther. 2011;24(3):267–71.
37. Greene SM, Simpson CB. Evidence for sensory neuropathy and pharmacologic management. Otolaryngol Clin North Am 2010;43(1):67–72, viii.
38. Niimi A. Cough and asthma. Curr Respir Med Rev. 2011;7(1):47–54.
39. Takemura M, Niimi A, Matsumoto H, Ueda T, Yamaguchi M, Matsuoka H, et al. Atopic features of cough variant asthma and classic asthma with wheezing. Clin Exp Allergy. 2007;37(12):1833–9.
40. Dicpinigaitis PV, Dobkin JB, Reichel J. Antitussive effect of the leukotriene receptor antagonist zafirlukast in subjects with cough-variant asthma. J Asthma. 2002;39(4):291–7.
41. Dicpinigaitis PV. Chronic cough due to asthma: ACCP evidence-based clinical practice guidelines. Chest. 2006;129(1 Suppl):75S–9S.
42. Matsumoto H, Niimi A, Takemura M, Ueda T, Tabuena R, Yamaguchi M, et al. Prognosis of cough variant asthma: a retrospective analysis. J Asthma. 2006;43(2):131–5.
43. Gibson PG, Dolovich J, Denburg J, Ramsdale EH, Hargreave FE. Chronic cough: eosinophilic bronchitis without asthma. Lancet. 1989;1(8651):1346–8.
44. Brightling CE, Ward R, Goh KL, Wardlaw AJ, Pavord ID. Eosinophilic bronchitis is an important cause of chronic cough. Am J Respir Crit Care Med. 1999;160(2):406–10.
45. Berry MA, Hargadon B, McKenna S, Shaw D, Green RH, Brightling CE, et al. Observational study of the natural history of eosinophilic bronchitis. Clin Exp Allergy. 2005;35(5):598–601.
46. Shi JH, Liu HR, Xu WB, Feng RE, Zhang ZH, Tian XL, et al. Pulmonary manifestations of Sjogren's syndrome. Respiration. 2009;78(4):377–86.
47. Bellido-Casado J, Plaza V, Diaz C, Geli C, Dominguez J, Margarit G, et al. Bronchial inflammation, respiratory symptoms and lung function in Primary Sjogren's syndrome. Arch Bronconeumol. 2011;47(7):330–4.
48. Belafsky PC, Postma GN. The laryngeal and esophageal manifestations of Sjogren's syndrome. Curr Rheumatol Rep. 2003;5(4):297–303.
49. La Corte R, Potena A, Bajocchi G, Fabbri L, Trotta F. Increased bronchial responsiveness in primary Sjogren's syndrome. A sign of tracheobronchial involvement. Clin Exp Rheumatol. 1991;9(2):125–130.
50. Black H, Mendoza M, Murin S. Thoracic manifestations of inflammatory bowel disease. Chest. 2007;131(2):524–32.
51. Henry MT, Davidson LA, Cooke NJ. Tracheobronchial involvement with Crohn's disease. Eur J Gastroenterol Hepatol. 2001;13(12):1495–7.
52. Storch I, Rosoff L, Katz S. Sarcoidosis and inflammatory bowel disease. J Clin Gastroenterol. 2001;33(4):345.

53. Hunder GG, Bloch DA, Michel BA, Stevens MB, Arend WP, Calabrese LH, et al. The American College of Rheumatology 1990 criteria for the classification of giant cell arteritis. Arthritis Rheum. 1990;33(8):1122–8.
54. Valstar MH, Terpstra WF, de Jong RS. Pericardial and pleural effusion in giant cell arteritis. Am J Med. 2003;114(8):708–9.
55. Karam GH, Fulmer JD. Giant cell arteritis presenting as interstitial lung disease. Chest. 1982;82(6):781–4.
56. Andres E, Kaltenbach G, Marcellin L, Imler M. Acute pulmonary embolism related to pulmonary giant cell arteritis. Presse Med. 2004;33(19 Pt 1):1328–9.
57. Zenone T, Puget M. Dry cough is a frequent manifestation of giant cell arteritis. Rheumatol Int. 2013;33(8):2165–8.
58. Becourt-Verlomme C, Barouky R, Alexandre C, Gonthier R, Laurent H, Vital Durand D, et al. Inaugural symptoms of Horton's disease in a series of 260 patients. Rev Med Interne. 2001;22 (7):631–7.
59. Carassou P, Aletti M, Cinquetti G, Banal F, Landais C, Graffin B, et al. Respiratory manifestations of giant cell arteritis: 8 cases and review of the literature. Presse Med. 2010;39 (9):e188–96.
60. Brightling CE. Chronic cough due to nonasthmatic eosinophilic bronchitis: ACCP evidence-based clinical practice guidelines. Chest. 2006;129(1_suppl):116S–21S.

Index

Note: Page numbers followed by f and t indicate figures and tables, respectively

© Springer International Publishing Switzerland 2016
A.C. Mehta et al. (eds.), *Diseases of the Central Airways*,
Respiratory Medicine, DOI 10.1007/978-3-319-29830-6

Mucor, 196, 209

Mucormycosis, 196. *See also* Zygomycosis treatment outcomes, 210

Mucosa-associated lymphoid tissue (MALT), 282

lymphomas, 283, 284*f*

Mucosal ischemia, 15

Mucous gland adenoma, 262

Multidetector computed tomography, 27 subglottic tracheal stenosis, 29*f*

Mycobacterium tuberculosis (MTB), 309 healed, 310*f*

Myeloperoxidase (MPO), 109

N

Narrow band imaging (NBI), 148

Nasal mucosal sarcoidosis, 72, 73*f*

NBI. *See* Narrow band imaging (NBI)

NEC. *See* Neuroendocrine cell (NEC)

Necator americanus, 239

Neoplastic disorders, 2, 3*t*

Neuroendocrine cells (NEC), 295
abnormalities, 296
hyperplasia, 295, 296, 297*f*, 298*f*
pulmonary (PNEC), 297

NIMV. *See* Non-invasive mechanical ventilation (NIMV)

NOD2. *See* Nucleotide-binding oligomerization domain containing 2 (NOD2)

Non-asthmatic eosinophilic bronchitis, 367

Non-Hodgkin's lymphoma
extranodal, 282
pulmonary, 289

Non-invasive mechanical ventilation (NIMV), 142

Non-neoplastic disorders, 2, 3*t*

Nucleotide-binding oligomerization domain containing 2 (NOD2), 90

O

Obstructive *Aspergillus* tracheobronchitis, 200*f*

Obstructive sleep apnea, 364–365

Ochronosis, 306–307. *See also* Alkaptonuria

P

Paclitaxel-coated balloon (PCB) dilation, 347

PAIR. *See* Puncture, aspiration, injection, and re-aspiration (PAIR)

Papillomas, 2, 216, 222, 223
CO_2 laser in, 219
juvenile recurrent, 5*f*
laryngeal, 215
mulberry-type texture of, 218, 217*f*

Papillomatosis, 215. *See also* Recurrent respiratory papillomatosis (RRP)

Paragonimiasis, 234*t*

Parasites infections, of lung
cestodes, 235*t*
mesomycetozoea, 235*t*
nematodes, key features, 233–234*t*
trematodes, key features, 234

Pattern recognition receptors (PRRs), 90

pCLE. *See* Probe-based confocal laser endomicroscopy (pCLE)

PCR. *See* Polymerase chain reaction (PCR)

PDT. *See* Photodynamic therapy (PDT)

PEEP. *See* Positive end-expiratory pressure (PEEP)

Pegylated interferon alpha 2a (Peg-IFNα-2a), 221

PFTs. *See* Pulmonary function tests (PFTs)

Photodynamic therapy (PDT), 220

Plasmodium falciparum, 236, 237

Plasmodium spp., 236

Pneumatodes, 231

Pneumonectomy
chest radiograph after, 184*f*
for fibrous EBTB, 183

Polymerase chain reaction (PCR), 179, 195
Aspergillus fumigatus-specific, 195

Positive end-expiratory pressure (PEEP), 330

Positive pressure ventilation, 330

Positron emission tomography (PET) scan, 241. *See also* Flurodeoxyglucose positron emission tomography (FDG-PET)

Post-tracheostomy stenosis, 15

Potassium titanyl phosphate (KTP) laser, 220

PPI. *See* Proton pump inhibitors (PPI)

PR3-ANCA, 107, 109

Primary epithelial-myoepithelial tumors, 263

Primary graft dysfunction, 330

Primary pulmonary candidiasis, 206

Primary pulmonary lymphoma, 281, 283

Primary tracheal lymphomas, 281

Probe-based confocal laser endomicroscopy (pCLE), 167

Proteinase-3 antineutrophil cytoplasm antibody (PR3-ANCA). *See* PR3-ANCA

Proton pump inhibitors (PPI), 360

Protozoal parasites
infections, 231
of lung, key features, 232*t*
pulmonary amebiasis, 236
pulmonary babesiosis, 237
pulmonary leishmaniasis, 236
pulmonary malaria, 236